Small Animal Orthopaedics

The Forelimb

Miguel Solano (editor)
Alan Danielski
Felipe de Vicente
Stephen Kalff

edra
PUBLISHING

This book was originally published in Spanish under the title:
Ortopedia en pequeños animales. El miembro anterior

ISBN Spanish edition: 978-84-18339-57-8

Small Animal Orthopaedics. The Forelimb
Miguel Solano Nicolás, Alan Danielski, Felipe de Vicente Collado, Stephen Kalff

ISBN: 978-1-957260-56-3
eISBN: 978-1-957260-89-1

Book Publishing Manager: Costanza Smeraldi
Paper, Printing and Binding Manager: Paolo Ficicchia
Translation: Chef du Monde SL (chs. Arthrocentesis, General concepts about arthrodesis, Ununited anconeal process, Pancarpal arthrodesis)
Illustrator and Cover: Jacob Gragera Artal
Layout: Raquel Fernández Bermúdez
Copyediting: Jorge Viejo Adiego

Edra Publishing US LLC
3309 Northlake Boulevard, Suite 203
Palm Beach Gardens, FL, 33403
EIN: 844113980
info@edrapublishing.com
www.edrapublishing.com

edra
PUBLISHING

Printed in Italy by "RGM printing" S.r.l. – January 2024

THE AUTHORS

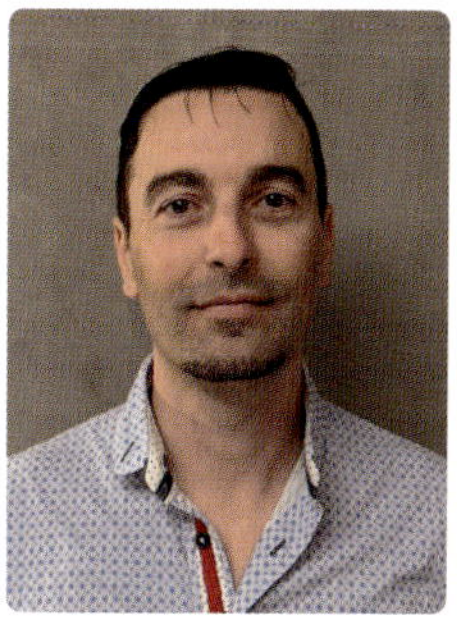

MIGUEL SOLANO (EDITOR)

Ldo Vet, DipECVS, MRCVS

Miguel Solano graduated in veterinary medicine from the Autonomous University of Barcelona, Spain, in 2007. He completed internships in surgery at Fitzpatrick Referrals and the University of Cambridge. In February 2015, he became a European diplomate in small animal surgery (DipECVS). Miguel has lectured internationally and reviews manuscripts for several scientific journals. He has published various articles with a particular focus on elbow and stifle conditions and neurosurgery. At the time of writing, he works as an orthopaedic specialist surgeon at The Ralph Veterinary Referral Centre, UK.

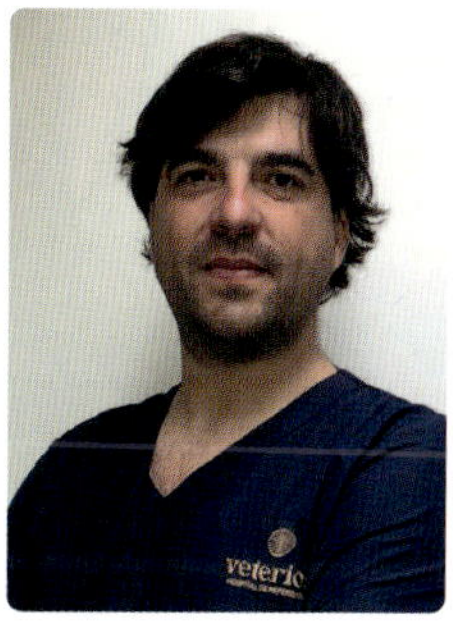

FELIPE DE VICENTE

Ldo Vet, PhD, PgCert VBM, DipECVS, FHEA, MRCVS

Felipe de Vicente holds a degree (2003) and a PhD (2009) in veterinary medicine from the Complutense University of Madrid, Spain. He completed an internship at the University of Glasgow, UK, in 2008 and a residency in small animal surgery at University College Dublin, Ireland, in 2012. He was awarded the ECVS diploma in small animal surgery in 2014 and the RCVS certificate in small animal surgery in 2016. Felipe has worked in several private veterinary hospitals throughout the UK and lectured in small animal surgery at Glasgow and Liverpool universities. He has also been the head of the Department of Trauma and Orthopaedics at the University of Liverpool. After working as a referral surgeon at Pride Veterinary Centre in Derby, UK, for almost 4 years, Felipe moved back to Spain in 2022. He currently works as head of small animal surgery and clinical director at Hospital Veterios in Madrid, Spain.

STEPHEN KALFF

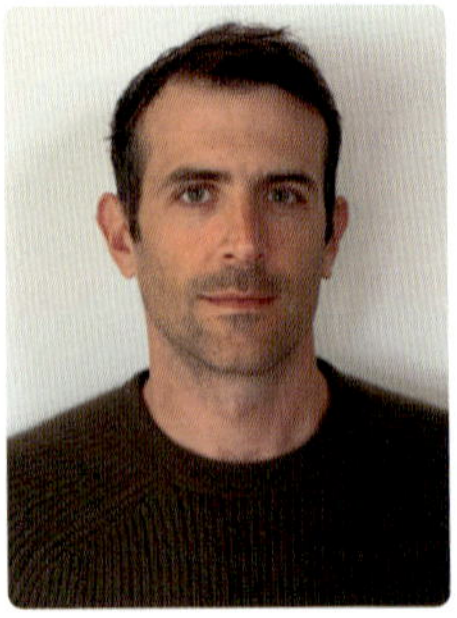

BVSc, MANZCVS(Surg), DSAS(Orth), MRCVS

Stephen Kalff graduated from the University of Melbourne, Australia, in 2003. In 2009, he attained membership of the Australian and New Zealand College of Veterinary Scientists (MANZCVS) by examination in small animal surgery. He then completed a private practice surgical internship in Melbourne in 2010, and a surgical residency at Willows Referrals, UK, in 2014. Stephen obtained the Royal College of Veterinary Surgeons (RCVS) diploma in small animal orthopaedics in 2014 and recognised specialist status in 2015. He continued working in the UK as a staff surgeon at Fitzpatrick Referrals until 2018, when he moved to the USA. He has been practising at Pacific and Santa Cruz Veterinary Specialists in California since then. Stephen continues to publish on a variety of orthopaedic topics and has been an AO VET faculty since 2015.

ALAN DANIELSKI

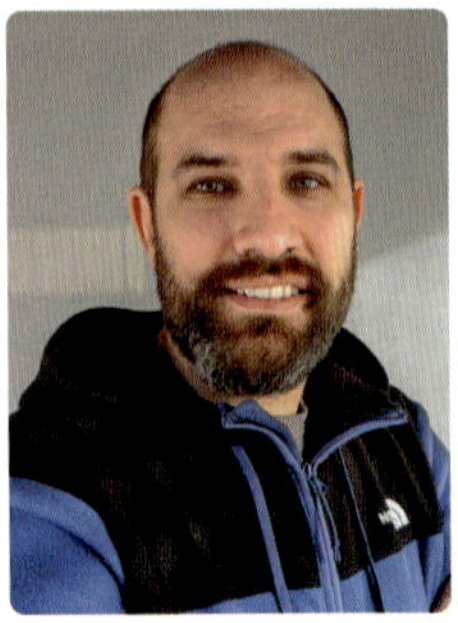

Med Vet, DipECVS, MRCVS

Alan Danielski graduated in veterinary medicine at the University of Parma, Italy. In 2007, he moved to the UK to continue his career in surgery and since then has pursued his goal of becoming a specialist in the field. He became an ECVS diplomate in small animal surgery in 2016 after completing a combined residency at Fitzpatrick Referrals and Cambridge University. Over the past 13 years, Alan has practised at two of the most important orthopaedic surgery referral centres in the UK, which has bestowed him with extensive experience in treating cases. Currently, he works as an orthopaedic surgeon at The Ralph Veterinary Referral Centre, UK. Alan has published scientific articles in the most important veterinary journals and is an international lecturer/instructor. His main areas of interest include elbow dysplasia, treatment of humeral intracondylar fissure and arthroscopy.

PREFACE

Small Animal Orthopaedics. The Forelimb has been conceived as a practical book that comprehensively describes the surgical treatment of the most common trauma injuries and orthopaedic diseases affecting the forelimb of cats and dogs.

The content of this book is divided into four parts. The first part focuses on arthrology; its goal is to provide the reader with a better understanding of the fundamentals, including general techniques, such as arthroscopy and arthrocentesis, and common diseases, such as septic arthritis and osteochondritis dissecans (OCD). The three subsequent parts describe various conditions and surgical treatments affecting the shoulder, elbow and carpal joints, respectively. Some of the surgical techniques covered in this book are specialised procedures, such as shoulder arthrodesis, synthetic osteochondral resurfacing of humeral OCD lesions using SynACART implants, and treatment of medial compartment disease of the elbow using the canine unicompartmental elbow (CUE) replacement, while other techniques, including management of shoulder/elbow joint luxation and carpal arthrodesis, are more commonly performed in veterinary practice.

Whether they be simple or complex, the different surgical techniques available for the treatment of forelimb diseases are thoroughly described. The description of each technique is structured around the following sections: introduction, indications, surgical planning, surgical procedure, postoperative management, prognosis, and complications. Text descriptions are complemented by photos and illustrations, along with videos in some chapters, to aid readers in understanding how to perform the technique. Our aim was to produce a book that benefited both the beginning veterinary practitioner who wants to delve deeper into trauma and orthopaedic surgery and the veterinary surgeon who is well-versed in this field. We hope that our experience in teaching ECVS residents pervades the pages of this book, making it a helpful tool and providing the reader with repeatable steps for the surgical procedures. We would like to take the opportunity to thank our families, friends and teachers.

We hope to never stop learning and sharing.

The authors

TABLE OF CONTENTS

FUNDAMENTALS AND PRACTICAL BASIS 1

Arthrocentesis 2
Felipe de Vicente

- Introduction 2
- Indications 3
- Clinical signs of the most common arthropathies 3
- Technique 3
  - Shoulder arthrocentesis 4
  - Elbow arthrocentesis 4
  - Carpal arthrocentesis 5
  - Hip arthrocentesis 5
  - Stifle arthrocentesis 5
  - Tarsal arthrocentesis 6
- Synovial fluid analysis 8
- Complications 12

Arthroscopy 17
Alan Danielski

- Introduction 17
- Elbow arthroscopy 17
  - Instrumentation 17
  - Preparation 19
  - Joint inspection 21
  - Postoperative management 27
- Shoulder arthroscopy 27
  - Instrumentation 27
  - Preparation 28
  - Joint inspection 28
  - Postoperative management 31

Generalities of osteochondritis dissecans 32
Alan Danielski

Introduction 32
Clinical presentation and diagnosis 32
Treatment 32
Conservative treatment 32
Surgical treatment 32

General concepts about arthrodesis 37
Felipe de Vicente

Introduction 37
Indications 37
Surgical technique 37
Postoperative Management 39
Outcome 39
Complications 39

SHOULDER 41

Traumatic shoulder luxation 42
Stephen Kalff

Introduction 42
Clinical presentation and diagnosis 42
Treatment 44
Conservative management 44
Surgical management 45
Postoperative management 46
Outcome and complications 47

Osteochondritis dissecans of the shoulder joint 48
Miguel Solano

Introduction 48
Clinical presentation and diagnosis 48

Treatment 50
Surgical management 50
Postoperative management 52
Outcome 56
Complications 56

Infraspinatus contracture (fibrotic myopathy) 58
Stephen Kalff

Introduction 58
Clinical presentation and diagnosis 58
Treatment 58
Surgical treatment 58
Postoperative management 59
Outcome 59

Biceps brachii tendinopathy 61
Alan Danielski

Introduction 61
Clinical presentation and diagnosis 61
Physical examination 62
Radiography 63
Ultrasonography 64
Magnetic resonance imaging 65
Treatment 66
Conservative treatment 66
Surgical treatment 66
Postoperative management 69
Outcome and complications 69

Supraspinatus tendinopathy 71
Miguel Solano

Introduction 71
Clinical presentation and diagnosis 71
Physical examination 71
Imaging 71

Treatment 73
Conservative treatment 73
Surgical treatment 73
Postoperative management 74
Outcome 74

Dorsal scapular luxation 75
Miguel Solano

Introduction 75
Clinical presentation and diagnosis 75
Treatment 76
Surgical treatment 76
Postoperative management 78
Outcome and complications 78

Shoulder arthrodesis 79
Miguel Solano

Introduction 79
Surgical planning 79
Surgical technique 80
Postoperative management 85
Outcome 86
Complications 86

ELBOW 89

Traumatic elbow luxation 90
Stephen Kalff

Introduction 90
Clinical presentation and diagnosis 90
Treatment 91
Joint reduction 91
Internal fixation 94

Outcome 97

Complications 97

Ununited anconeal process 98

Felipe de Vicente

Introduction 98

Clinical presentation and diagnosis 98

Treatment 100

Treatment in young animals 100

Treatment in adult animals 100

Surgical technique 100

Postoperative management 104

Patients treated via excision of the anconeal process 104

Patients treated to achieve union of the anconeal process 104

Outcome 105

Complications 105

Medial compartment disease 106

Alan Danielski

Introduction 106

Treatment 106

Conservative treatment 106

Surgical treatment 106

Osteochondrosis of the elbow joint 117

Alan Danielski

Introduction 117

Treatment 117

Conservative treatment 117

Surgical treatment 117

Postoperative management 120

Outcome and complications 121

Short ulna syndrome ... 122
Miguel Solano

Introduction ... 122
Clinical presentation and diagnosis ... 122
Treatment ... 126
Surgical treatment ... 126
Outcome ... 130

CARPUS ... 133

Abductor pollicis longus tenosynovitis ... 134
Stephen Kalff

Introduction ... 134
Clinical presentation and diagnosis ... 134
Treatment ... 135
Outcome ... 135

Pancarpal arthrodesis ... 137
Felipe de Vicente

Introduction ... 137
Indications ... 137
Clinical presentation and diagnosis ... 138
Surgical planning ... 139
Surgical technique ... 139
Postoperative management ... 143
Outcome ... 144
Complications ... 144

REFERENCES AND FURTHER READING ... 147

01

FUNDAMENTALS AND PRACTICAL BASIS

ARTHROCENTESIS

Felipe de Vicente

INTRODUCTION

The purpose of arthrocentesis is to obtain a sample of synovial fluid from a joint. Arthrocentesis and synovial fluid analysis allow for differentiation between the different types of joint disease. In general terms, arthropathies in small animals can be inflammatory (Fig. 1) or noninflammatory (Fig. 2). The former may be infectious, immune-mediated or crystal-induced (e.g. hydroxyapatite) in origin. Immune-mediated arthropathies are in turn classified into erosive and nonerosive.

The most common joint diseases in small animals are noninflammatory in nature, and most often are degenerative arthropathies (osteoarthritis) secondary to degenerative joint conditions. It has been estimated that 20 % of adult dogs and more than 60 % of cats suffer from osteoarthritis (Johnston, 1997; Hardie et al., 2002). Other less common types of noninflammatory joint diseases are arthropathies associated with trauma, tumours or coagulopathies.

The most common cause of infectious inflammatory arthropathy is bacterial infection. Other causes of infectious inflammatory joint disease have been described, such as rickettsiae (*Ehrlichia*), protozoa (*Leishmania*), fungi (*Aspergillus*, *Cryptococcus*), mycoplasmas, viruses (feline calicivirus, feline coronavirus) and spirochetes (*Borrelia*), among others.

The most common cause of noninfectious inflammatory arthropathy is immune mediated. In addition to immune-mediated polyarthritis, other causes of nonerosive immune-mediated joint disease include arthropathies associated with certain breeds (e.g. Akita and Shar Pei), osteoarthritis associated with systemic lupus erythematosus and lymphoplasmacytic synovitis.

Finally, erosive immune-mediated inflammatory arthropathies include rheumatoid arthritis, erosive polyarthritis of greyhounds, feline chronic progressive polyarthritis and periosteal proliferative arthropathy.

Figure 1. Classification of inflammatory arthropathies.

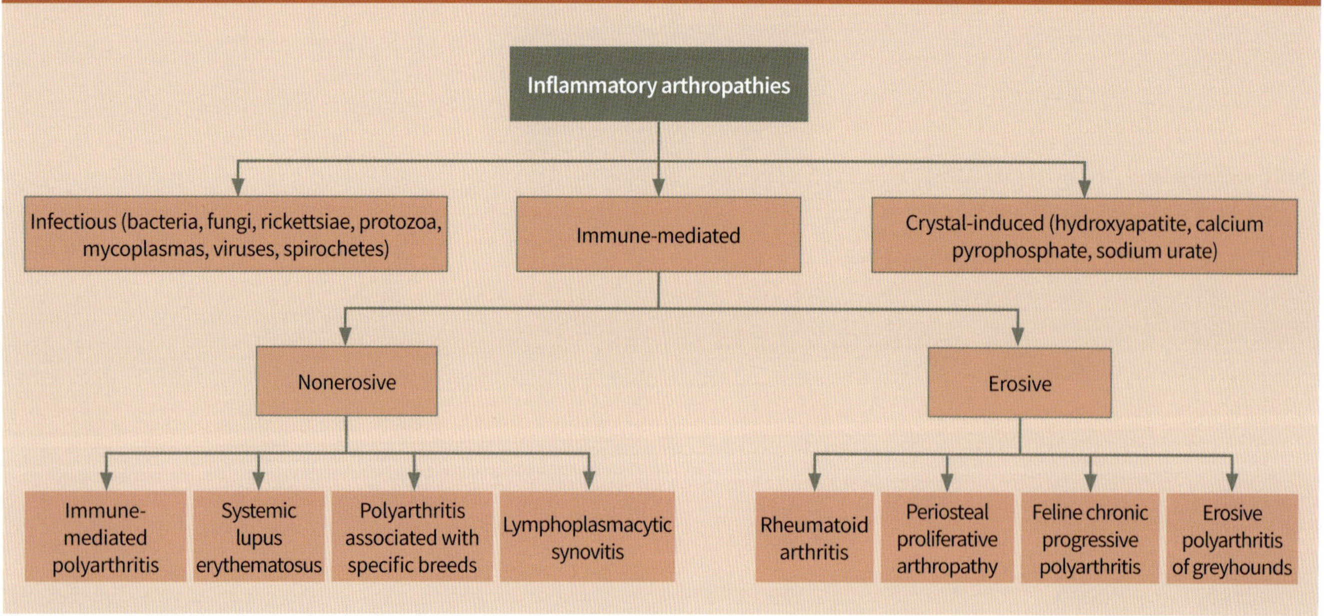

Adapted from Johnston SA, Tobias KM, *Veterinary Surgery: Small Animal Expert Consult*, 2nd ed. (2018).

Figure 2. Classification of noninflammatory arthropathies.

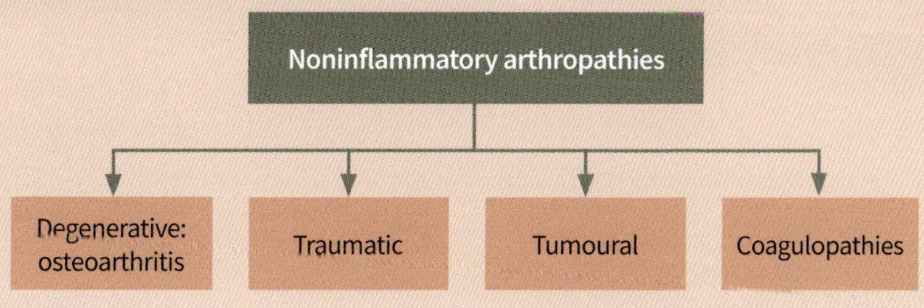

Adapted from Johnston SA, Tobias KM, *Veterinary Surgery: Small Animal Expert Consult*, 2nd ed. (2018).

INDICATIONS

Arthrocentesis is a technique indicated to evaluate synovial fluid in patients with suspected arthropathy.

> Synovial fluid analysis should be interpreted in conjunction with the patient's clinical signs, physical and orthopaedic examination findings and results of imaging of the affected joints.

CLINICAL SIGNS OF THE MOST COMMON ARTHROPATHIES

Clinical signs in animals with arthropathies vary from stiffness when walking to acute or chronic lameness. Lameness can occur with varying degrees of severity and can affect one or more limbs. Depending on the chronicity of the lameness, patients may have muscular atrophy or asymmetry in the affected limb. Some patients with inflammatory joint disease may present with fever (especially those with immune-mediated arthropathies) and nonspecific clinical signs of systemic disease (e.g. malaise, anorexia, enlarged lymph nodes).

Upon orthopaedic examination, it is possible to detect joint effusion in the affected limbs, and patients may show pain or discomfort upon palpation or when moving the joint. Also, when moving the joint throughout its range of motion, crepitus may be felt or the range of motion may be reduced.

It is very common to perform imaging tests on joints suspected of arthropathy. Although advanced diagnostic techniques can be performed (usually a CT scan, and less frequently an MRI), it is more common to perform orthogonal radiographs of the affected joint. Radiological findings depend on the cause of the arthropathy, and sometimes joints are radiologically normal even with disease. Nonspecific radiological changes, such as of effusion, distension of the joint capsule, osteophytosis, enthesiophytosis, subchondral sclerosis or thickening of periarticular soft tissues, are very frequent. These nonspecific radiographic findings are common in degenerative arthropathies (e.g. secondary to elbow dysplasia or rupture of the cranial cruciate ligament of the stifle). In contrast, in inflammatory arthropathies, changes such as lysis or sclerosis of the subchondral bone can be observed in some infectious conditions, whereas joint collapse with lysis and destruction of the subchondral bone can be observed in erosive inflammatory arthropathies.

TECHNIQUE

Arthrocentesis is performed by puncturing the joint with a hypodermic needle. The anatomical locations for this puncture have already been described for each joint (Clements, 2006; Torres and Duerr, 2020). This technique may cause discomfort and pain to the patient; therefore, sedation or anaesthesia is recommended for the procedure. Sedating the patient also decreases the probability of causing iatrogenic damage to the joint during sampling. Since most patients suspected of having joint disease undergo a diagnostic imaging study, it is common to perform arthrocentesis immediately after the imaging study, under the same sedation or anaesthesia.

The arthrocentesis technique must be performed aseptically, using sterile syringes, needles and gloves.

The patient is positioned in lateral recumbency and the area where the arthrocentesis is to be performed (usually a 5 × 5 cm square) is clipped and aseptically prepared. It is common to note an increase in resistance when passing through the joint capsule and inserting the hypodermic needle into the joint. The size of the hypodermic needle depends on the size of the joint to be tapped and on the size of the patient. Generally speaking, a 20–22-gauge needle is used in medium to large patients, and a 22–25-gauge needle is used in cats and small dogs. Once the joint has been punctured and synovial fluid has been obtained, it is important to cease aspirating with the syringe while leaving the joint to avoid contaminating the sample with peripheral blood.

Although there may be minor variations in the arthrocentesis technique, the current recommendations for each joint are described below.

SHOULDER ARTHROCENTESIS

Arthrocentesis of the shoulder joint can be performed through a lateral or cranial approach. A 22-gauge hypodermic needle 40 mm long is usually used for the procedure, although an 80 mm long needle may be necessary in giant-breed dogs.

Palpating the shoulder joint may be difficult, so anatomical landmarks are used to locate it. To perform lateral arthrocentesis, the shoulder is held in a neutral position, the acromial process of the scapula is taken as a landmark and the hypodermic needle is inserted immediately distal to it, directing the needle perpendicular to the scapula (Fig. 3).

The other option is to perform the technique via a cranial approach. In this case, the greater tubercle of the humerus is used as an anatomical landmark and the needle is introduced immediately medial to it (and distal to the supraglenoid tubercle of the scapula) in a craniocaudal direction (Fig. 4).

ELBOW ARTHROCENTESIS

Arthrocentesis of the elbow joint is usually performed with a 22-gauge needle, 40 mm in length. This technique is performed with the patient in lateral recumbency, and the sample is taken from the lateral aspect of the elbow. The author usually places the patient's elbow in a slightly flexed position (approximately 15–25 degrees of angulation). The lateral part of the humeral condyle and the olecranon of the ulna are located and used as anatomical landmarks. The hypodermic needle is introduced caudal and medial to the lateral condyle of the humerus, proximal to the olecranon, in a proximodistal direction between the most distal part of the lateral supracondylar crest of the humerus and the anconeal process of the ulna (Fig. 5).

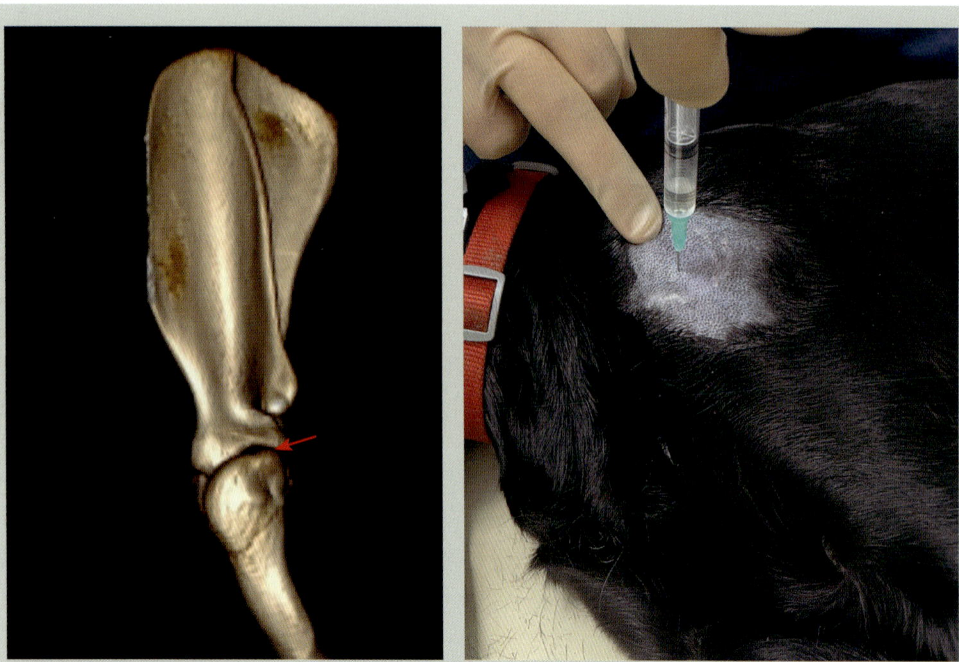

Figure 3. Shoulder arthrocentesis via lateral approach. The acromial process of the scapula is used as an anatomical landmark. The hypodermic needle is introduced immediately distal to the acromial process and directed perpendicular to the scapula. In the image, the surgeon is indicating the acromial process with their index finger.

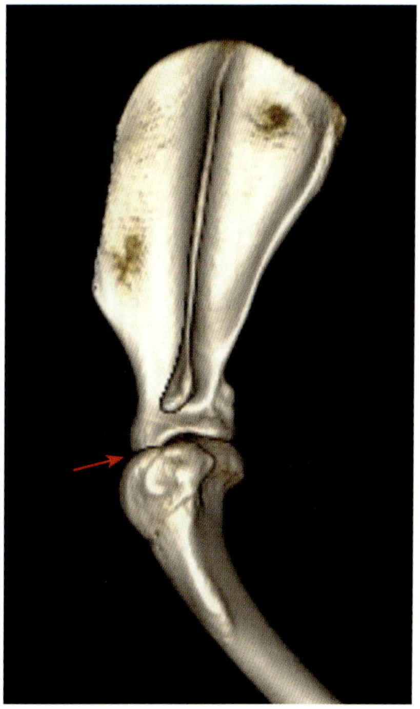

Figure 4. Shoulder arthrocentesis via cranial approach. The greater tubercle of the humerus is used as anatomical landmark. The needle is introduced immediately medial to the greater tubercle (and distal to the supraglenoid tubercle of the scapula) in a craniocaudal direction.

CARPAL ARTHROCENTESIS

To perform arthrocentesis of the carpal joint, a 25-gauge hypodermic needle 20–40 mm in length is usually utilised. The radiocarpal joint can be localised by palpating the cranial aspect of the carpus while flexing/extending the joint. In healthy patients, a depression can easily be identified when the joint is palpated; however, this may be more difficult in patients with joint disease due to intra-articular effusion.

Once the carpal joint has been located, the joint is flexed 90 degrees, the hypodermic needle is inserted perpendicular to the joint (Fig. 6) and synovial fluid is aspirated. When inserting the needle, the cephalic vein crossing the joint dorsally should be avoided; therefore, the needle should be inserted medial to said vein and to the tendon of the common digital extensor muscle. Sometimes a synovial fluid sample can be taken from the intercarpal joint using the same technique (Fig. 7).

HIP ARTHROCENTESIS

Locating the coxofemoral joint to perform arthrocentesis can be challenging, as it has a small joint space that is found several centimetres deep. Using the greater trochanter of the femur as an anatomical landmark, the hypodermic needle is introduced slightly craniodorsal to it. A 22-gauge, 80 mm long needle is usually used, and the needle is directed somewhat ventrally as it is advanced in the direction of the joint (Fig. 8). Sometimes it is useful to rotate internally, apply traction distally and abduct the limb to introduce the needle into the coxofemoral joint.

STIFLE ARTHROCENTESIS

The two most commonly used techniques to perform arthrocentesis of the stifle joint are the lateral technique and

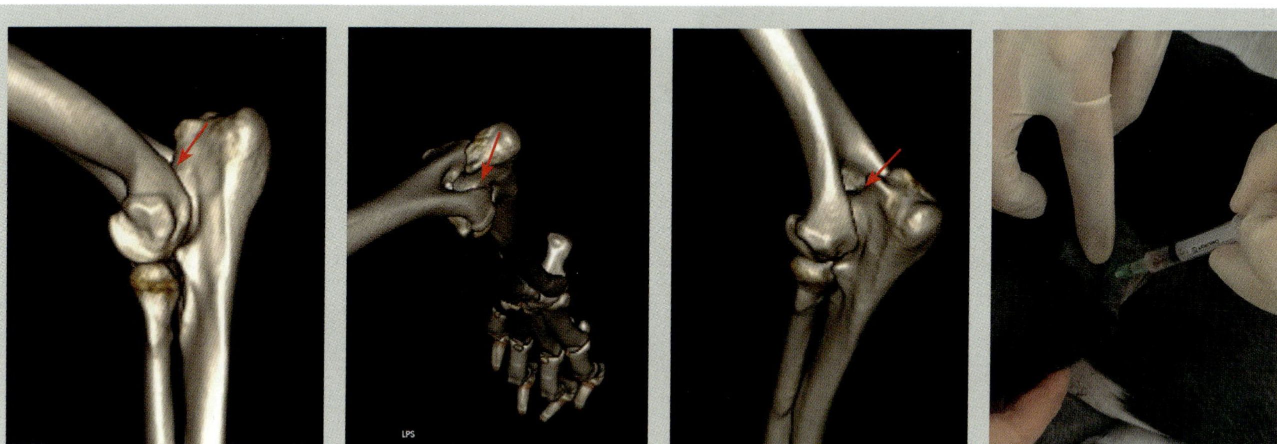

Figure 5. Elbow arthrocentesis via lateral approach. The needle is directed in a proximodistal direction between the most distal part of the lateral supracondylar crest of the humerus (indicated by the surgeon in the image) and the anconeal process of the ulna.

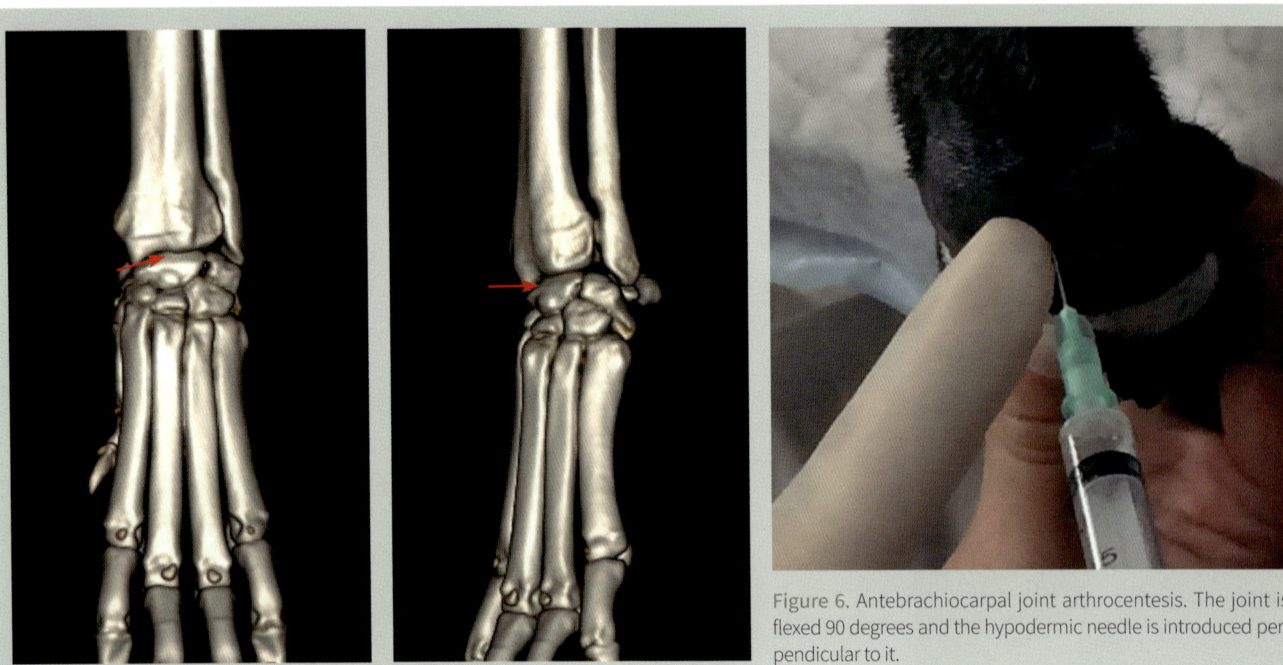

Figure 6. Antebrachiocarpal joint arthrocentesis. The joint is flexed 90 degrees and the hypodermic needle is introduced perpendicular to it.

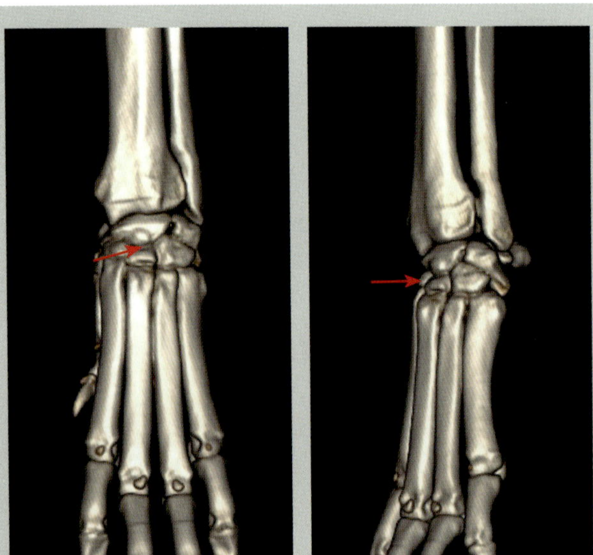

Figure 7. Intercarpal joint arthrocentesis. The hypodermic needle is introduced perpendicular to the joint.

the dorsal technique (the latter is preferred and routinely applied by the author). In both cases, the patient is placed in lateral recumbency, and a 22-gauge hypodermic needle, 40 mm in length, is usually used.

In the lateral technique, the limb is flexed slightly and the patellar ligament is used as an anatomical reference to introduce the needle. The needle is inserted immediately lateral to the patellar ligament, at the midpoint between the patella and the tibial tuberosity, with an orientation perpendicular to the joint (Fig. 9).

In the dorsal technique, the limb is extended or very slightly flexed. The hypodermic needle is introduced immediately lateral to the patellar ligament, in its distal third, in a distoproximal direction. Therefore, the hypodermic needle enters the joint immediately caudal to the patella, in the trochlear groove of the femur (Fig. 10).

TARSAL ARTHROCENTESIS

Arthrocentesis of the tarsal joint can be performed via a cranial or a caudolateral approach. A 25-gauge needle, 20–40 mm in length, is used regardless of the approach.

In the cranial approach, the tibiotarsal joint should be palpated and located via flexion and extension movements. Once the joint has been identified, the hypodermic needle is directed in a craniocaudal direction perpendicular to the joint (Fig. 11).

In the caudolateral approach, the lateral malleolus of the fibula and the calcaneus are used as anatomical landmarks. In this case, the tarsal joint should be slightly flexed and the hypodermic needle inserted immediately medial to the lateral malleolus of the fibula (Fig. 12).

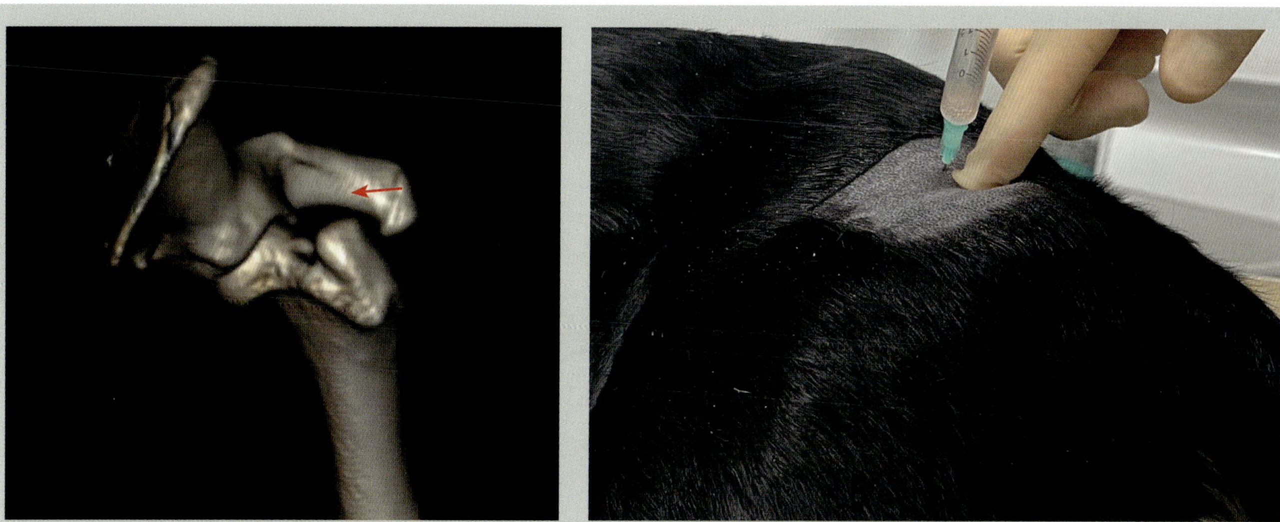

Figure 8. Coxofemoral joint arthrocentesis. The greater trochanter of the femur (indicated by the surgeon in the image) is used as anatomical landmark. The hypodermic needle is introduced slightly craniodorsal to the greater trochanter and directed with a slightly ventral orientation.

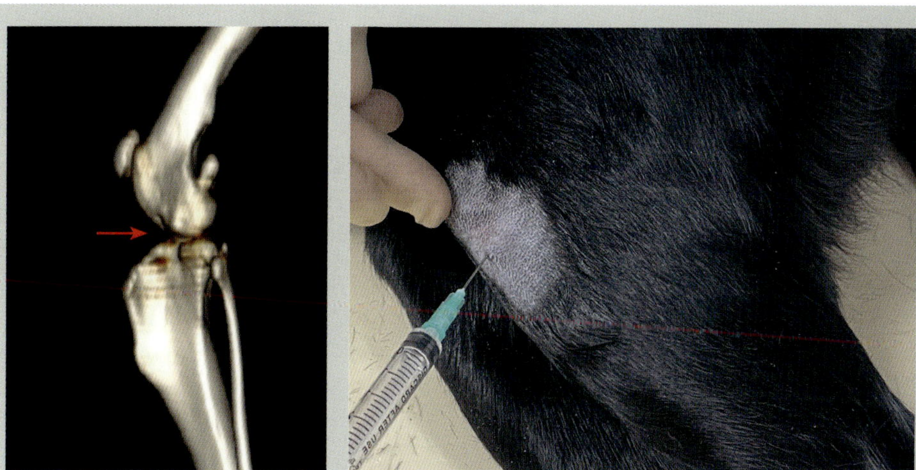

Figure 9. Stifle arthrocentesis via lateral approach. The needle is inserted immediately lateral to the patellar ligament, at the midpoint between the patella and the tibial tuberosity, with an orientation perpendicular to the joint.

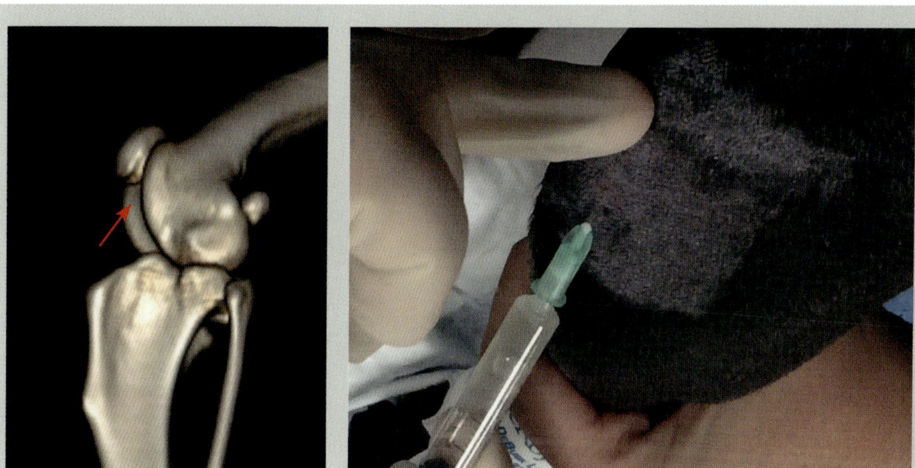

Figure 10. Stifle arthrocentesis via dorsal approach. The hypodermic needle is introduced immediately lateral to the patellar ligament, in its distal third, and is directed immediately caudal to the patella (indicated by the surgeon in the image), in the trochlear groove of the femur.

SYNOVIAL FLUID ANALYSIS

Synovial fluid is an ultrafiltrate of plasma with hyaluronic acid. Analysis of synovial fluid is based on subjective qualitative assessment and on cytological and microbiological evaluation (culture and antibiogram). When synovial fluid is analysed in an external laboratory, it is recommended to transport it at 4 °C within 24 hours (Harris and Santangelo, 2020).

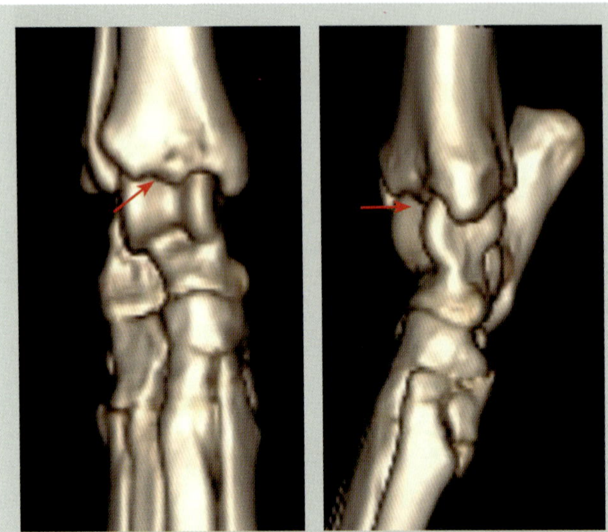

Figure 11. Tibiotarsal joint arthrocentesis via cranial approach. The hypodermic needle is directed in a craniocaudal direction perpendicular to the joint.

The cytological analysis includes determining the total cell count, the differential cell count and the proportion of mononuclear cells (lymphocytes, macrophages and synoviocytes) and polymorphonuclear cells (neutrophils). Once the synovial fluid has been obtained, the sample can be smeared on slides and placed in sterile tubes (glucose, lactate, total protein, mucin clot test and microbiological analysis), EDTA tubes (total cell count, cytology and total protein), heparin tubes (total cell count, total protein and mucin clot test) and culture media (if septic arthritis is suspected).

The number of samples that need to be sent for analysis depends on the amount of synovial fluid obtained and on the clinical suspicion. If a very small sample is available (1–2 drops), the author performs at least a smear on a slide for cytological examination. If the sample quantity is more abundant, the author routinely sends fresh smears on several slides, a sample preserved in EDTA, a sample in a sterile tube and a sample in a culture medium with blood (if septic arthritis is suspected).

The following parameters should be considered when analysing synovial fluid:

- **Volume.** The normal volume of synovial fluid in a joint depends on the size of the patient and the size of the joint. In general terms, the volume of synovial fluid should be very low and a volume greater than 0.5–1 ml is considered suggestive of arthropathy (Clements, 2006).

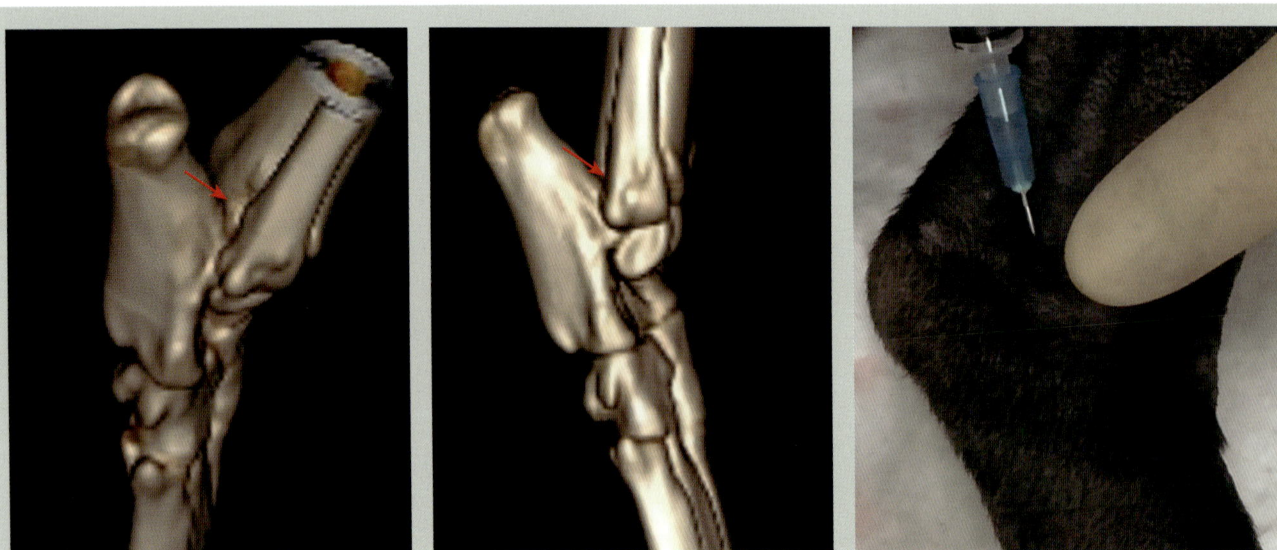

Figure 12. Tibiotarsal joint arthrocentesis via caudolateral approach. The hypodermic needle is introduced immediately medial to the lateral malleolus of the fibula (indicated by the surgeon in the image).

- **Colour.** Normal synovial fluid should be clear (although it may occasionally have a pale yellow colour). In the presence of joint disease, the synovial fluid may be sero-haemorrhagic or haemorrhagic, have a yellow orange colour (xanthochromia indicative of previous bleeding) or have a yellow white colour (suggestive of inflammatory arthropathy). A sample free of iatrogenic blood contamination should be obtained in order to differentiate whether the colour change is due to a pathological condition or due to sample collection (Fig. 13).
- **Viscosity.** Normal synovial fluid is viscous. Its degree of viscosity can be assessed subjectively by placing a drop of synovial fluid between two fingers and assessing the length of the thread the fluid forms when spreading the fingers apart before it breaks (Fig. 14). Normal synovial fluid should be able to spread about 2–4 cm before breaking. In joint disease, the synovial fluid is less viscous, so the length of fluid thread between the fingers is less than 2 cm.
- **Turbidity.** Synovial fluid is clear/transparent, so increased turbidity is considered pathologic. An increase in synovial fluid turbidity indicates an increase in cellularity (Fig. 15).

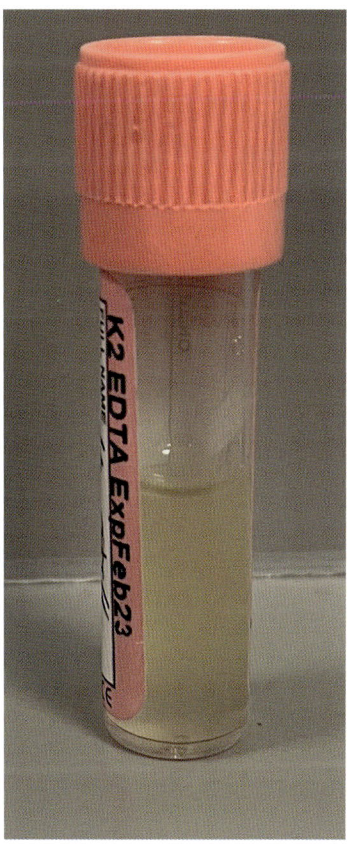

Figure 13. Synovial fluid sample of whitish colour, suggestive of joint disease.

- **Laboratory analysis:**
  - Total cell count:

  Normal synovial fluid has a very low total cellularity, of less than 2×10^9/l. Increased cellularity in the synovial fluid suggests the presence of joint disease. In inflammatory arthropathies, the increase in synovial fluid cell count can be very marked, reaching a cellularity of $250–350 \times 10^9$/l.

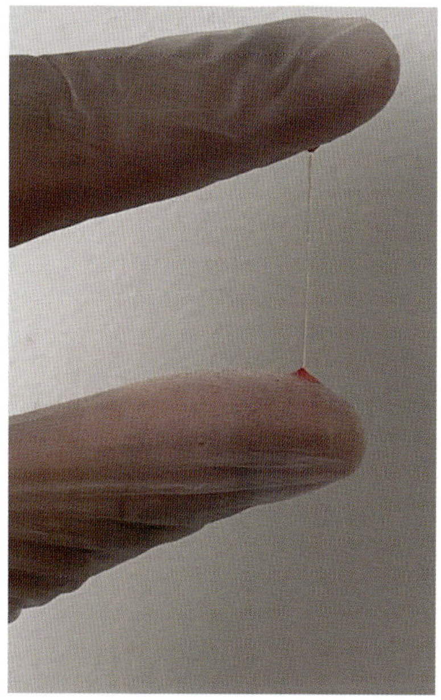

Figure 14. Subjective assessment of the degree of viscosity of the synovial fluid. A drop is placed between the fingers and, when they are separated, the length of the fluid thread is measured before it breaks.

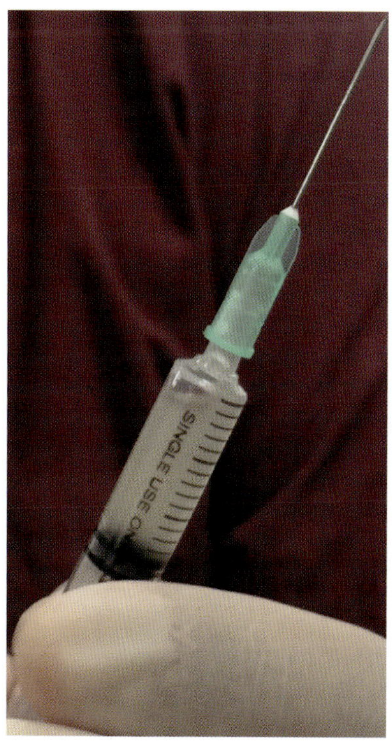

Figure 15. Synovial fluid sample with an increased degree of turbidity, suggestive of joint disease.

Total cell count can be carried out with an automatic analyser. To estimate this cell count, however, a direct smear of synovial fluid can be performed and the mean number of cells in 10 microscopic fields can be counted with a high-power objective lens (40×). Multiplying the average number of cells per microscopic field by 1000 gives an estimated number of cells per microlitre (Harris and Santangelo, 2020). Estimating with a direct smear is less accurate, so this value should only be used as a guideline in cases where an automatic analyser is not available.

- Differential cell count:

If sufficient sample volume is obtained, it should be placed in an EDTA tube to preserve cell morphology for subsequent analysis. If the volume is very small, 1–2 drops of synovial fluid are smeared on a slide and stained with a Diff-Quik-type rapid stain.

> Cytological analysis of the synovial fluid sample is probably the most important factor in differentiating the various types of arthropathy.

When a cytological study of the synovial fluid is performed, the proportion of each cell type must be determined, which makes it possible to differentiate whether an arthropathy has an inflammatory or noninflammatory origin. Noninflammatory joint diseases have a predominance of mononuclear cells (lymphocytes, macrophages and synoviocytes) (Fig. 16a), whereas inflammatory arthropathies have an increased number of polymorphonuclear cells (neutrophils) (Fig. 16b). If these are immune-mediated inflammatory arthropathies, the neutrophils have a nondegenerate appearance, whereas in case of infectious inflammatory joint diseases, neutrophils with a degenerated appearance may be present.

Although uncommon, the cytological analysis of synovial fluid can be pathognomonic when cells of a tumoural origin or intracellular bacteria are present in the sample.

- Microbiological culture:

A microbiological culture of synovial fluid should be performed whenever septic arthritis is suspected. The false negative rate of synovial fluid cultures is very high in septic arthritis, so it is recommended to culture synovial fluid in blood media (Fig. 17).

- **Mucin clot test.** The purpose of this test is to semiquantitatively determine the hyaluronic acid content of synovial fluid. To do so, acetic acid is mixed with the synovial fluid, causing a polymerisation of the hyaluronic acid. The result is the formation of a precipitate, which is evaluated for its quantity and consistency. Slower precipitate formation is associated with pathological or inflammatory conditions in the joint. This test is rarely used.
- **Lactate.** A recent study (Proot et al., 2015) evaluated the lactate concentration in the synovial fluid of patients with joint disease. This study found that patients with septic arthritis had higher lactate levels in their synovial fluid

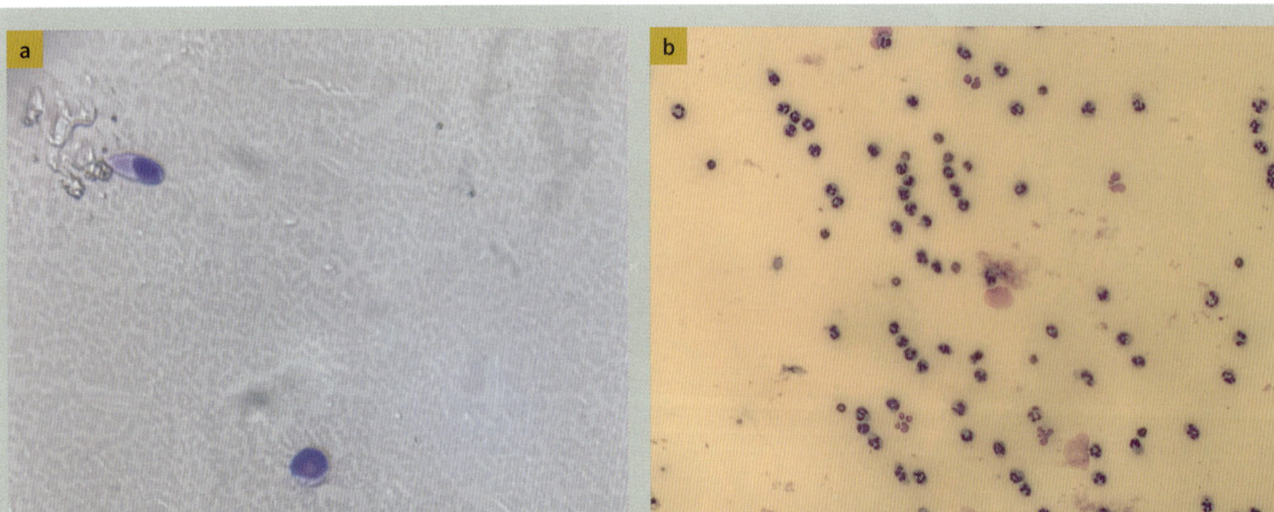

Figure 16. Cytological image of two synovial fluid samples. Sample from a patient with a noninflammatory arthropathy that has a predominance of mononuclear cells (a). Sample from a patient with an inflammatory arthropathy that has a predominance of neutrophils (b).

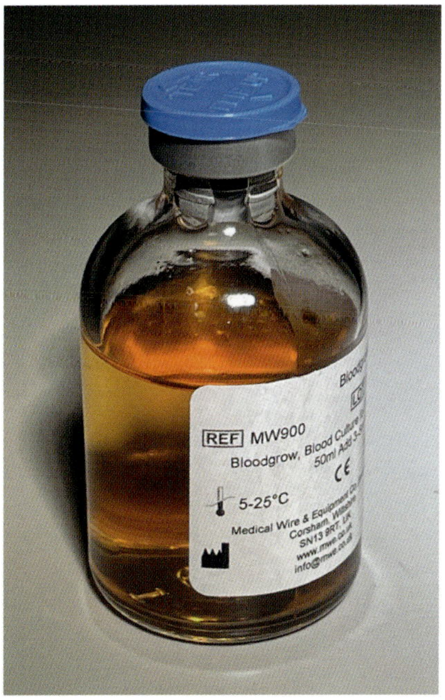

Figure 17. Blood culture medium used for the microbiological analysis of synovial fluid.

than was found in other types of arthropathies or in normal synovial fluid. Thus, a synovial fluid lactate result higher than 6.5 mmol/l was established as a predictive value for septic arthritis.

- **Total protein.** A determination of the protein content of synovial fluid can be performed using a refractometer or automatic counts. Values between 1.5 and 3 g/dl are considered normal (MacWilliams and Friedrichs, 2003). Its clinical use is limited, although an increase in this value is considered indicative of the presence of arthropathy. When assessing this result, it should be considered whether the blood:EDTA ratio in the collection tube was adequate, as an excess of EDTA due to a low volume of blood in the tube will lead to a false positive result.

The common findings observed in the synovial fluid of patients with the most common arthropathies are summarised in Table 1. Normal synovial fluid is viscous, and has a clear or pale yellow colour. From a cytological point of view, the synovial fluid in a normal joint has a very low cellularity (<2 × 10^9/l) and the cell population is predominantly mononuclear (94–100 %), with a low population of nondegenerate neutrophils (0–6 %).

In the presence of noninflammatory degenerative joint disease (osteoarthritis), the synovial fluid is usually also clear or pale yellow, but it is present in greater volume and has lower viscosity and higher cellularity (2–5 × 10^9/l). The predominant cell population in degenerative arthropathies is also mononuclear (88–100 %), and there may be a low population of nondegenerative neutrophils (0–12 %).

When a patient has a noninfectious inflammatory arthropathy, the synovial fluid is denser, with greater volume, lower viscosity and very high cellularity (4–370 × 10^9/l). Regarding the percentage of mononuclear cells and neutrophils, very variable ranges have been described (5–85 % and 15–95 %, respectively). It should be noted that it is very common for noninfectious inflammatory arthropathies to have an immune-mediated origin and affect several joints. Therefore, it is necessary to take samples from several joints if an immune-mediated arthropathy is suspected (it is recommended to take samples from at least four different, preferably distal, joints).

> If immune-mediated joint disease is suspected, it is recommended to take samples from at least four different joints, preferably distal.

In the presence of an infectious inflammatory arthropathy (septic arthritis), the synovial fluid is denser, with greater volume and lower viscosity. From a cytological point of view, the synovial fluid in these cases is largely composed of neutrophils (>90 %), both degenerated and nondegenerated.

TABLE 1. Common findings in synovial fluid in the most frequent arthropathies.

	Volume	Viscosity	Colour	Turbidity	Proteins	Total cell count	Mononuclear cells	Neutrophils
Normal	<0.5–1 ml	Viscous	Colourless, pale yellow	Clear, transparent	1.5–3 g/dl	2 × 10^9/l	>94 %	<6 %
Osteoarthritis	Normal/↑	Viscous/↓	Colourless, pale yellow	Clear, transparent	>3 g/dl	2–5 × 10^9/l	>88 %	<12 %
Immune-mediated arthritis	↑/↑↑	↓	Yellow, white, serosanguineous	Transparent, turbid	>3 g/dl	4–370 × 10^9/l	5–85 %	15–95 %
Septic arthritis	↑/↑↑	↓	Yellow, white, serosanguineous	Turbid	>3 g/dl	40–267 × 10^9/l	<10 %	>90 %

Occasionally, the presence of bacteria can be seen in the cytological examination, although this is not common. If bacteria are present in the sample, they are only pathognomonic of septic arthritis if they are located intracellularly; otherwise, they could be due to sample contamination.

COMPLICATIONS

The complication rate of arthrocentesis is extremely low when the technique is performed properly.

The most frequent complication is iatrogenic blood contamination of the sample. If mild, the results may be interpretable, as the pathologist can sometimes assess the cell count by comparing it to the peripheral blood count.

Although very rare, another potential complication is iatrogenic septic arthritis. When performing an arthrocentesis, it is essential to follow a strict aseptic protocol and avoid performing this test if the patient presents signs of dermatitis or pyoderma. The incidence of this complication when performing arthrocentesis in small animals is unknown, but in horses it has been reported in less than 0.1 % of cases (Steel et al., 2013).

Septic arthritis *(by Miguel Solano)*

Septic arthritis is an active joint infection, usually of bacterial origin, which typically results in inflammation, swelling, pain and lameness (Mielke et al., 2018) (Videos 1 and 2). Infection can occur by direct inoculation, by haematogenous spread or by extension of a local infection. The majority of bacterial septic arthritis cases manifest as an acute or chronic monoarthropathy.

Several different bacteria, most commonly *Staphylococcus intermedius*, *Staphylococcus aureus* and beta-haemolytic streptococci, have been implicated in bacterial infective arthritis in dogs (Mielke et al., 2018). Males of large-breed dogs are predisposed. The degree of lameness at presentation is variable but can be severe. Joint effusion and a variable periarticular swelling are seen (Fig. 19). Some dogs may present with severe clinical signs of cellulitis.

Video 1. Dog with clinical signs of right thoracic limb lameness related to septic arthritis.

Previous joint surgery has been reported as the most common cause of septic arthritis in a study of 31 dogs (Clements, 2006). Septic arthritis, even in the absence of pyrexia, should be considered as a major differential diagnosis in middle-aged, large-breed dogs with preexisting elbow arthritis that suffer an acute onset of lameness with elbow joint effusion and discomfort (Mielke et al., 2018).

Synovial fluid sampling is strongly recommended (Figs. 18 and 20). Samples for cytology, culture (inoculated into a blood culture medium) and lactate analysis (if available) should be taken. Mielke et al. (2018) reported positive culture results in only 50 % of dogs with suspected septic arthritis. Considering the high number of false negative results, it is recommended to incubate the synovial fluid sample in blood culture media for 24 hours to increase the sensitivity of the test (Miller et al., 2018).

> Synovial fluid samples should be taken for cytology, culture and lactate analysis. Incubating the sample in blood culture media improves the sensitivity of culture.

A presumptive diagnosis of bacterial infective arthritis can be made when the synovial fluid collected from a monoarthropathy shows very high nucleated cell counts (>50 × 10^9 cells/ml), predominantly polymorphonuclear cells (Fig. 21), the presence of intracellular bacteria on cytology or a combination of both findings. Synovial fluid lactate concentration is significantly increased in septic arthritis and can be used to rule out this condition in a quick and cost-effective manner (Proot et al., 2015) (Fig. 22).

Septic arthritis *(by Miguel Solano)*

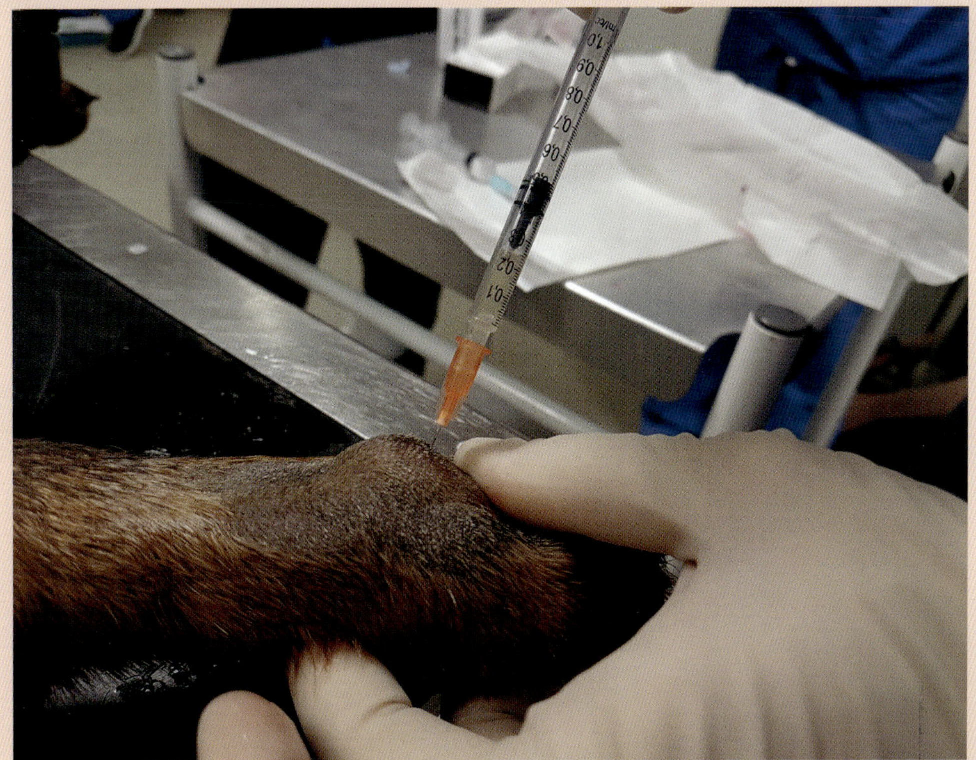

Figure 18. Arthrocentesis in the same dog as in Video 1. Note the yellow, milky appearance of the synovial fluid in the syringe.

> Synovial fluid analysis results consisting of very high polymorphonuclear leukocyte counts, intracellular bacteria on cytology and/or high lactate concentrations are indicative of bacterial septic arthritis.

Video 2. Dog with right pelvic limb lameness and an enlarged right hock.

Video 3. Low viscosity of the synovial fluid shown in Figure 20.

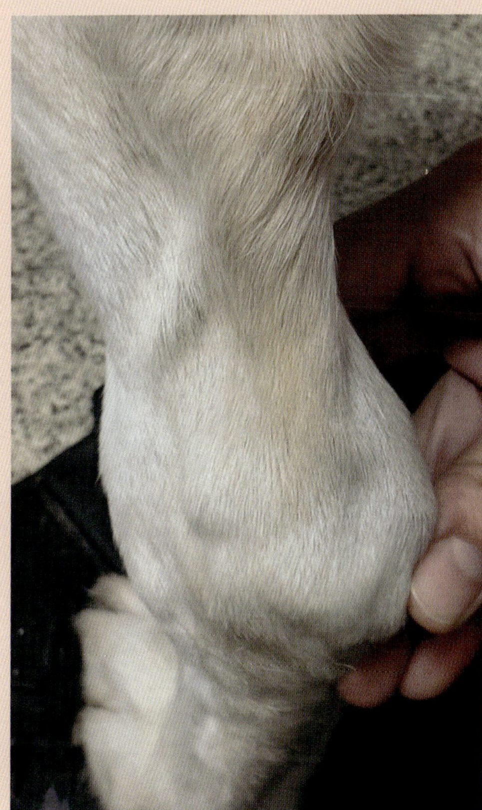

Figure 19. Same patient as in Video 2. Enlarged right hock, with palpable effusion and periarticular thickening.

Septic arthritis *(by Miguel Solano)*

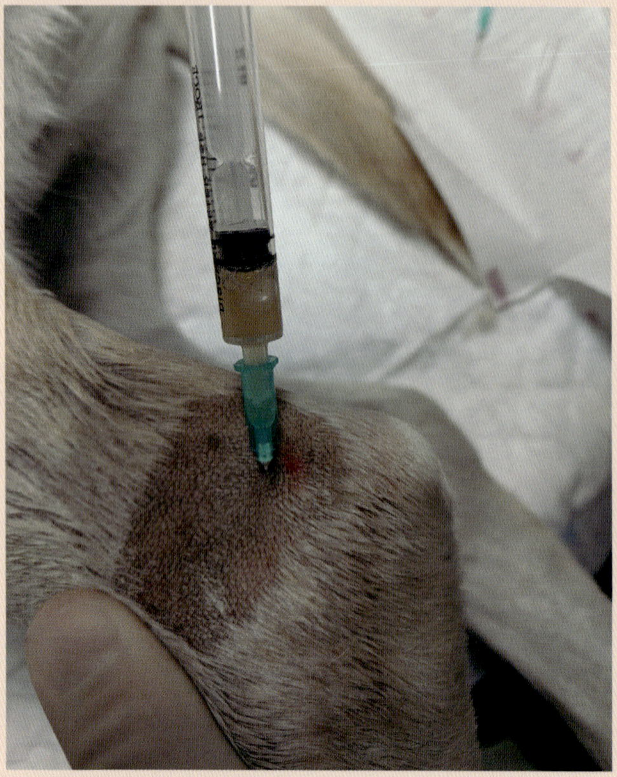

Figure 20. Arthrocentesis of the right hock in the same dog as in Video 2. Note the yellow, milky appearance of the synovial fluid.

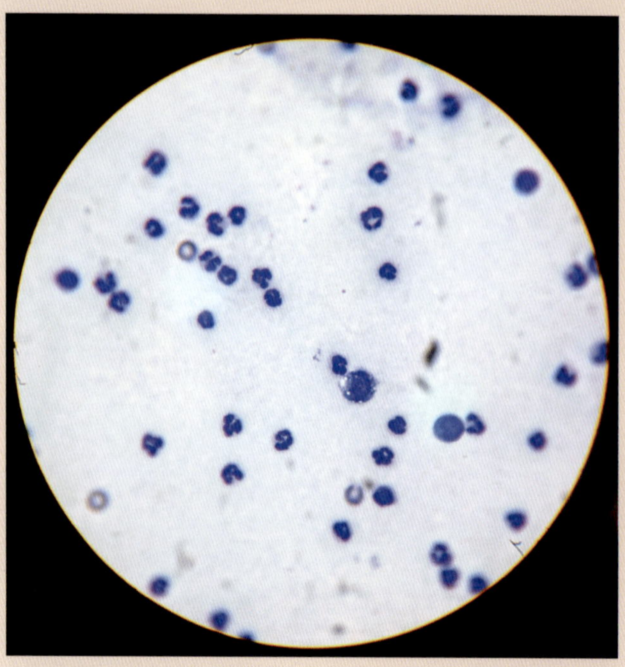

Figure 21. Synovial fluid cytology from the right hock of the same patient as in Video 2. High numbers of polymorphonuclear neutrophils can be seen.

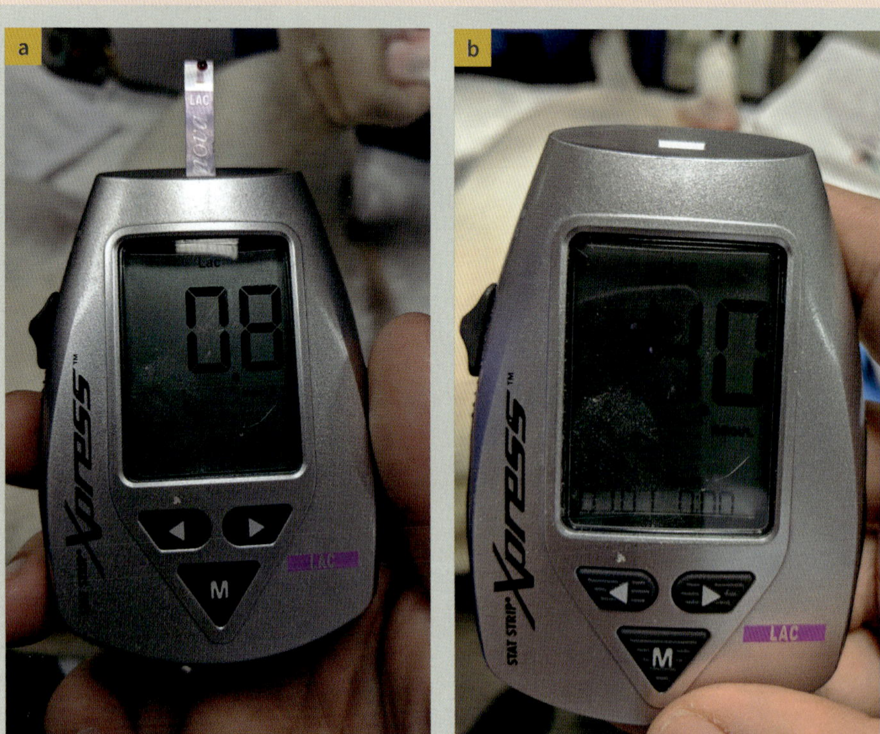

Figure 22. Lactate concentrations in the same patient as in Video 2. Peripheral blood lactate concentration (a). Lactate concentration in the synovial fluid of the right hock (b). Note the high intrasynovial lactate values. Sepsis cannot be ruled out based on these results.

Septic arthritis *(by Miguel Solano)*

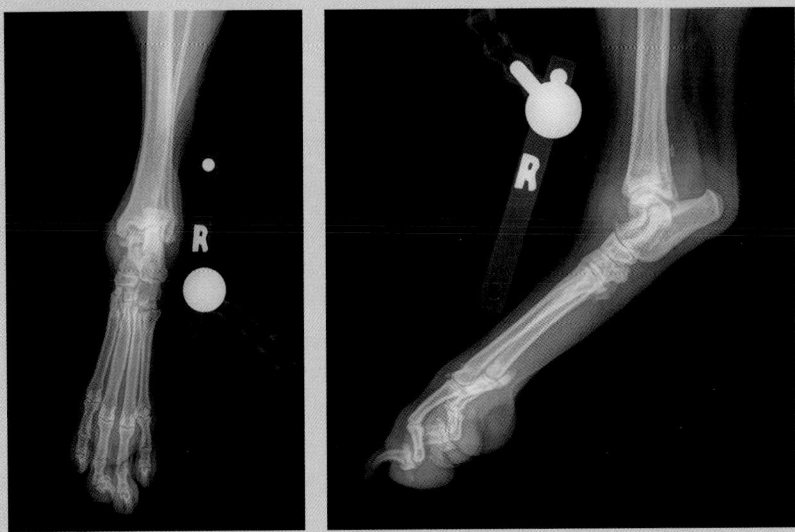

Figure 23. Orthogonal radiographs of the same dog as in Video 2 showing signs of an irregular medial talar ridge with concurrent periarticular degenerative changes and a soft tissue opacity around the talocrural joint suggestive of effusion and periarticular thickening. The changes seen on the talus are likely related to a chronic osteochondritis dissecans lesion.

The vast majority of affected dogs improve after antibiotic therapy for 4–6 weeks based on culture and sensitivity testing, if available, with no difference in the outcomes of dogs that had joint lavage and/or arthrotomy in addition to antibiotic therapy (Mielke et al., 2018; Clements, 2006). The most commonly prescribed antibiotics were potentiated amoxicillin, cephalexin or potentiated amoxicillin with enrofloxacin (Mielke et al., 2018). After treatment, dogs with preexisting joint osteoarthritis and a previous history of lameness may be similarly or more severely lame when compared to the lameness prior to the septic episode.

Joint neoplasia *(by Miguel Solano)*

Tumours of the joints should be suspected in older, large-breed dogs with periarticular swelling and radiographic evidence of osteolysis on both sides of the affected joint (Craig et al., 2002) (Fig. 24; Video 4). This generally helps to differentiate joint tumours from primary bone tumours, which typically involve one of the bones surrounding the affected joint.

Common periarticular tumours are histiocytic sarcoma, synovial cell sarcoma, synovial myxoma/myxosarcoma and malignant fibrous histiocytoma. The most common joint neoplasia reported in a study of 35 dogs was histiocytic sarcoma (51 %), followed by synovial myxoma (17 %), synovial cell sarcoma (14 %) and others (17 %) (Craig et al., 2002). Rottweilers were overrepresented in the histiocytic sarcoma group, and Dobermans in the synovial myxoma group. The most common affected joint overall was the stifle, and 54 % of dogs with histiocytic sarcoma in the stifle had clinical signs of cranial cruciate ligament disease. This is important to remember when dogs present to veterinary practices for management of cranial cruciate ligament disease with an atypical level of periarticular swelling and diffuse lytic changes. It is strongly recommended to take synovial samples for analysis when encountering a potentially pathological synovium.

One study reported a median survival time for dogs with periarticular histiocytic sarcoma (5.3 months) that

Joint neoplasia *(by Miguel Solano)*

was shorter than the median survival time for dogs with synovial cell sarcoma or synovial myxoma (>30 months) (Craig et al., 2002). Staging is strongly recommended. The surgical and medical management of joint neoplasia is beyond the scope of this book.

Video 4. Frontal, sagittal and transverse plane CT scan of the same dog as in Figure 24 diagnosed with a periarticular sarcoma. Note the additional detail on the lytic changes observed in the femur and tibia when compared with the radiographs.

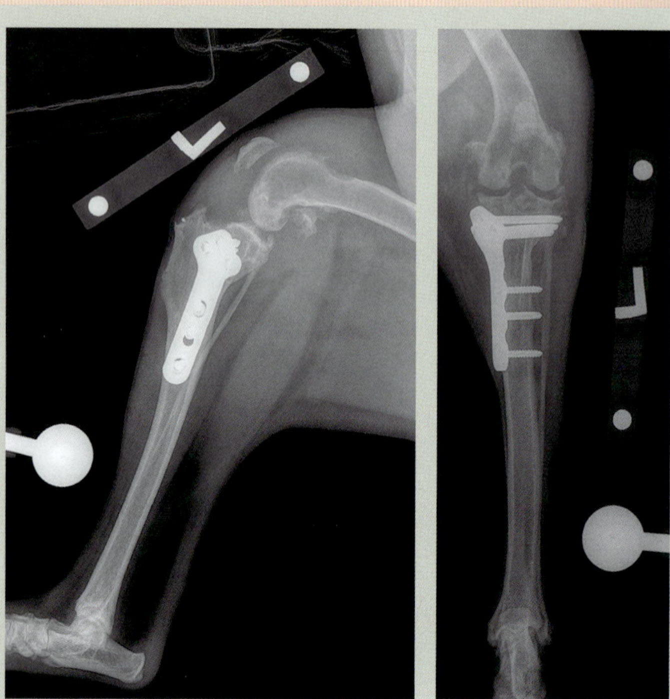

Figure 24. Orthogonal radiographs of the stifle of a dog 6 months after tibial plateau levelling osteotomy showing multiple lytic lesions in the distal femur and proximal tibia. Note the increased soft tissue opacity surrounding the proximal, cranial and caudal aspects of the stifle joint.

ARTHROSCOPY

Alan Danielski

INTRODUCTION

Arthroscopy is considered a minimally invasive procedure that offers the advantages of enhanced visualisation of intra-articular structures, increased precision, minimal soft tissue trauma, reduced postoperative pain and, therefore, faster postoperative recovery. Disadvantages include a relatively steep learning curve and the cost associated with the purchase of the equipment and consumables used during surgery (Schulz, 2012).

Given the possibility of severely damaging the articular cartilage at the time of performing arthroscopy, especially in small joints, it is highly advisable to first practice on cadaveric joints before attempting to perform arthroscopy in clinical cases.

As the indications for performing arthroscopy of the carpus are very limited, only arthroscopy of the elbow and shoulder joints will be discussed in this chapter.

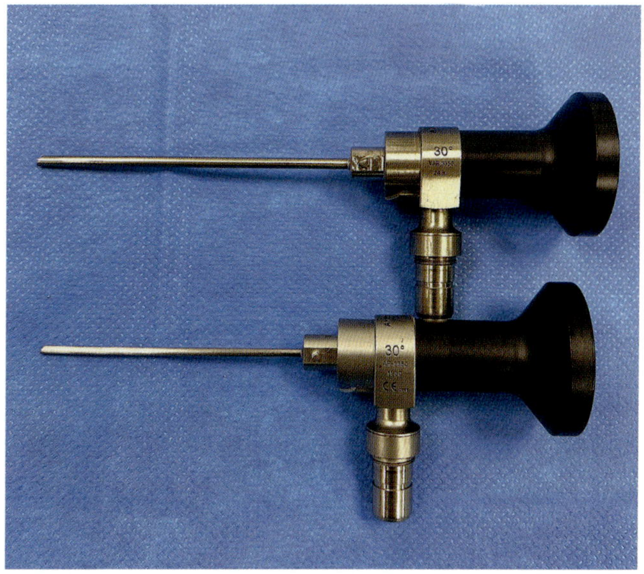

Figure 1. 2.4 mm short 30-degree oblique arthroscope (top) and 1.9 mm short 30-degree oblique arthroscope (bottom) (Arthrex Vet Systems, Munich, Germany).

ELBOW ARTHROSCOPY

The elbow is the joint of the thoracic limb in which arthroscopy is most commonly performed. Depending on the size of the animal, elbow arthroscopy is relatively easy to perform because of the clearly recognisable bony landmarks and the relatively thin soft tissue coverage.

When combined with preoperative CT scan assessment, arthroscopy allows the surgeon to fully examine the joint and reach a meaningful diagnosis.

INSTRUMENTATION

Arthroscopy of the elbow joint is usually performed using a 2.4 mm 30-degree rigid arthroscope in medium- and large-breed dogs and a 1.9 mm 30-degree rigid arthroscope in small-breed dogs (Figs. 1 and 2).

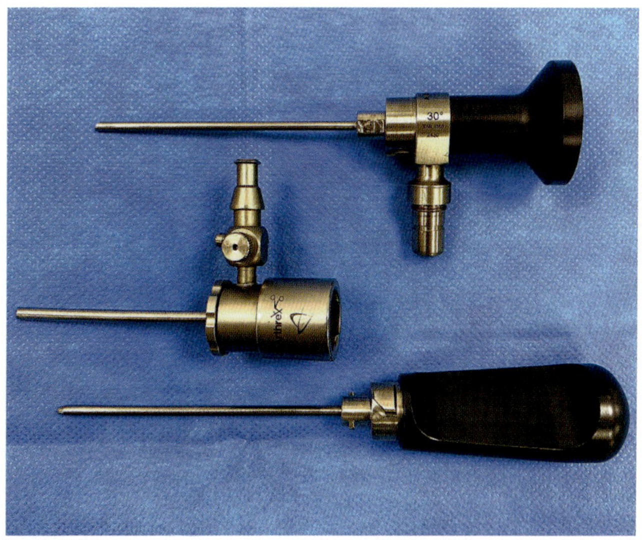

Figure 2. 2.4 mm short arthroscope (top), stopcock sheath for the 2.4 mm arthroscope (middle) and relatively blunt trocar (bottom) (Arthrex Vet Systems, Munich, Germany).

The author prefers to use a short arthroscope in order to be able to fully control the depth of insertion of the sheath

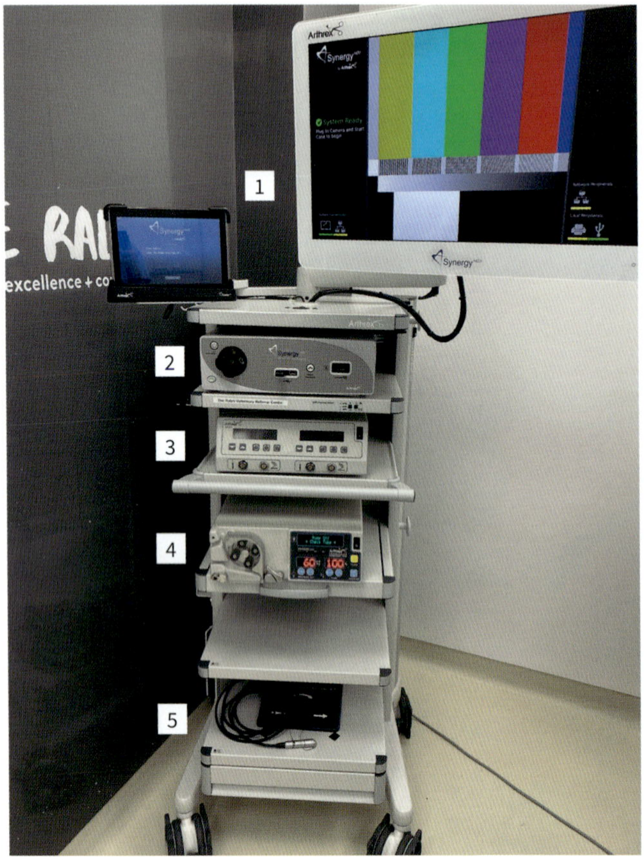

Figure 3. Arthroscopy tower (Arthrex Vet Systems, Munich, Germany). 1, display and tablet; 2, HD console, which combines HD camera, LED lighting and image management; 3, shaver box; 4, fluid pump; 5, shaver pedal control.

and of the arthroscope by keeping one or two fingers of the left hand on the skin whilst holding the camera with the rest of the hand and using the right hand to move the light post around to change the view direction inside the joint. A 1080p HD three-chip camera coupled with a LED light cable allows to achieve the best image definition (Figs. 3 and 4).

Basic instrumentation for joint inspection and treatment of the main conditions affecting the elbow includes an arthroscope and sheath, a smooth and sharp trocar, two Gordon's coronoid osteotomes (2 and 4 mm), a right-angle probe, a hand burr, an arthroscopic knife, a 40-degree micropick and at least two different types of grasping forceps (Figs. 5–8). These forceps vary in size and length; the selection depends on the joint being inspected, the size of the dog and the surgeon's preference. Small forceps are preferable in the joints of small animals, but their fragility and high cost should be taken into account.

The fluids used to distend the joint can be administered via a gravity flow system (with or without the use of a compression bag) or a fluid pump. Using a fluid pump is recommended, as this permits selection of the flow rate and pressure of the fluid, and it also maintains a constant desired pressure inside the joint. The ideal fluid pressure for the elbow joint is 60–70 mmHg (with the flow rate kept at 10–20 %).

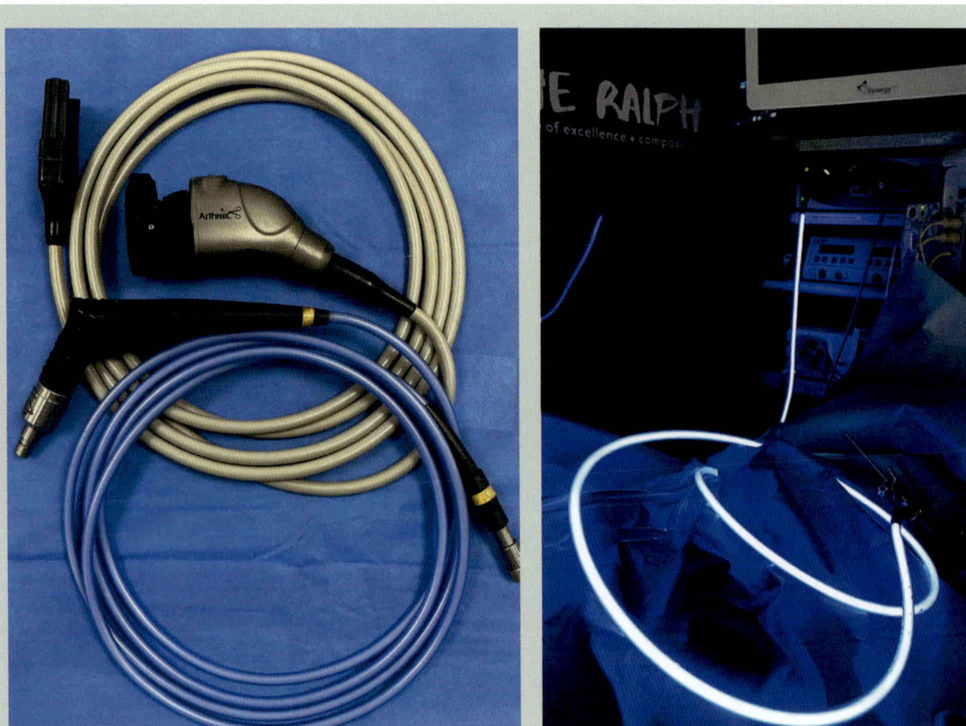

Figure 4. 1080p HD autoclavable camera head and LED light cable (Arthrex Vet Systems, Munich, Germany).

PREPARATION

Meticulous preparation and the help of a good surgical assistant are key to a successful surgery. The limb is clipped and aseptically prepared from the most proximal aspect of the scapula to the distal carpus. A plastic glove and a cohesive bandage are used to wrap the foot distal to the carpus. The patient is then placed on the operating table in dorsal recumbency with a hanging limb technique. Large sandbags or a trough are placed under the lumbar spine to keep the patient well positioned and straight during surgery. A sandbag or a custom-made brace is positioned adjacent to the affected elbow to be used as a fulcrum for initial joint distraction. Some surgeons prefer to use the table edge as a fulcrum to distract the joint. It is the author's preference to place a narrow sandbag, rather than a wide one, next to the patient's body under the sterile drapes in order to allow correct placement of the sandbag under the distal humerus (Fig. 9). This facilitates limb leverage and subsequent joint distraction.

The assistant then holds the distal limb such that the humerus is parallel to the floor and externally rotates the distal extremity (pronation) to allow additional opening of the medial aspect of the joint space (Fig. 10). It is crucial that the assistant does not move from that position during surgery, as this will cause the medial compartment of the

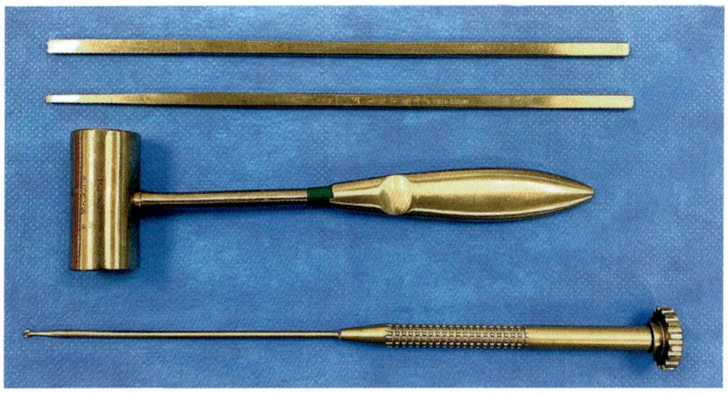

Figure 5. Instrumentation (top to bottom): 2 mm Gordon's osteotome, 4 mm Gordon's osteotome, mallet and hand burr (Veterinary Instrumentation, Sheffield, UK).

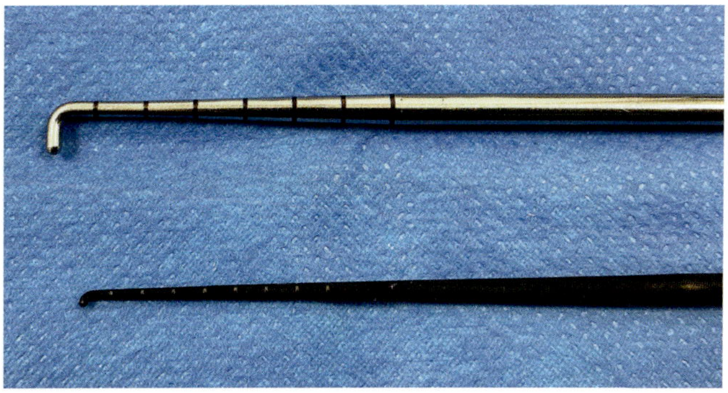

Figure 6. Arthroscopic probes with measuring marks for large and small joints (Arthrex Vet Systems, Munich, Germany).

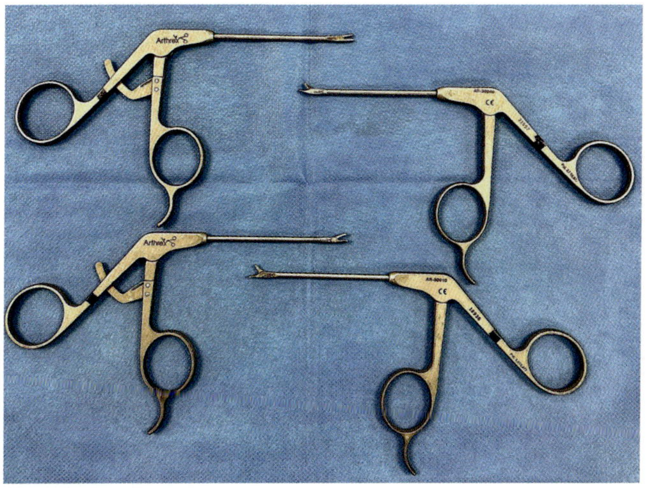

Figure 7. Locking (left) and non-locking (right) arthroscopic grasping forceps (Arthrex Vet Systems, Munich, Germany).

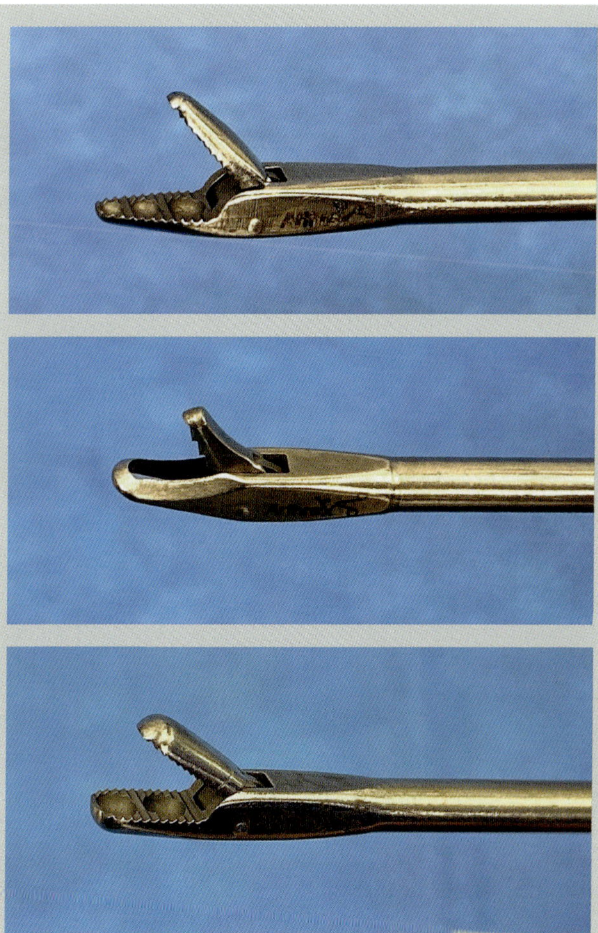

Figure 8. Detail of the grasping ends of the different arthroscopic grasping forceps of Figure 7.

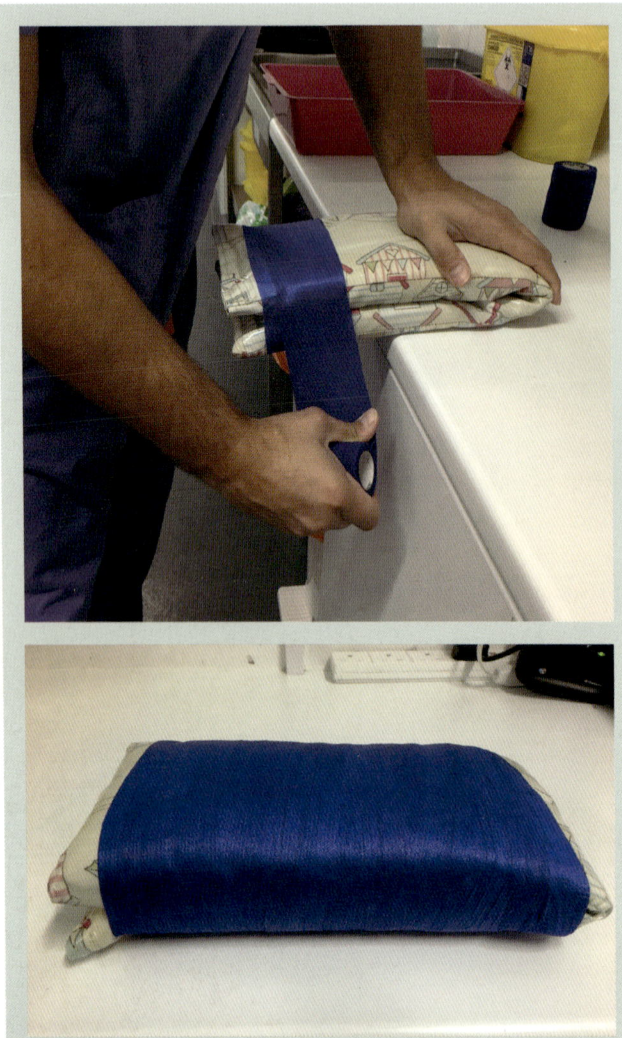

Figure 9. A sandbag is tightly wrapped with a cohesive bandage.

elbow to collapse, will impede inspection and may lead to iatrogenic cartilage damage.

> The assistant should not push the limb too further down to avoid tearing the medial collateral ligament

Figure 10 shows the correct positioning of the patient on the surgical table and the correct placement of the sandbag used to distract the elbow joint.

The egress portal (Fig. 11) is established first by inserting an 18-gauge needle (connected to a 10 ml syringe filled with sterile lactated Ringer's solution) craniomedially into the elbow joint (ideally aiming to insert it just caudal to the medial collateral ligament and the median nerve) in a caudolateral direction. Once synovial fluid is aspirated, confirming intra-articular placement, sterile lactated Ringer's solution is instilled to distend the joint.

The arthroscopic portal is established next. The author prefers to use a more caudal arthroscopic portal rather than the traditional medial portal (Beale et al., 2003), as it allows a better visualisation of the medial and caudal elbow compartments. After making a small skin incision with a number 11 scalpel blade, the arthroscope cannula with the attached blunt obturator is inserted caudal to the medial epicondyle and the ulnar nerve, in a craniolateral direction, parallel to the medial surface of the anconeal process of the ulna (Fig. 12). Typically, the skin incision is made along the

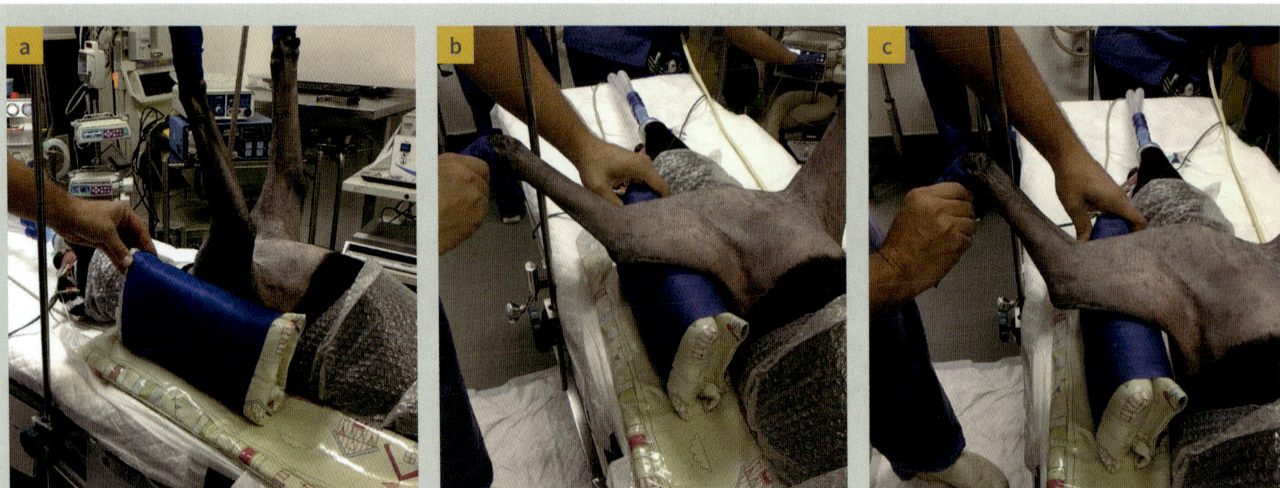

Figure 10. The wrapped sandbag is placed adjacent to the affected elbow, on the top of another sandbag (a). The limb is extended, taking care to keep the humerus parallel to the table, and the sandbag is used as a fulcrum to help with joint distraction (b). The distal extremity is externally rotated to point down, achieving pronation of the elbow joint and therefore additional joint distraction (c).

palpable and visible line of indentation between the cranial border of the triceps muscle and the caudal aspect of the medial humeral epicondyle, taking care to avoid the ulnar nerve in this region.

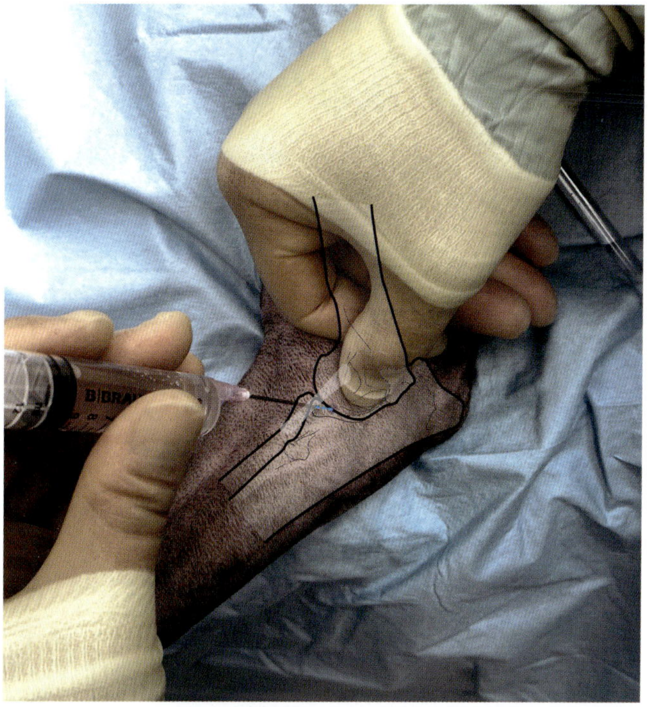

Figure 11. The egress portal is established with an 18-gauge needle on a 10 ml syringe. The needle is inserted in a craniomedial to caudolateral direction immediately caudal to the medial collateral ligament.

JOINT INSPECTION

The camera head needs to be always maintained in an upright position (in order to keep the proximal aspect of the joint at the top of the screen), and the light post is rotated to inspect the joint. This helps immensely in maintaining orientation and spatial awareness. The assistant should achieve adequate medial joint distraction to facilitate the movement of the arthroscope inside the joint and avoid iatrogenic cartilage damage. A systematic thorough exploration of the joint is recommended.

The nontraditional caudal portal allows inspection of the entirety of the medial coronoid process (MCP), the radial head, the medial collateral ligament, the biceps brachii insertion on the medial aspect of the MCP, the medial humeral condyle, the abaxial aspect of the lateral humeral condyle (from the most cranial aspect to the most caudal aspect by simply extending and flexing the elbow under visualisation), the lateral coronoid process, the entirety of the medial aspect of the ulnar notch, the anconeal process and, in some cases, the most caudal aspect of the supratrochlear foramen (Fig. 14).

It is important to get used to what is normal in order to be able to recognise what is abnormal. This is why practicing on sound cadaveric joints is essential, as the lack of blood and synovitis (Fig. 15) will provide a better understanding of the normal joint anatomy. A grading system derived from the original Outerbridge classification was proposed by Farrell et al. in 2014 to classify the degree of articular cartilage damage based on the arthroscopic appearance (Table 1).

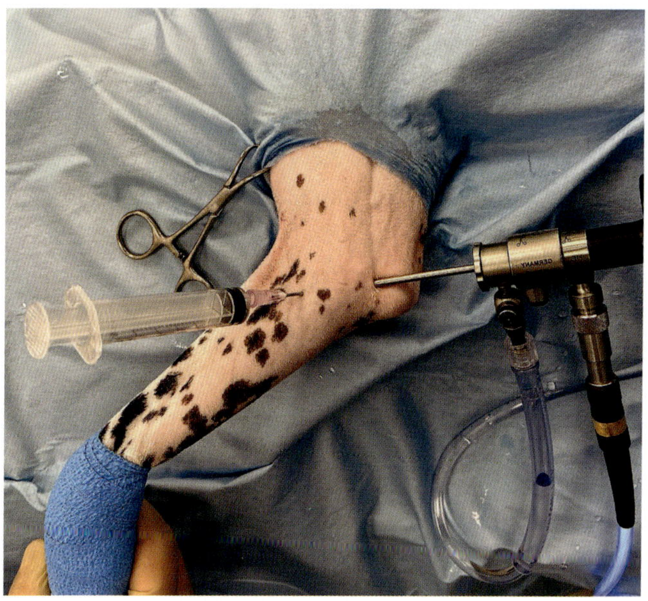

Figure 12. The arthroscopic portal is usually created in the little depression at the cranial border of the triceps muscle and immediately caudal to the caudal aspect of the medial humeral epicondyle.

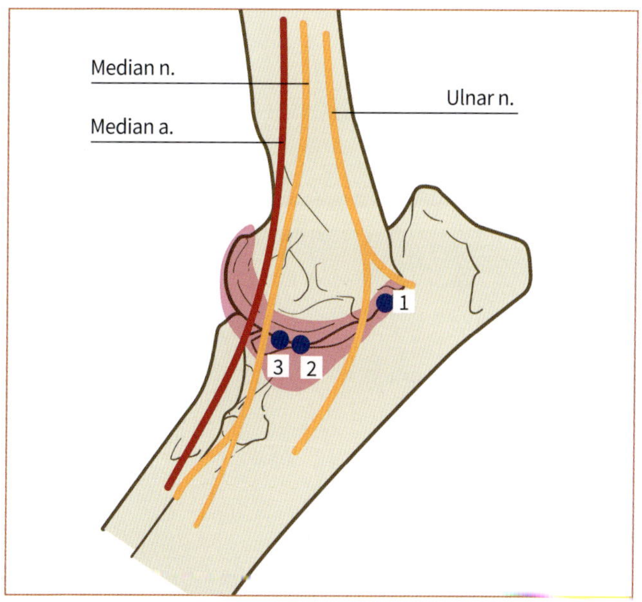

Figure 13. Medial view of the elbow joint: anatomical landmarks and portal locations for arthroscopy. 1, arthroscopic portal; 2, instrument portal; 3, egress portal.

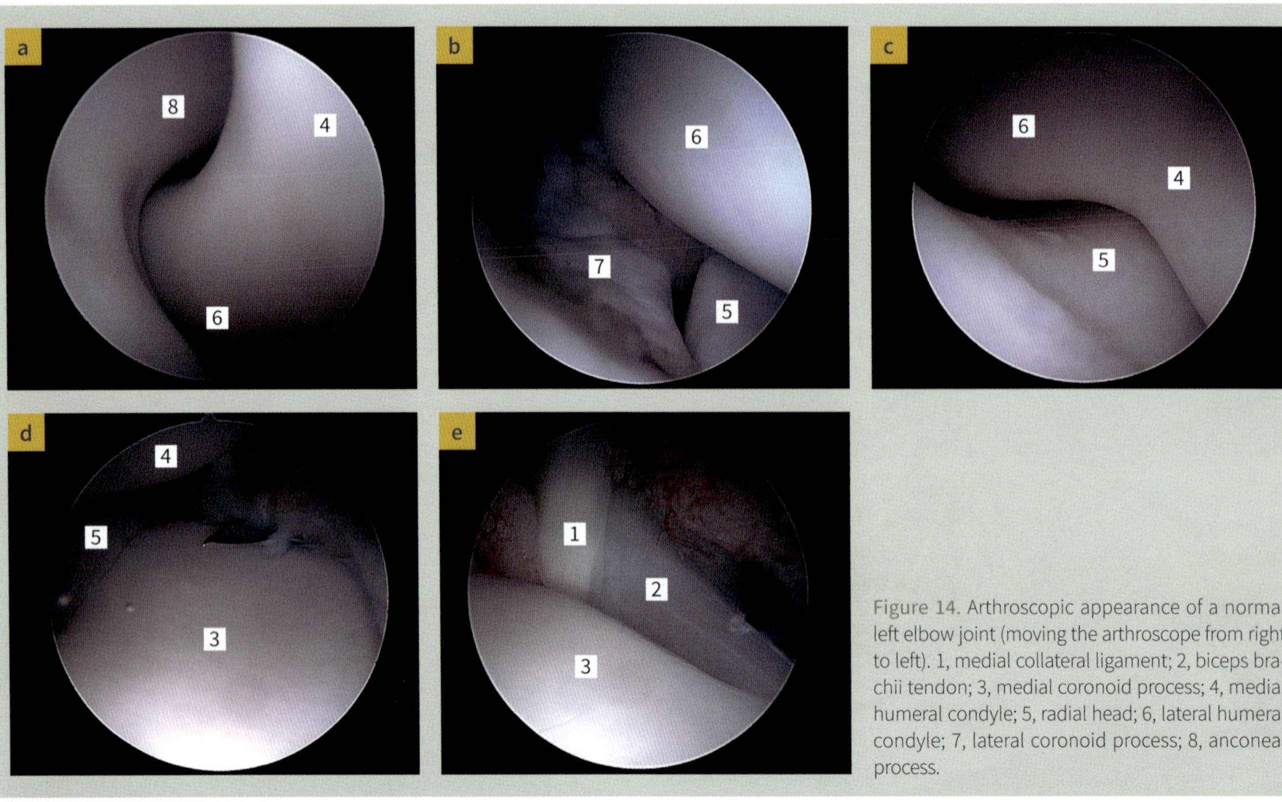

Figure 14. Arthroscopic appearance of a normal left elbow joint (moving the arthroscope from right to left). 1, medial collateral ligament; 2, biceps brachii tendon; 3, medial coronoid process; 4, medial humeral condyle; 5, radial head; 6, lateral humeral condyle; 7, lateral coronoid process; 8, anconeal process.

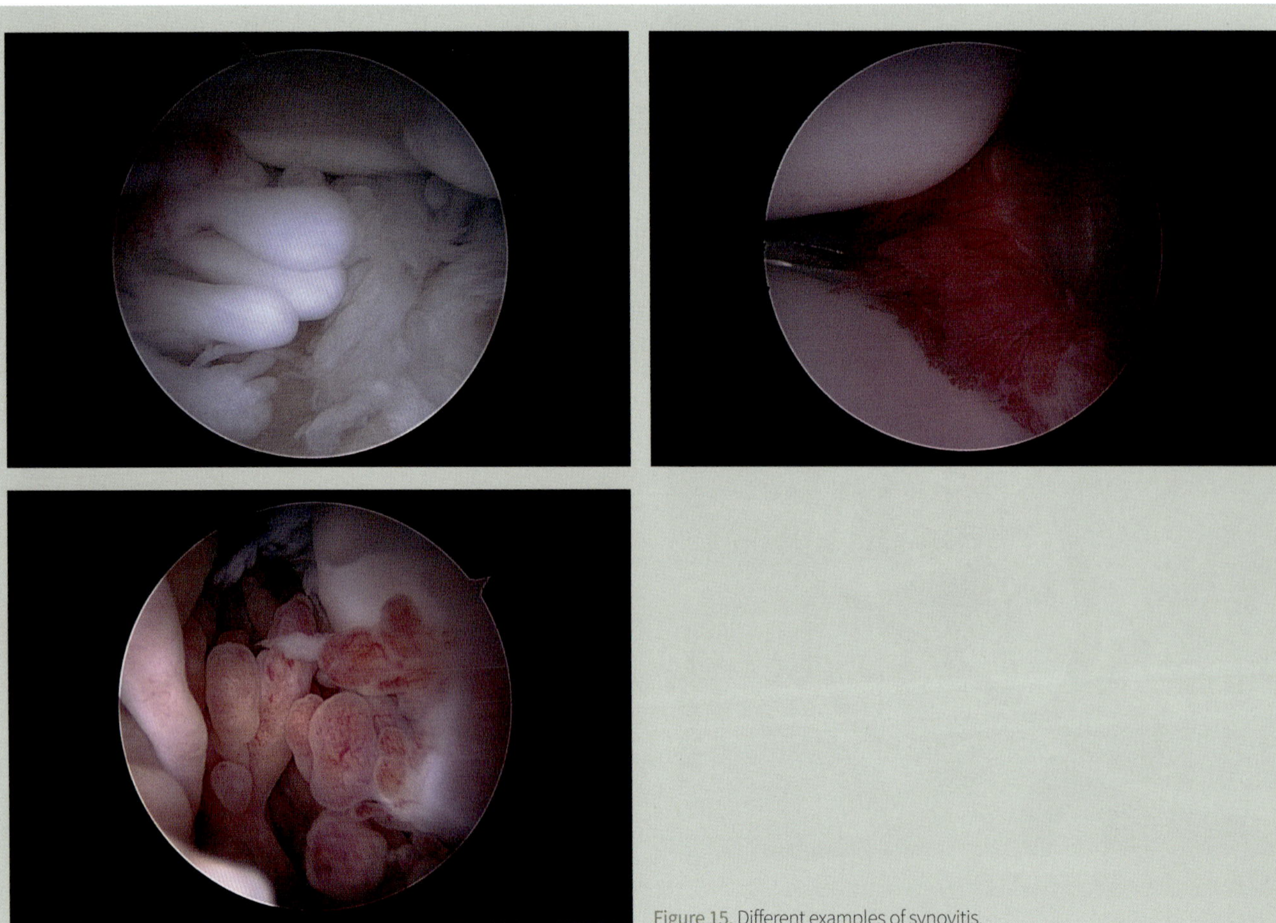

Figure 15. Different examples of synovitis.

TABLE 1. Modified Outerbridge score system for the classification of articular cartilage damage.

Grade	Description	Examples
I	Cartilage softening and swelling (the cartilage appears thicker, or its surface appears dull/less translucent than that of the adjacent cartilage)	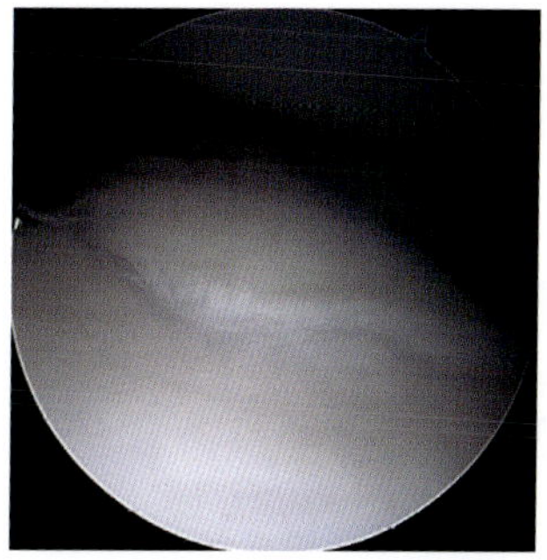 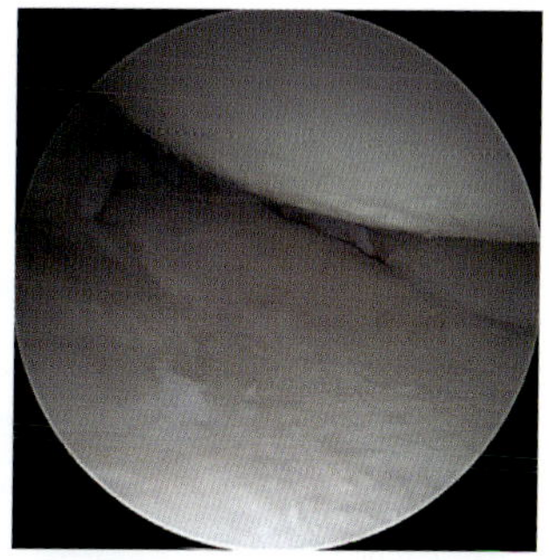
II	Partial-thickness surface defects, cartilage fibrillation that does not reach the subchondral bone	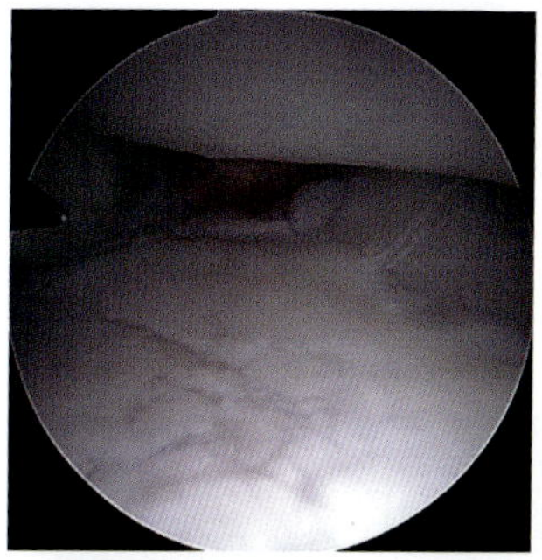 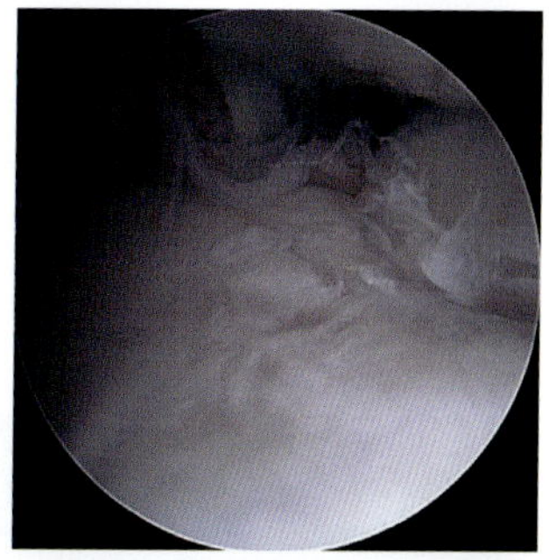
III	Deep cartilage fibrillation to the level of the subchondral bone, with poor-quality flocculent cartilage	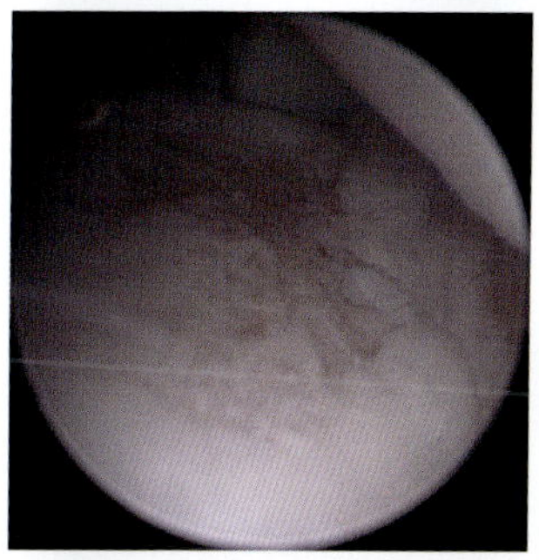 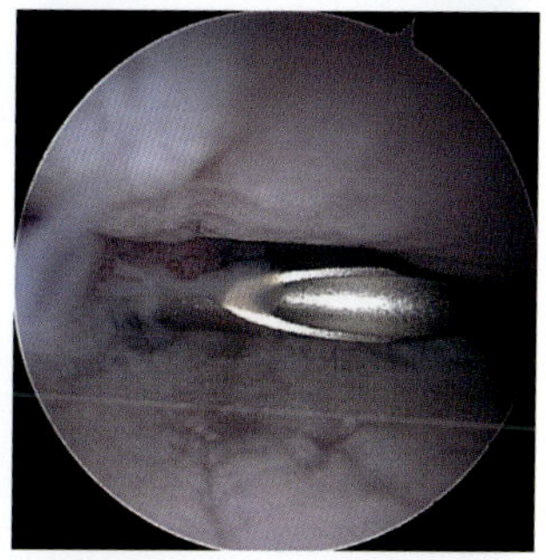
IV	Full-thickness cartilage erosion	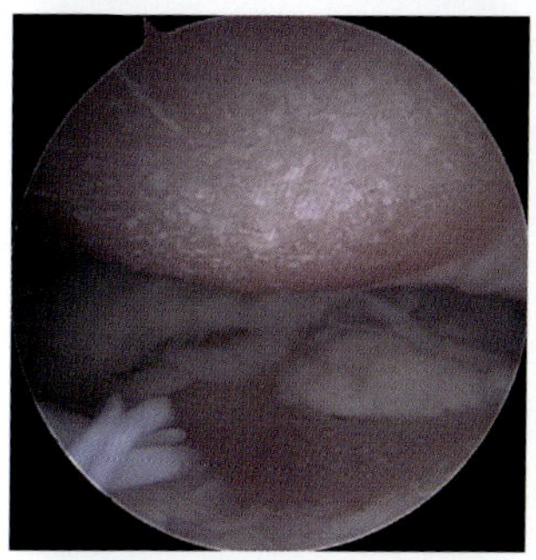 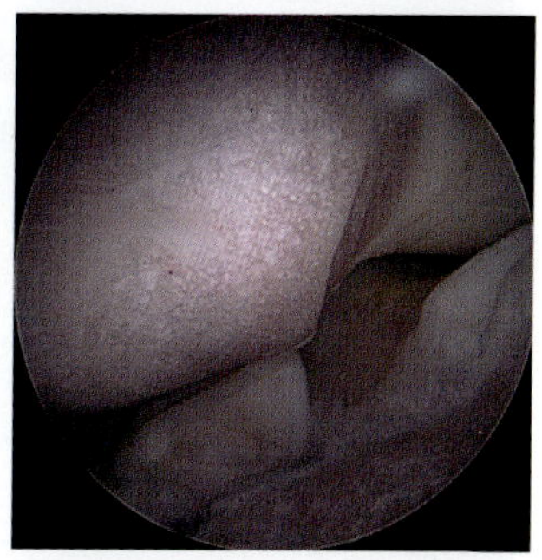
V	Full-thickness cartilage erosion, subchondral bone eburnation (the bone appears more of an orange colour rather than pink/light purple)	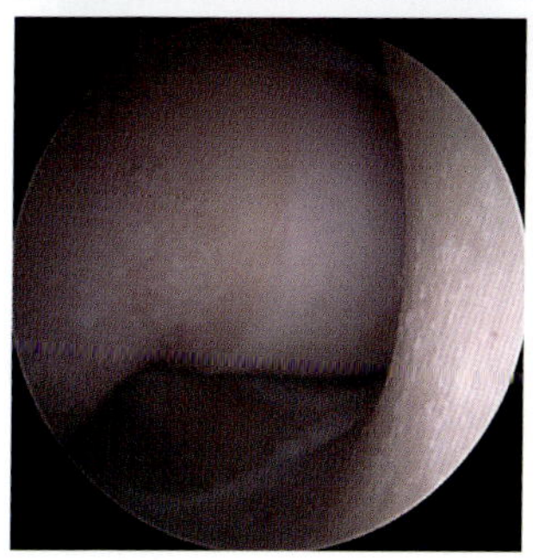 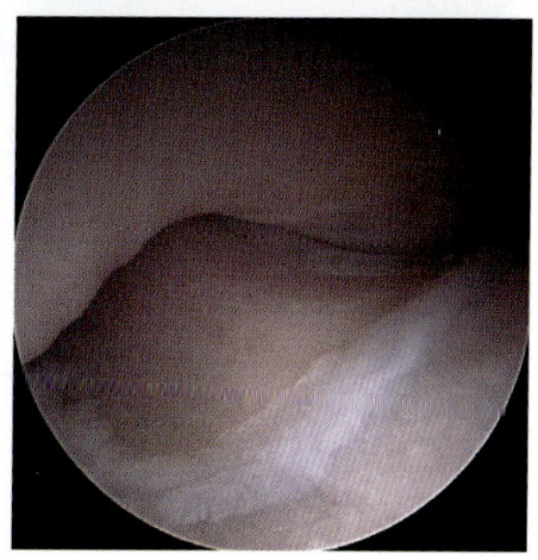

The most common indications to perform elbow arthroscopy are:

- Diagnosis and treatment of fragmentation/fissuring of the MCP.
- Diagnosis and treatment of a humeral osteochondritis (dissecans) lesion.
- Assessment of the stability of an ununited anconeal process (UAP) prior to deciding to perform fragment removal or UAP reattachment.
- Assessment of joint incongruence (Fig. 16).
- Assessment of the degree of cartilage damage prior to deciding whether to perform more invasive procedures, such as bi-oblique proximal ulnar osteotomy, proximal abducting ulnar osteotomy (PAUL; Kyon) or canine unicompartmental elbow (CUE) replacement (Arthrex).

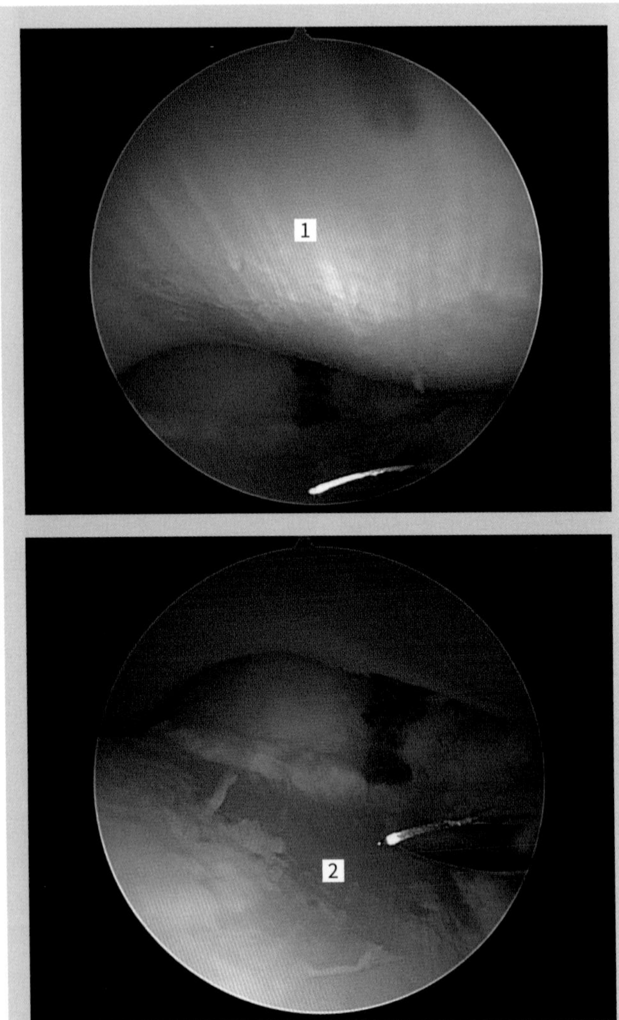

Figure 16. Typical arthroscopic appearance of "kissing lesions" caused by humeroulnar incongruence. 1, medial humeral condyle; 2, medial coronoid process.

Fragmentation of the medial coronoid process

Fragmentation of the medial coronoid process (MCP) represents the most common component of the elbow dysplasia complex, and it is the most important cause of thoracic limb lameness in young dogs. Its aetiopathogenesis is not completely understood but, due to the presence of histomorphometric lesions affecting the entire subchondral bone adjacent to the radial incisure, radio-ulnar incongruence is believed to be the cause of the fissuring/fragmentation process. This "earthquake-like" phenomenon across the MCP can result in arthroscopic MCP pathology such as radial incisure fragmentation/fissuring, tip fragmentation/fissuring or a combination of the two (Figs. 17 and 18).

Traditional treatment includes removal of the fragment combined with a varying degree of abrasion or excision of the surrounding structures based on their appearance. However, this traditional technique does not take into account the presence of subchondral microcracks (as shown by Danielson et al. in 2006), potentially leading to further fragmentation of the MCP and the subsequent need for additional surgery.

Subtotal coronoid ostectomy (SCO) has recently been proposed for the treatment of this pathology, and it is the preferred technique used by the author to treat fragmentation/fissuring of the MCP (Fig. 19a). Using the aforementioned caudal portal, the instrument portal is created immediately cranial and adjacent to the egress needle by using a number 11 Bard-Parker scalpel blade to make a 5–10 mm soft tissue tunnel (Fig. 19b).

A 2 or 4 mm Gordon's osteotome is then placed immediately caudal to the insertion of the medial collateral ligament (Fig. 19c). The assistant starts tapping the osteotome whilst the surgeon looks at the monitor and directs the osteotomy cut to the most caudal aspect of the fragmentation/fissuring line (Fig. 19d). It is important not to remove a too large section of the MCP, as this could destabilise the medial humeral condyle (that is partially supported by the MCP) and lead to severe humeroulnar incongruence and, therefore, severe cartilage damage.

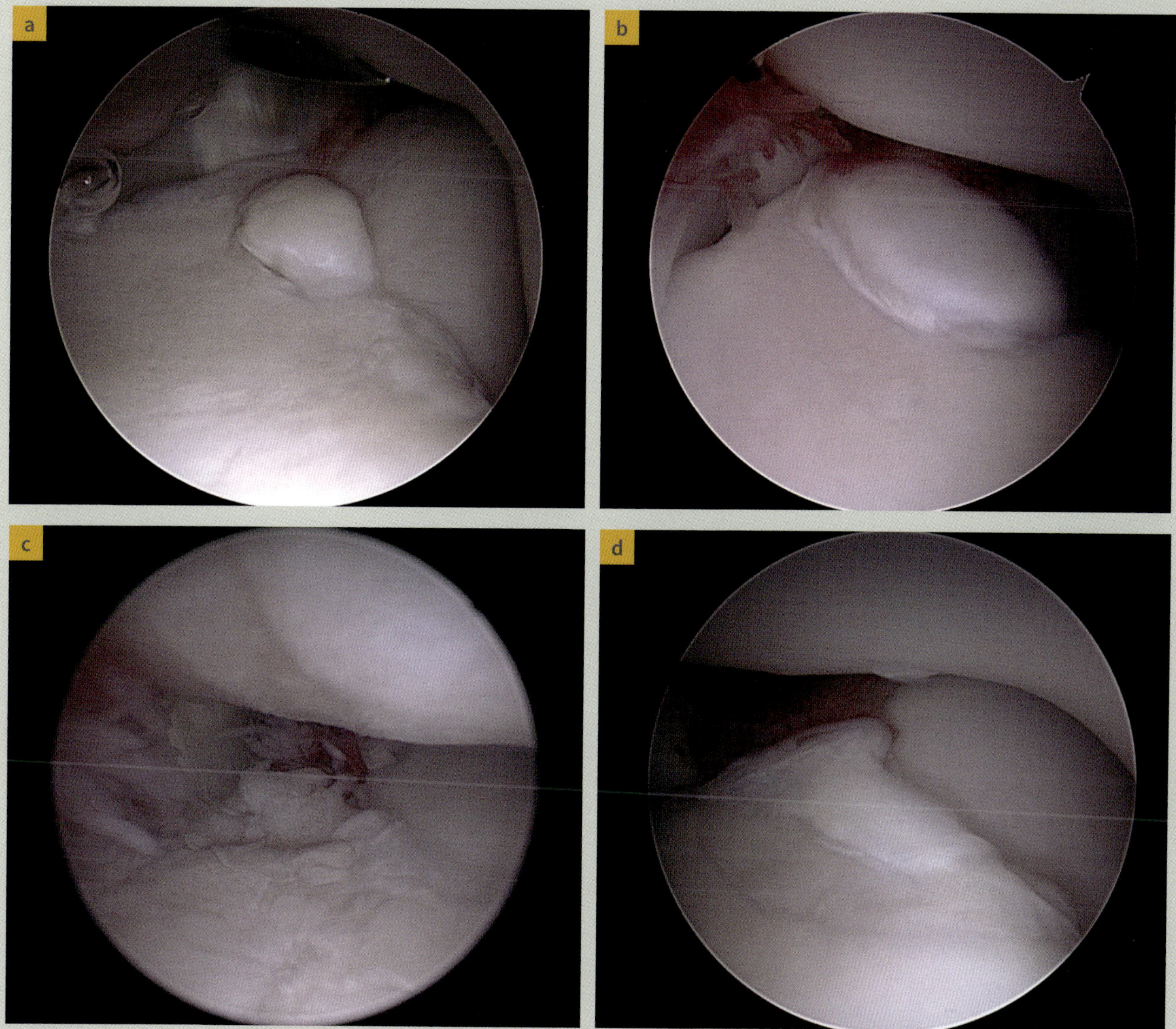

Figure 17. Fragmentation of the medial coronoid process. Radial incisure fragments (a, b). Tip fragment (c). Combination of a tip and radial incisure fragment (d). An obvious step is present at the cleavage plane, with the fragment being elevated/separated from the rest of the remaining ulnar coronoid process.

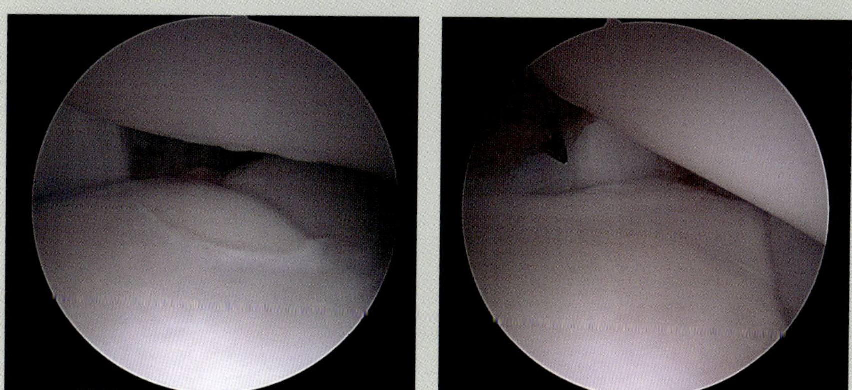

Figure 18. Fissuring of the medial coronoid process. There is no obvious step at level of the cleavage plane.

Fragmentation of the medial coronoid process

When performing a subtotal coronoid ostectomy procedure, care should be taken not to make the osteotomy cut too superficial; otherwise, radioulnar incongruence will persist at a deeper level, with the risk of future microcrack formation and medial coronoid process fragmentation.

One of the advantages of the caudal arthroscopic portal is the ability to visualise the entire MCP. This helps the surgeon evaluate if the SCO procedure about to be performed will remove an adequate or excessive amount of coronoid process.

An arthroscopic grasping forceps of the appropriate size is then inserted through the instrument portal, and the piece or pieces of subchondral bone are removed (Fig. 19e). The bone fragment has soft tissue attachments, particularly to the annular ligament immediately cranial to the radial head, that can complicate its retrieval. The sharp end of the osteotome or of the egress needle, or a Beaver blade, can be used to cut these attachments and free the fragment. After the fragment is grasped by the forceps, a "crocodile manoeuvre" can be performed (rotating the fragment several times over itself) to detach any residual soft tissue attachment. Should the fragment be too large, it can be broken in a few smaller fragments using the osteotome and a mallet. Bupivacaine 0.5 % (0.5 mg/kg) is injected intra-articularly (after evacuation of the extra fluid present in the joint) to provide additional local analgesia.

Small grasping forceps should not be used to grab large bone fragments, as the forceps may break. It is preferable to break the large fragment into smaller pieces first.

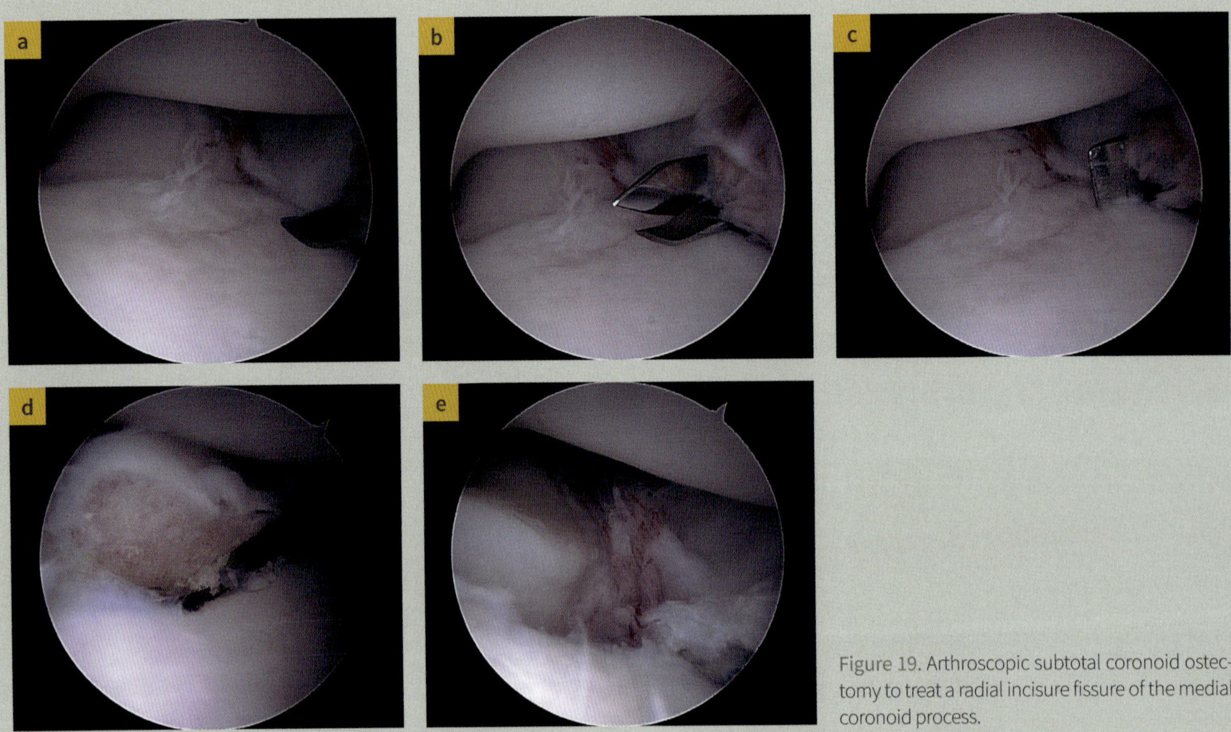

Figure 19. Arthroscopic subtotal coronoid ostectomy to treat a radial incisure fissure of the medial coronoid process.

POSTOPERATIVE MANAGEMENT

Postoperative analgesia is provided by administration of methadone (0.2 mg/kg) followed by buprenorphine (0.02 mg/kg, after 6–12 hours). Perioperative antibiotic therapy is administered, and it is discontinued after the surgical procedure has been completed. Nonsteroidal anti-inflammatory drugs are given orally for 3 weeks. The patient is discharged with instructions of crate confinement for 6 weeks followed by room confinement for 6 additional weeks. Very short (5 minutes) walks at a slow pace using a lead are allowed from day one postoperatively up to four times a day. The duration of each walk can be increased on a weekly basis by 5–10 minutes. Hydrotherapy is usually recommended 6 weeks after surgery to increase the muscle tone of the thoracic limbs and eliminate any residual joint stiffness. The use of joint supplements containing omega-3 fatty acids is recommended to reduce local inflammation and delay the progression of osteoarthritis.

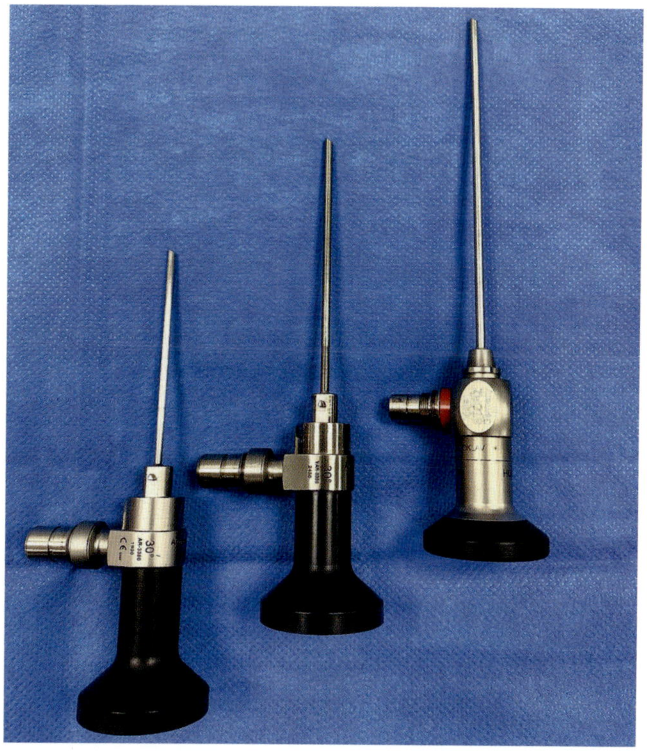

Figure 20. 1.9 mm short 30-degree oblique arthroscope (left) and 2.4 mm short 30-degree oblique arthroscope (middle) (Arthrex Vet Systems, Munich, Germany). 2.7 mm long 30-degree oblique arthroscope (right) (Storz, Slough, UK).

SHOULDER ARTHROSCOPY

Shoulder arthroscopy has gained popularity for the minimally invasive management of shoulder osteochondritis dissecans, bicipital tendinopathy and medial glenohumeral ligament injury, for arthroscopy-assisted stabilisation or simply as a diagnostic tool for intra-articular pathology.

Introducing an arthroscope into the shoulder joint is far more challenging than doing so in the elbow joint because of the bulky musculature that surrounds the joint. Thorough knowledge of the anatomy of the shoulder joint is mandatory.

Biomechanically, the shoulder joint is stabilised by passive (static) and active (dynamic) mechanisms that work together to provide joint stability. Passive mechanisms include limited joint volume, concavity compression and capsuloligamentous restraints (glenohumeral ligaments, joint capsule, biceps brachii tendon and labrum). Active mechanisms include the supraspinatus, infraspinatus, subscapularis, teres minor and biceps brachii muscles.

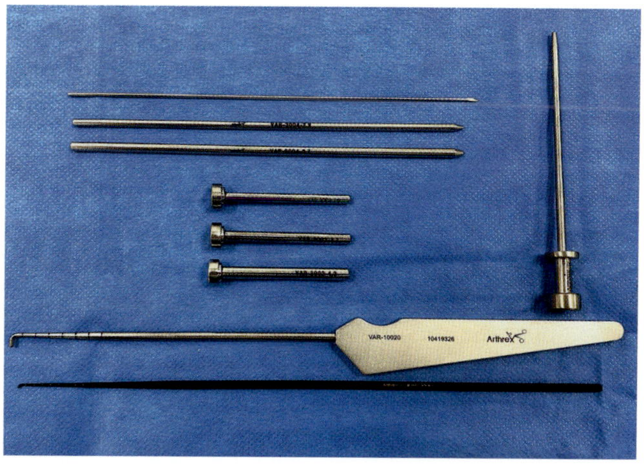

Figure 21. Canine arthroscopy cannula and switching stick set (Arthrex Vet Systems, Munich, Germany). This system permits progressive dilation of the portal and subsequent insertion of larger cannulas. The use of cannulas depends on the joint, the instruments being used and surgeon's preference.

INSTRUMENTATION

A 2.7 mm 30-degree arthroscope is normally inserted relatively easily in the shoulder joint of medium- and large-breed dogs, but in smaller dogs a 2.4 mm (or even a 1.9 mm) arthroscope may be necessary to avoid iatrogenic damage to the articular cartilage (Fig. 20). A blunt obturator (rather than a sharp one) is usually recommended in order to prevent this kind of damage.

Instruments can be inserted through an open portal or through instrument cannulas. If the latter technique is used, a selection of different diameter and length cannulas and switching sticks is necessary (Fig. 21). The recommended handheld instruments include a probe to assist in the inspection of intra-articular structures, grasping forceps for removal of free bodies or cartilaginous flaps, biopsy forceps and instruments for surface abrasion (handheld burrs, curettes or a motorised shaver).

PREPARATION

The skin is clipped from the dorsal midline of the patient to the carpal joint. The surgeon, especially beginning surgeons, needs to be prepared to perform an open arthrotomy in case it is not possible to correctly place the arthroscope or if fluid extravasation impedes correct visualisation and placement of instrument portals. The patient is placed in lateral recumbency with a hanging limb technique, with the limb to be examined uppermost, and final aseptic skin preparation is performed. The assistant maintains the limb with the humerus parallel to the ground (neutral position) or with the shoulder mildly adducted.

The spine of the scapula is palpated down to its most distal aspect (i.e. the acromion). Preoperative radiographs help to recognise the location of the distal tip of the acromion in relationship to the joint line (the imaginary line between the tip of the acromion and the greater tubercle).

An 18-gauge spinal needle is inserted just distal to the acromion vertically into the joint. When the needle enters the joint, a "pop" should be felt (Fig. 23a). The correct location of the needle within the joint can be confirmed by aspirating synovial fluid through a syringe connected to the needle (the fluid can be kept for analysis). A 10 ml syringe is then filled with sterile saline and the shoulder joint is distended. Once the joint is distended and there is back pressure on the syringe, the arthroscopic portal can be established by using a number 11 scalpel blade to cut down immediately next to the needle (Fig. 23b). When the joint is entered, fluid will flow from the portal and the needle can be removed. The arthroscope is inserted directly vertical until the joint is felt (this requires some controlled pressure) (Fig. 23c).

The blunt trocar is removed, and the camera is inserted to confirm correct placement within the joint. The egress cannula is then placed at the cranial aspect of the joint under arthroscopic guidance. Its location is adjacent to the biceps brachii tendon on the medial aspect of the joint. This can be located by palpation over the craniomedial aspect of the joint or by visualisation of the light source from the arthroscope through the skin. A 16-gauge intravenous catheter (or an 18-gauge needle) is then inserted, and the stylet is removed leaving only the soft catheter inside the joint (safe and without the risk of damaging the cartilage) (Fig. 23d).

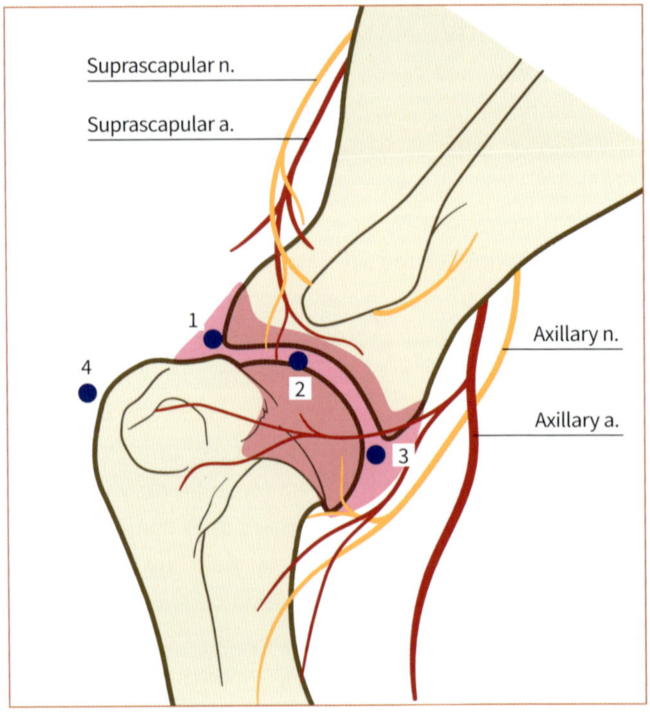

Figure 22. Lateral view of the shoulder joint: anatomical landmarks and portal locations for arthroscopy. 1, egress portal; 2, arthroscopic portal; 3, instrument portal; 4, additional portal to access the biceps brachii tendon.

Using a shoulder distraction device such as the Leipzig distractor may help improve the outcomes of shoulder arthroscopy by decreasing arthroscopy time and the risk of iatrogenic articular cartilage lesions.

JOINT INSPECTION

Since the arthroscope is located between the humeral head and the glenoid, it is important to be careful not to move the trocar too much in order to avoid iatrogenic damage to the articular surface; instead, the joint should be inspected by changing the field of view by moving the light post from right to left and vice versa. The camera head should always be maintained in an upright position. Orientation is correct when left is to the left, right is to the right, dorsal is up and ventral is down. A systematic inspection of all intra-articular structures of the joint is recommended.

Moving the camera head towards the caudal aspect of the joint (i.e. to the right in the left shoulder) and keeping the light post directed caudally (i.e. to the right in the left shoulder) allows visualisation of the cranial compartment of the shoulder joint and inspection of the biceps brachii tendon at its attachment on the supraglenoid tuberosity and the cranial joint capsule (Fig. 24). The supraspinatus muscle

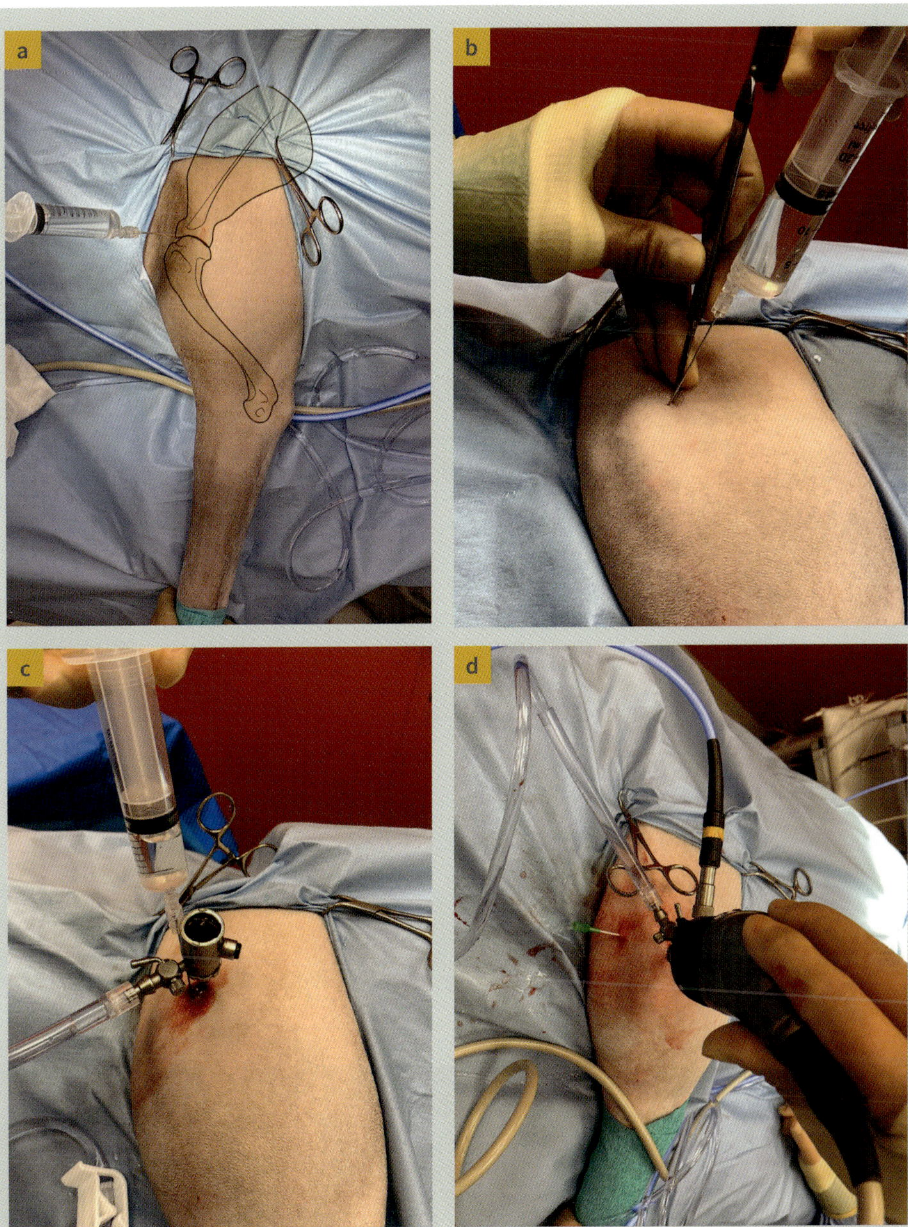

Figure 23. The acromion is palpated, and the egress portal is established with an 18-gauge spinal needle connected to a 10 ml syringe inserted distal to the acromion (a). The joint is distended with sterile solution, and the skin incision is performed with a number 11 scalpel blade immediately caudal to the needle (b). The arthroscopic portal is established using a blunt trocar, taking care to control the depth of insertion in order to avoid iatrogenic cartilage damage (c). Once the joint is entered, correct placement within the joint is confirmed by efflux of saline from the arthroscope sheath. The egress portal is established under arthroscopic guidance by using a 16-gauge intravenous catheter inserted through the craniomedial aspect of the shoulder joint (immediately medial to the biceps brachii tendon) (d).

insertion is visible as a soft tissue bulging immediately lateral to the biceps brachii tendon only when mineralisation/thickening of the insertion of the supraspinatus muscle is present (leading, in some cases, to secondary impingement of the biceps brachii tendon).

Inspection of the central part of the shoulder joint is possible by keeping the camera head vertical to the table, in an upright position, and by moving the light post from up to down and vice versa. At the bottom of the image (light post up), the status of the cartilage of the humeral head can be assessed. At the top of the image (light post down), the status of the cartilage of the glenoid cavity can be assessed. At the centre of the image, between the articular surface of the humeral head and the glenoid, the cranial arm of the glenohumeral ligament (running from caudal to cranial immediately ventral to the glenoid) and the subscapularis tendon of insertion (running from dorsal to ventral immediately behind the cranial arm of the glenohumeral ligament) can be seen (Fig. 25). The glenohumeral ligament can be assessed in its entirety by moving the light post from caudal to cranial; it presents as a Y-shaped figure, with the cranial arm looking like a thin band attached to

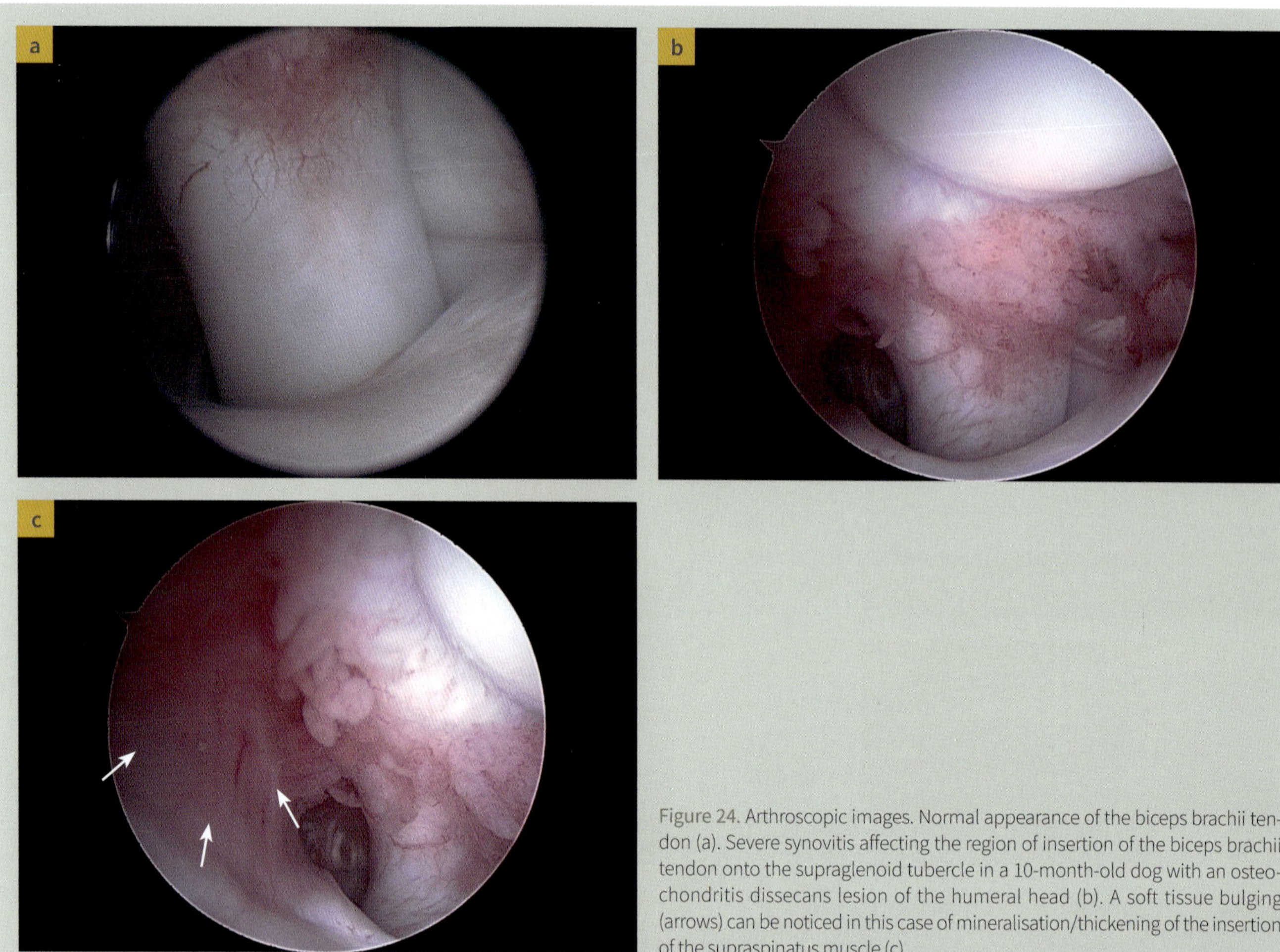

Figure 24. Arthroscopic images. Normal appearance of the biceps brachii tendon (a). Severe synovitis affecting the region of insertion of the biceps brachii tendon onto the supraglenoid tubercle in a 10-month-old dog with an osteochondritis dissecans lesion of the humeral head (b). A soft tissue bulging (arrows) can be noticed in this case of mineralisation/thickening of the insertion of the supraspinatus muscle (c).

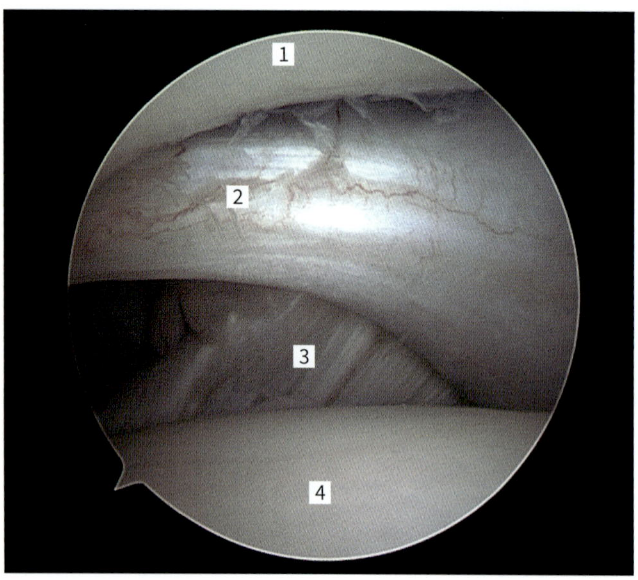

Figure 25. Normal arthroscopic appearance of the central part of the shoulder joint (the cranial aspect of the joint is on the left side of the image and the caudal aspect is on the right). 1, glenoid; 2, cranial arm of the glenohumeral ligament; 3, subscapularis tendon; 4, humeral head.

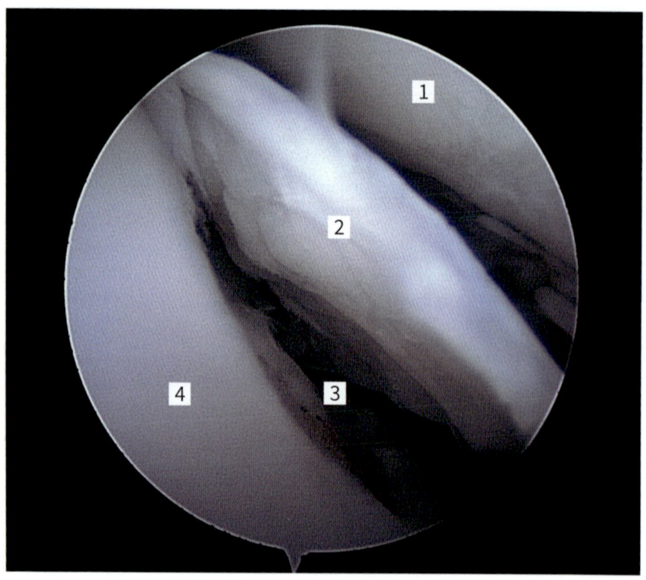

Figure 26. Arthroscopic appearance of an osteochondritis dissecans lesion present in the caudomedial region of the humeral head. Note that the cartilaginous flap is still attached and the subchondral bone is exposed. 1, caudal aspect of the glenoid; 2, detached cartilaginous flap; 3, exposed subchondral bone; 4, caudal aspect of the humeral head.

the medial surface of the supraglenoid tubercle (dorsal) at its most cranial attachment and, as the light post is rotated from right to left in the left shoulder and from left to right in the right shoulder, it progressively becomes wider. The caudal arm of the medial glenohumeral ligament in fact originates from the medial surface of the scapular neck and inserts onto the medial aspect of the humeral neck.

Then, it is possible to inspect the most caudocentral aspect of the humeral head by moving the camera head towards a more cranial position and keeping the light post cranial and slightly dorsal (between the 9 and 11 o'clock positions when examining the left shoulder joint). It is sometimes necessary to adjust the depth and position of the arthroscope by adducting and internally rotating the shoulder joint. Osteochondritis dissecans lesions are generally localised in this area or slightly more medial (Fig. 26). The most caudal aspect of the shoulder joint is inspected by gently moving the tip more caudally and medially, sliding the arthroscope on the humeral head until the caudal gutter (where the joint capsule inserts on the humerus) becomes visible. Joint mice have a tendency to end up in this location, and a caudal instrument portal would allow their retrieval.

It is challenging to thoroughly inspect the lateral collateral ligament using this arthroscopic portal, and a caudal portal is recommended if damage to the lateral collateral ligament is suspected on clinical examination. However, partial inspection is possible by returning the camera head and light post to the original entry position and by slowly withdrawing the arthroscope and rotating the light post. The tip of the arthroscope can be easily displaced out of the joint, and fluid extravasation is likely to happen; this is why the lateral compartment is inspected last.

The most common indications to perform shoulder arthroscopy are:

- Diagnosis and treatment of osteochondritis dissecans lesions.
- Diagnosis and treatment of bicipital tenosynovitis.
- Diagnosis of shoulder instability (in some cases, partial tears of ligamentous structures can be treated arthroscopically by ablation/radiofrequency).
- Diagnosis of incomplete fusion of the caudal glenoid ossification centre.
- Shoulder joint inspection.

Excessive fluid extravasation can occur and usually resolves within the first 24 hours. If an open arthrotomy is being considered and excessive fluid extravasation is noticed during arthroscopy, it is preferable to abort the arthroscopic procedure sooner rather than later; otherwise, the extravasated fluids will severely distort the anatomy and hinder the surgical approach to the joint.

POSTOPERATIVE MANAGEMENT

Postoperative analgesia is provided by administration of methadone (0.2 mg/kg) followed by buprenorphine (0.02 mg/kg, after 6–12 hours). Perioperative antibiotic therapy is administered, and it is discontinued after the surgical procedure has been completed. During recovery, cryotherapy is applied to the operated shoulder for 3–5 days to provide additional analgesia and reduce local swelling. Nonsteroidal anti-inflammatory drugs are given orally for 3 weeks. Passive physiotherapy and massages can be started 3–5 days after the arthroscopic procedure; hydrotherapy, on the other hand, is usually recommended 6 weeks after the procedure (to increase the muscle tone of the thoracic limbs and eliminate any residual joint stiffness). The patient is discharged with instructions of crate confinement for 6 weeks followed by room confinement for 6 additional weeks. Very short (5 minutes) walks at a slow pace using a lead are allowed from day one postoperatively up to four times a day. The duration of each walk can be increased on a weekly basis by 5–10 minutes. To increase the range of motion of the shoulder when out for a walk, the owner is asked to walk the dog in high grass or over small steps. The duration of the walk should be reduced if the patient becomes particularly lame at the end of the exercise period, and it should be increased again only after the patient copes well with that set amount of exercise.

GENERALITIES OF OSTEOCHONDRITIS DISSECANS

Alan Danielski

INTRODUCTION

Osteochondrosis is a disturbance of the normal process of endochondral ossification whereby the growth cartilage in epiphyses and growth plates is gradually turned into bone through a sequence of matrix mineralisation, chondrocyte death, vascularisation and ossification.

Neither the aetiology nor the pathogenesis of osteochondrosis is completely understood. It has been suggested that the primary lesion of osteochondrosis is a focal necrosis of epiphyseal cartilage canals, resulting in areas of cartilage ischaemia and necrosis. Fissures, clefts and cracks may then start at the necrotic cartilage lesion and, if they extend to the joint surface, form a cartilage flap off the underlying subchondral bone (hence the name osteochondritis dissecans – OCD –). This usually results in typical signs of synovitis, joint effusion, arthralgia, lameness and osteoarthritis progression. In humans, the most popular hypothesis is that there is a combined effect of acute or chronic repetitive microtrauma and disturbance of the local blood supply. The heritability of canine osteochondrosis has not yet been established, but it is likely that there are genetic risk factors and environmental influences, including diet and exercise.

CLINICAL PRESENTATION AND DIAGNOSIS

This disease tends to affect mainly large and giant breeds of dogs (e.g. Labrador, Rottweiler, Mastiff, Great Dane), with males being more commonly affected than females. Shoulder and elbow osteochondrosis are usually diagnosed between 4 and 8 months of age, but it is occasionally seen in skeletally mature dogs. Affected dogs usually present for assessment of unilateral thoracic limb lameness.

Dogs with shoulder OCD tend to show moderate pain on joint manipulation and pressure application over the caudal aspect of the shoulder joint. Crepitus and palpable joint effusion are rarely present.

Dogs with elbow OCD show moderate discomfort on joint flexion and supination of the antebrachium. Obvious joint effusion can sometimes be evident as a puffiness / soft tissue swelling on the lateral aspect of the elbow joint.

Radiography is the most widely available imaging modality in veterinary centres. In dogs with OCD, the disrupted endochondral ossification process is identified by a change in shape of the subchondral bone. This appears as a flattened or irregular margin of the caudal humeral head or of the medial humeral condyle. Regional subchondral sclerosis is often a concurrent finding. Joint effusion, mineralised flaps and fragments, gas and secondary degenerative changes may also be present. These lesions are most reliably identified on a mediolateral projection of the shoulder joint and on a craniocaudal projection of the elbow joint.

Advanced imaging (CT and MRI) is considered a superior diagnostic tool, as it provides the exact location and size of the osteochondral defect for preoperative planning (Figs. 1–3).

TREATMENT

CONSERVATIVE TREATMENT

Conservative treatment is only indicated when the lesion is small and the patient is asymptomatic or very mildly lame. It consists of the use of nonsteroidal anti-inflammatory drugs, exercise restriction, nutraceutical supplementation with glucosamine, chondroitin sulphate and omega-3 fatty acids, body weight control, and administration of a well-balanced diet with reduced caloric density.

SURGICAL TREATMENT

This is the treatment of choice and the one preferred by the author. Establishment of portals is described in chapter "Arthroscopy".

Most surgeons prefer to simply remove the cartilaginous flap and perform curettage and abrasion arthroplasty of the lesion. The technique involves careful debridement of necrotic cartilage and diseased bone under arthroscopic

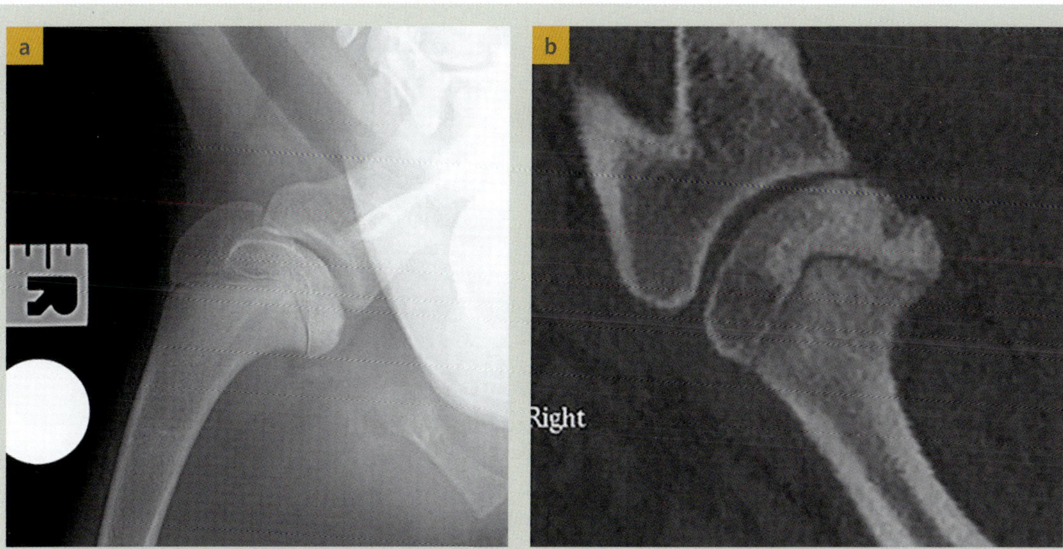

Figure 1. Radiographic (a) and CT (b) images of an OCD lesion present on the caudal aspect of the humeral head. CT images offer significantly better details of the lesions, in particular regarding lesion size and depth.

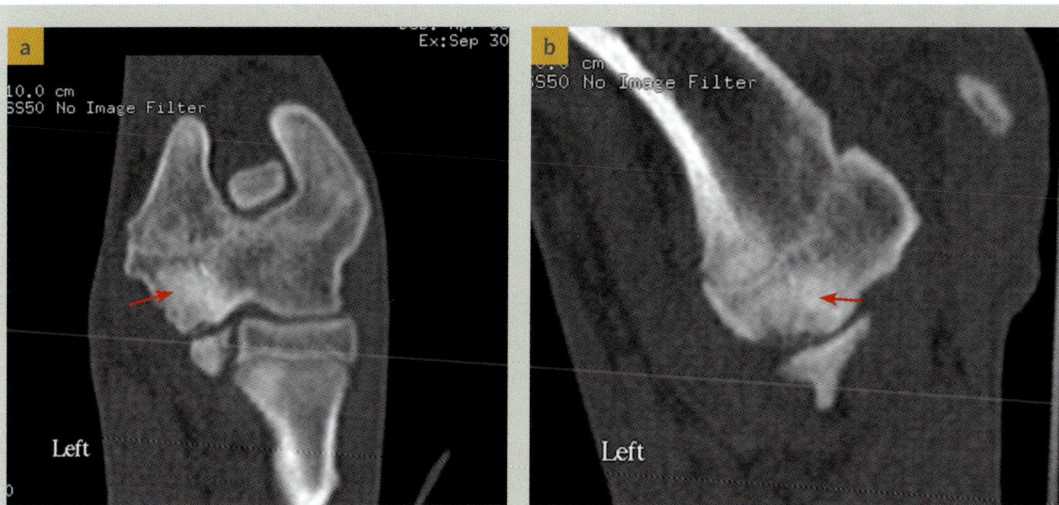

Figure 2. Frontal (a) and sagittal (b) plane CT images of the elbow of a dog with an OCD lesion on the medial humeral condyle. Note the intense sclerosis of the subchondral bone (white area indicated by arrows) surrounding the subchondral defect (black area at the level of the articular surface).

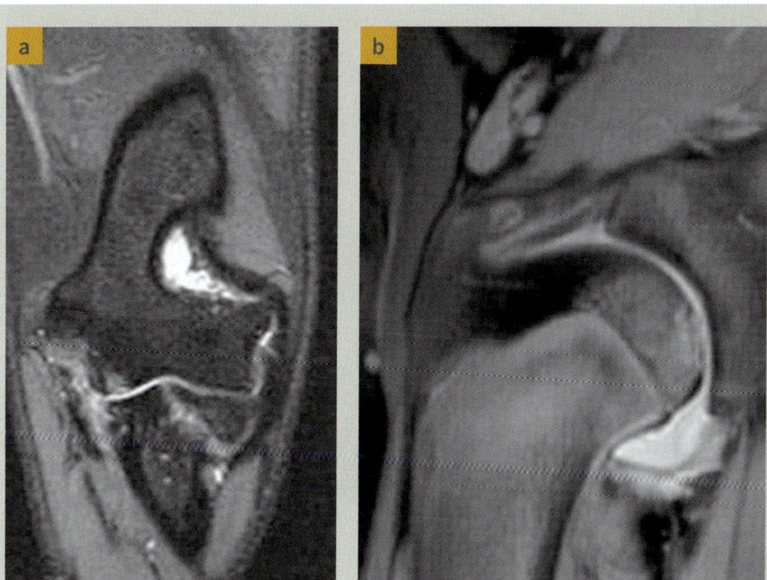

Figure 3. T2-weighted MRI sequences of two dogs with OCD lesions. Frontal view of an elbow joint (a) and sagittal view of a shoulder joint (b), showing an OCD lesion and markedly hyperintense fluid density between the subchondral bone and the lesion.

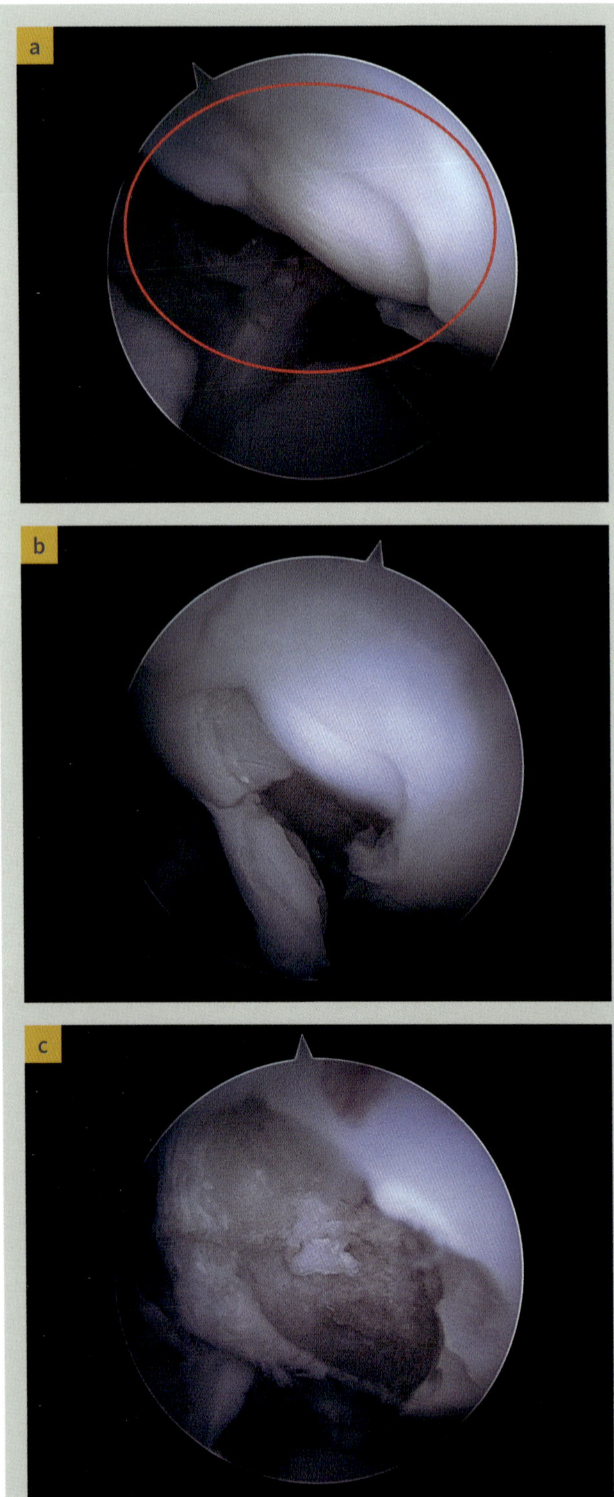

Figure 4. Treatment of an OCD lesion on the medial humeral condyle. The lesion (circle) appears as a soft, irregular area of cartilage (a). After partially detaching the cartilage with the aid of a grasper locked on the flap, a crater, caused by the absence of normal subchondral bone thickness, becomes apparent (b). The dead cartilage is peeled off the underlying bone, and the edges of the lesion are palpated with a probe to identify and remove any additional loose cartilage. Abrasion with a manual burr and microfracture with a pick is then performed until the bone starts bleeding (c).

guidance to expose healthy subchondral bone. This is achieved with graspers (to remove the necrotic cartilage or the cartilage around the lesion that is not firmly attached to the underlying subchondral bone) and a hand burr (to remove the necrotic subchondral bone) (Fig. 4).

> Care must be taken not to enlarge the lesion too much and not to make it too deep. Otherwise, the normal healing process will be impaired, resulting in poor fibrocartilage infilling of the lesion.

Other surgeons prefer to combine the above technique with forage (also called osteostixis) and microfracture, which consist in making numerous small holes into the subchondral bone of the lesion bed to achieve active bleeding. This can be performed with fine Kirschner wires or small picks and awls. These techniques are particularly useful in those cases in which the subchondral bone is very sclerotic (hard) and burring achieves no bleeding.

The increased intra-articular pressure caused by fluids when performing arthroscopy may impede bleeding from the subchondral bone, which can erroneously be interpreted as being due to insufficient curettage of the lesion. To avoid this, after performing debridement and forage/microfracture, the ingress of fluids into the joint should be stopped for a few minutes and the lesion bed should be checked for bleeding.

The most recent study analysing the results of arthroscopy combined with debridement and osteostixis as a treatment for shoulder OCD in dogs reported lameness resolution in 91 % of the affected limbs (Olivieri et al., 2007). Dogs presenting with a lesion located more medially on the humeral head had a better functional outcome compared to those dogs with a more central lesion.

Osteochondral autologous grafts have been used to immediately restore the cartilaginous defect with durable hyaline cartilage. Osteochondral grafts with the shape of a cylinder are harvested from healthy, non-weight-bearing portions of the same or different joints of the same patient and implanted into the recipient site (after being appropriately prepared). The main disadvantages of this procedure include donor site morbidity and the fact that the cartilage of the harvested graft does not have the same uniform thickness and biomechanical properties as the cartilage surrounding the recipient site.

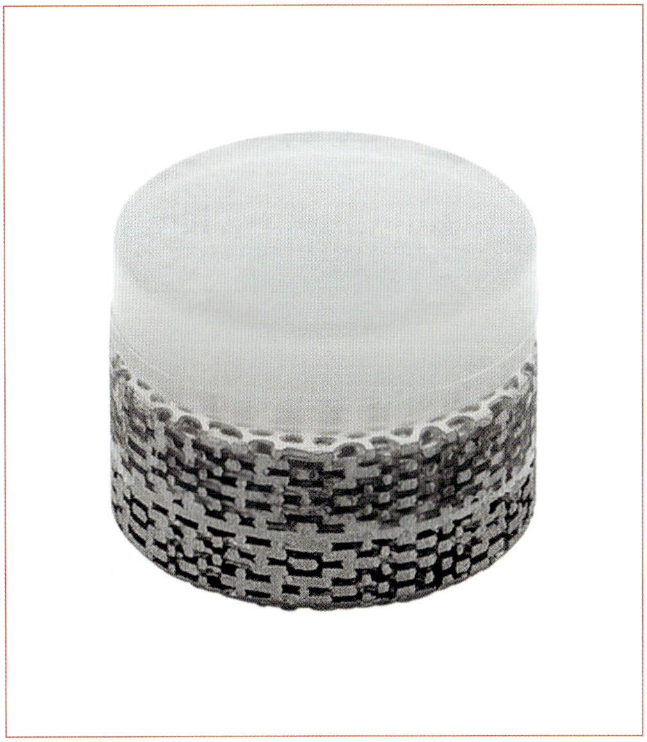

Figure 5. Osteochondral implant. The deep layer is composed of lattice-type titanium to facilitate bone growth. The surface layer, which is composed of polycarbonate urethane, is secured within the upper half of the titanium base and is smooth and rounded to function as a synthetic articular surface.

Consequently, research has focused on synthetic osteochondral implants in humans, horses and dogs. The use of a synthetic implant consisting of a surface layer of polycarbonate urethane and a deep layer of lattice-type titanium that facilitates bone ingrowth (SynACART, Arthrex Vet Systems) is the author's preferred method to treat OCD lesions (Figs. 5–7). These implants allow the surgeon to immediately reconstruct the normal topography of the articular surface, they eliminate the risk of donor site morbidity, and bypass the problem regarding the difference in cartilage thickness and uniformity. In fact, the polycarbonate surface layer has been designed and tested to resist surface degradation and fissuring, and it has been reported to be biocompatible and have excellent wear and bearing properties in in vivo studies (Cook et al., 2014; Husby et al., 2016). This implant is 8 mm deep and is available in different diameter sizes (8, 10, 15, 20 and 25 mm). A recent study demonstrated that the use of these implants in shoulders with central OCD lesions was successful in leading to clinical resolution of lameness in 13 dogs (15 affected shoulders) (Egan et al., 2018). The clinical application of these implants is described in chapters "Osteochondritis dissecans of the shoulder joint" and "Osteochondrosis of the elbow joint".

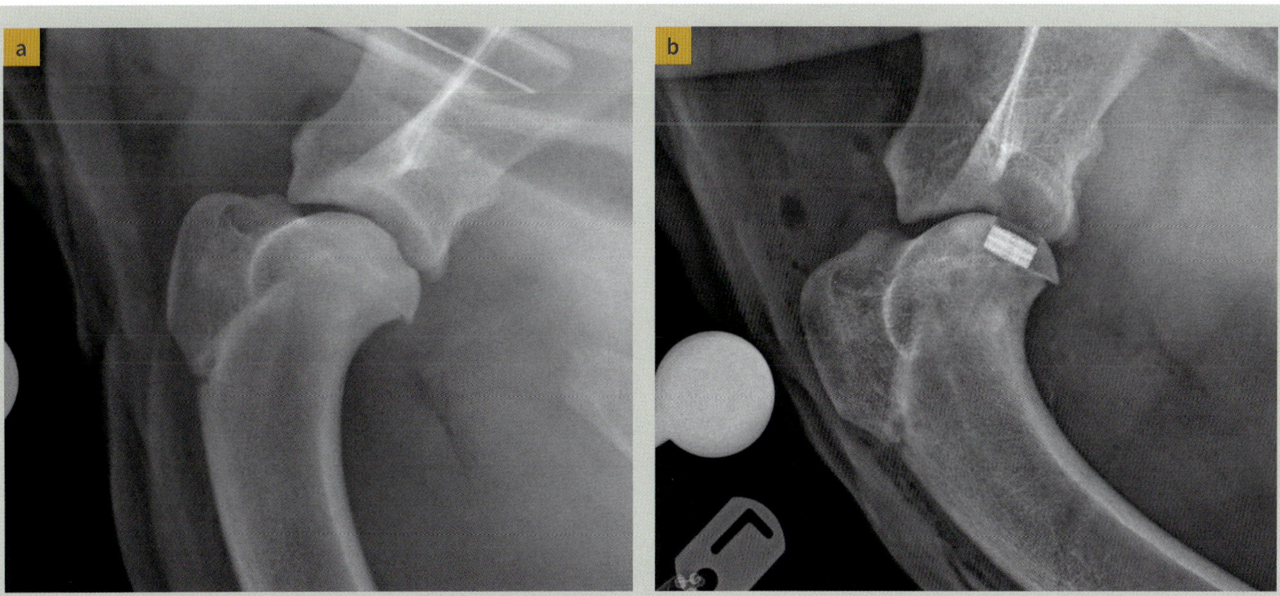

Figure 6. Mediolateral radiographs of the shoulder of an 8-month-old Bullmastiff with a large OCD lesion on the caudal aspect of the humeral head, before (a) and after (b) placement of an osteochondral implant (10 × 8 mm).

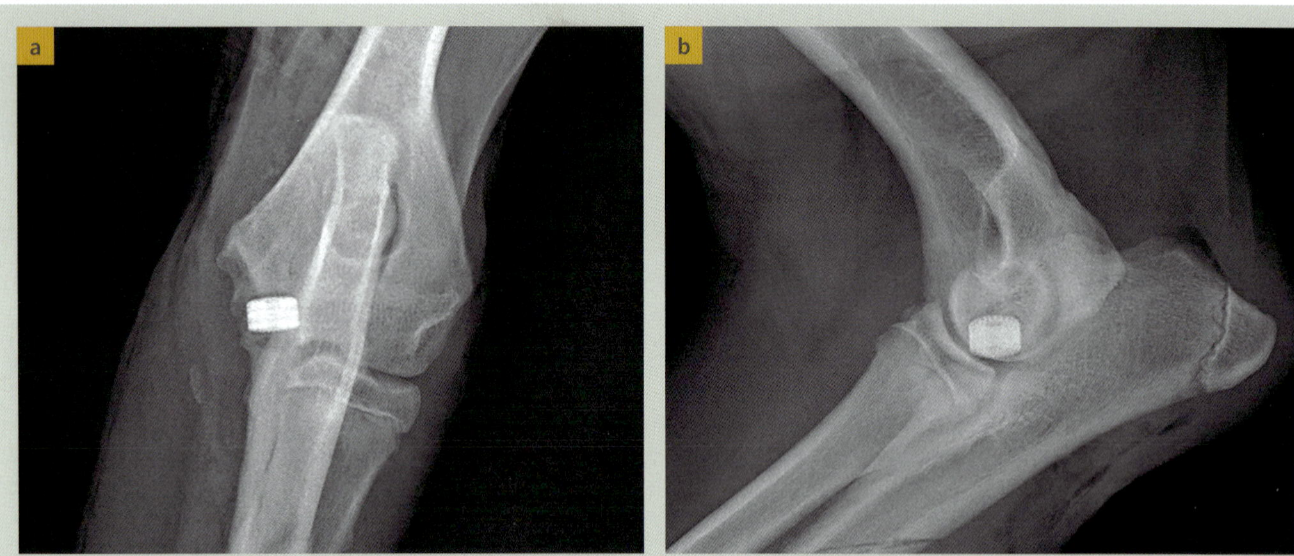

Figure 7. Craniocaudal (a) and mediolateral (b) radiographs of the elbow of a 7-month-old Labrador presenting with an OCD lesion on the medial humeral condyle treated by placement of an osteochondral implant (8 × 8 mm).

GENERAL CONCEPTS ABOUT ARTHRODESIS

Felipe de Vicente

INTRODUCTION

Arthrodesis is the surgical fusion of a joint. Considered a salvage procedure, it should be used when there are no other surgical interventions that can achieve a satisfactory functional result in the patient.

This procedure can be performed in joints in which eliminating mobility is tolerable for the functionality of the limb and, therefore, of the patient. The joints in which arthrodesis is most frequently performed are the carpus and tarsus. It is performed less frequently in cases involving the shoulder, elbow, stifle and proximal interphalangeal joints.

> Arthrodesis can be performed on all appendicular joints except the hip and distal interphalangeal joints.

INDICATIONS

The indications for joint arthrodesis are:

- Severe joint instability.
- Nonreducible joint luxation.
- Severe pain in range of motion (e.g. due to advanced osteoarthritis).
- Nonreconstructible intra-articular fracture.
- Malunion (consolidation defect).
- Loss of function due to nonrepairable tendon injuries (common calcaneal tendon or triceps tendon).
- Certain neurological lesions that affect the functionality of the limb (especially the functionality of the carpus or tarsus).

SURGICAL TECHNIQUE

The following factors should be considered when performing arthrodesis:

1. The joint must be fixed in an anatomical position that is functional for the patient's locomotion, thus avoiding significant limb length loss. In general, the angle of fixation of a joint can be determined by measuring the angle of the contralateral joint (provided it is normal) in stance. If this is not possible, recommended fixation angles for the different joints can be used as a reference (Table 1).
2. Arthrodesis should be performed only in the absence of infection.
3. The articular cartilage should be removed and the subchondral bone exposed (Fig. 1). Osteostixis can be performed to create vascular channels and the cartilage can be removed using a pneumatic burr, which preserves the contour of the bone, using gouges or by performing ostectomies.
4. A bone graft (preferably autogenous) is used to accelerate bone consolidation (Fig. 2). The graft is placed both inside and around the joint.
5. Rigid internal fixation in compression should be applied, usually using compression plates (Fig. 3) or compression screws and neutralisation plates. In the case of long bones, the plates should be placed with a minimum of three or four screws. Kirschner wires, tension bands or external fixators may be used as a fixation method in some patients. Ideally, the implants should be placed on the tension side of the joint.

TABLE 1. Recommended angles for the various joints.

Joint	Recommended angle (degrees)
Shoulder	105–110
Elbow	110
Carpus	10–12 (15–20 cats)
Stifle	135–140 (120–125 cats)
Tarsus	135–145 (115–125 cats)

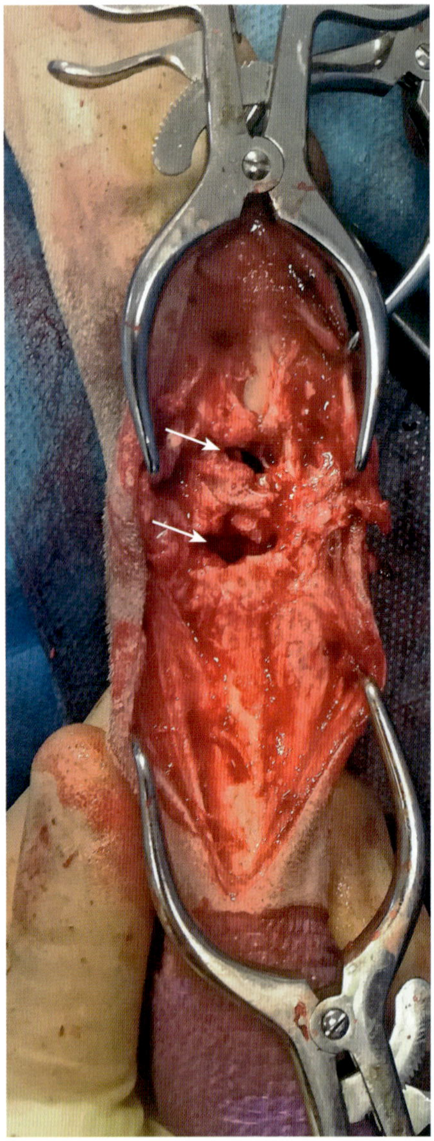

Figure 1. Patient with intertarsal instability. Partial tarsal arthrodesis is performed. The articular cartilage was removed with a pneumatic burr, exposing the subchondral bone at the level of the proximal intertarsal (tarsocalcaneal) and tarsometatarsal joints (arrows).

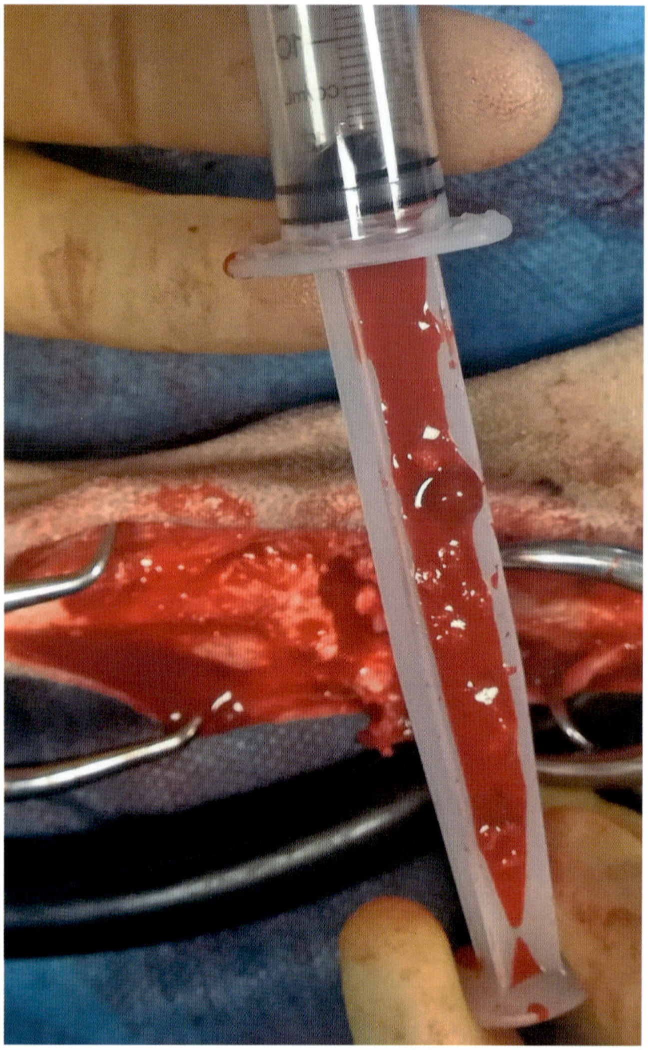

Figure 2. Autogenous bone graft harvested to perform a partial tarsal arthrodesis. Enough graft should be harvested so as to fill the joint cavity and to place graft around the joint.

Box 1. Bone graft functions.

- Osteogenesis: ability to form bone directly, due to the presence of osteoblasts and bone precursors in the graft.
- Osteoinduction: ability to release growth factors that stimulate mesenchymal cells and bone production.
- Osteoconduction: ability to provide structural support for bone production by mesenchymal cells.
- Osteointegration: ability to produce a union between the graft and the patient's bone.
- Osteopromotion: ability to stimulate the bone regeneration that is occurring.

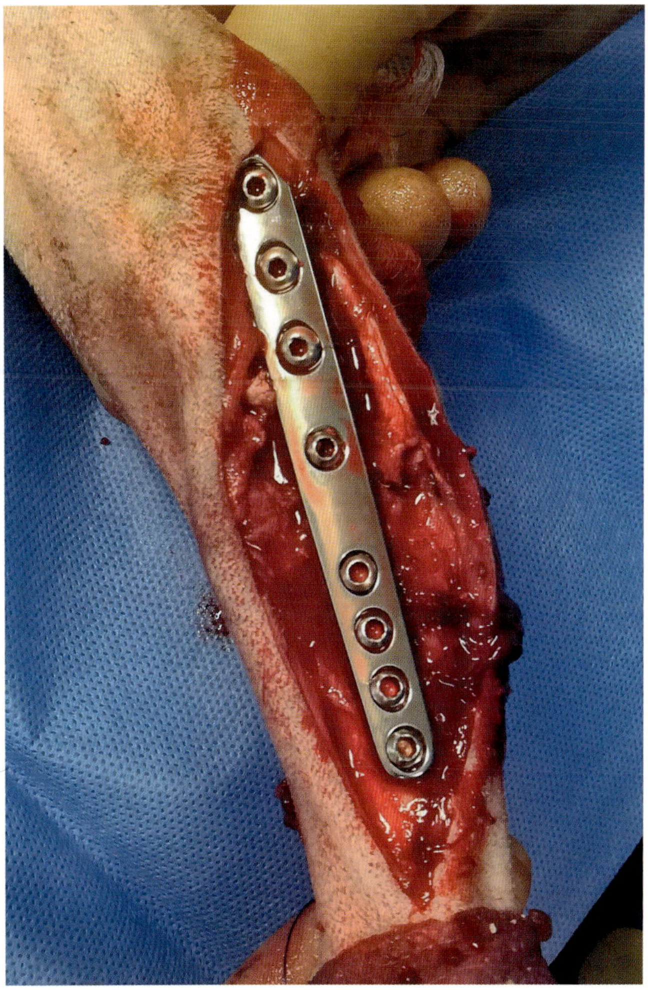

Figure 3. Partial tarsal arthrodesis by compression plate fixation.

POSTOPERATIVE MANAGEMENT

Traditionally, the use of splints and supportive bandages has been recommended for the first 4–8 weeks after arthrodesis. Long-term dressings should be changed whenever they become wet or loose. In any case, they should be changed periodically (1–2 times per week) to check if the dressing is causing any injury to the skin. Recent studies have questioned the need for these in some locations such as the carpus (see chapter "Pancarpal arthrodesis"), when sufficiently rigid fixation has been achieved.

> It is essential to restrict postoperative exercise to minimise the risk of complications. Prolonging this restriction is advised until there is radiographic evidence of joint fusion.

OUTCOME

The degree of limb functionality impairment depends on the joint in which arthrodesis has been performed. Carpal and tarsal arthrodesis cause milder changes in limb functionality, and patients with carpal/tarsal arthrodesis maintain an excellent quality of life. In contrast, stifle and elbow arthrodesis cause significant changes in the functionality of the limb. Shoulder arthrodesis results in mild changes in limb functionality, and good to excellent outcomes have been reported.

> The functionality of a limb in which joint arthrodesis has been performed will never be completely normal.

COMPLICATIONS

The most frequent complications when performing arthrodesis are:

- Lack of joint fusion. This complication is usually due to an error in the surgical technique (e.g. insufficient debridement of the articular cartilage).
- Implant loosening or breakage. This complication may be due to inadequate implant size selection or implant fatigue if nonunion or delayed union of the arthrodesis occurs.
- Angular limb deformities. Angular deformities after arthrodesis are due to a surgical technique error, wherein the surgeon created this deformity while fixing the joint.
- Postoperative infection.

02
SHOULDER

TRAUMATIC SHOULDER LUXATION

Stephen Kalff

INTRODUCTION

Although a detailed description of the anatomy and biomechanics of the shoulder (glenohumeral) joint is beyond the scope of this book, in brief, like all joints, physiological movement of the shoulder is maintained by coordination of active (muscle–tendon units and proprioceptive pathways) and passive (joint capsule, glenohumeral ligaments and moderately congruent, concave articular surface) stabilisers. It should be noted that in addition to providing active support to the shoulder, the biceps brachii tendon provides some passive stability.

There is a high degree of passive laxity in the normal shoulder, with a wide range of cranial, caudal, medial and lateral translation possible. This passive laxity is most evident during flexion and reduces in a linear pattern until the joint is in full extension. Given this degree of passive laxity, coordination of the active stabilisers probably provides primary stabilisation during the physiological range of motion, with the passive stabilisers only being engaged at the extreme range of this motion. Failure of this active glenohumeral balance will result in supraphysiological loading of the passive stabilisers, the failure of which may result in shoulder instability and/or luxation.

Whilst shoulder instability syndromes, including subluxation and congenital luxation, have been widely discussed in the literature, this chapter focuses on traumatic shoulder luxation.

Traumatic shoulder luxation is an uncommon injury in dogs that occurs when one or both glenohumeral ligaments fail (Sidaway et al., 2004; Vasseur et al., 1982). Although this is usually a soft tissue injury, medial luxation following avulsion fracture of the lesser tubercle (insertion site of the medial glenohumeral ligament) has been reported (Huck and Bergh, 2011). Medial luxation is reportedly most commonly, followed by lateral and then, rarely, cranial and caudal.

CLINICAL PRESENTATION AND DIAGNOSIS

Definitive diagnosis requires orthogonal radiographs (Figs. 1 and 2), although physical examination and observation of the patient will usually raise suspicion.

Physical examination findings can include palpable displacement of the acromion relative to the greater tubercle of the humerus with variable degrees of instability. These findings may be limited by patient pain and localised swelling. Most dogs will be non-weight-bearing, with the elbow flexed and with the distal limb abducted in case of medial luxation and adducted in case of lateral luxation (Video 1; Fig. 3). Concurrent brachial plexus injuries are not uncommon in lateral luxations. Medial displacement of the biceps brachii tendon is also common in cranial luxations.

Video 1. Dog with a traumatic luxation of the left shoulder.

Video 2. Medial luxation of the left shoulder in a dog when hyperflexion of the shoulder is performed.

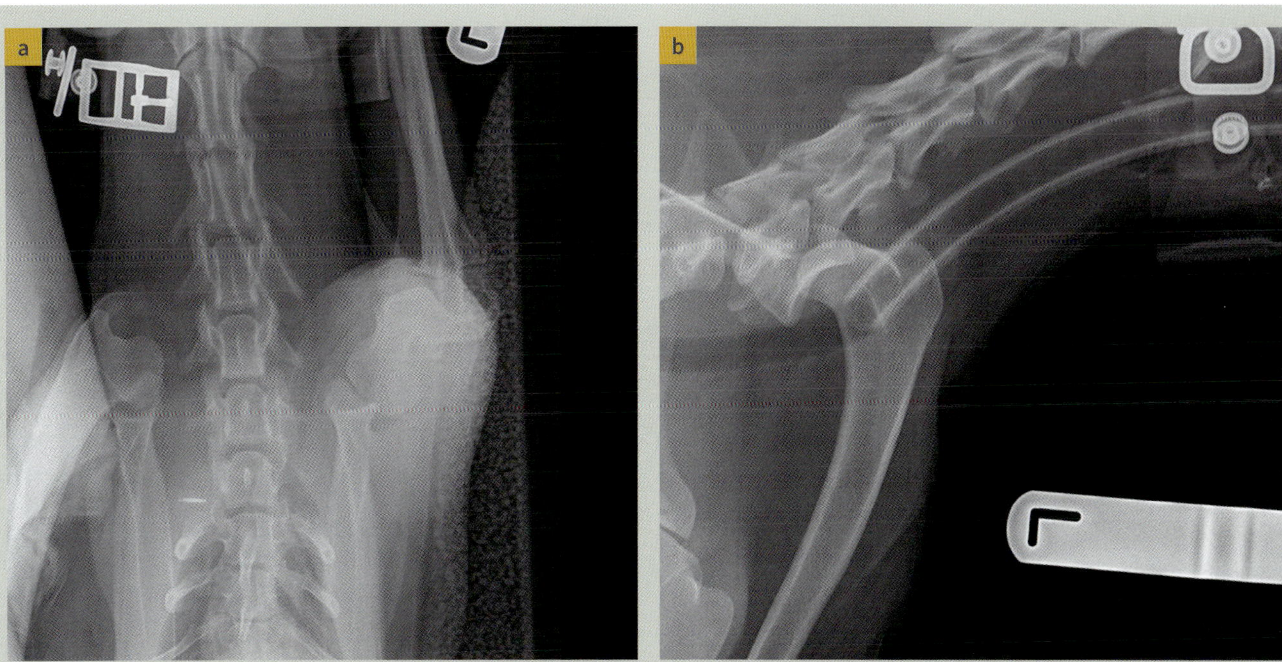

Figure 1. Preoperative craniocaudal (a) and mediolateral (b) radiographs showing lateral luxation of the left shoulder.

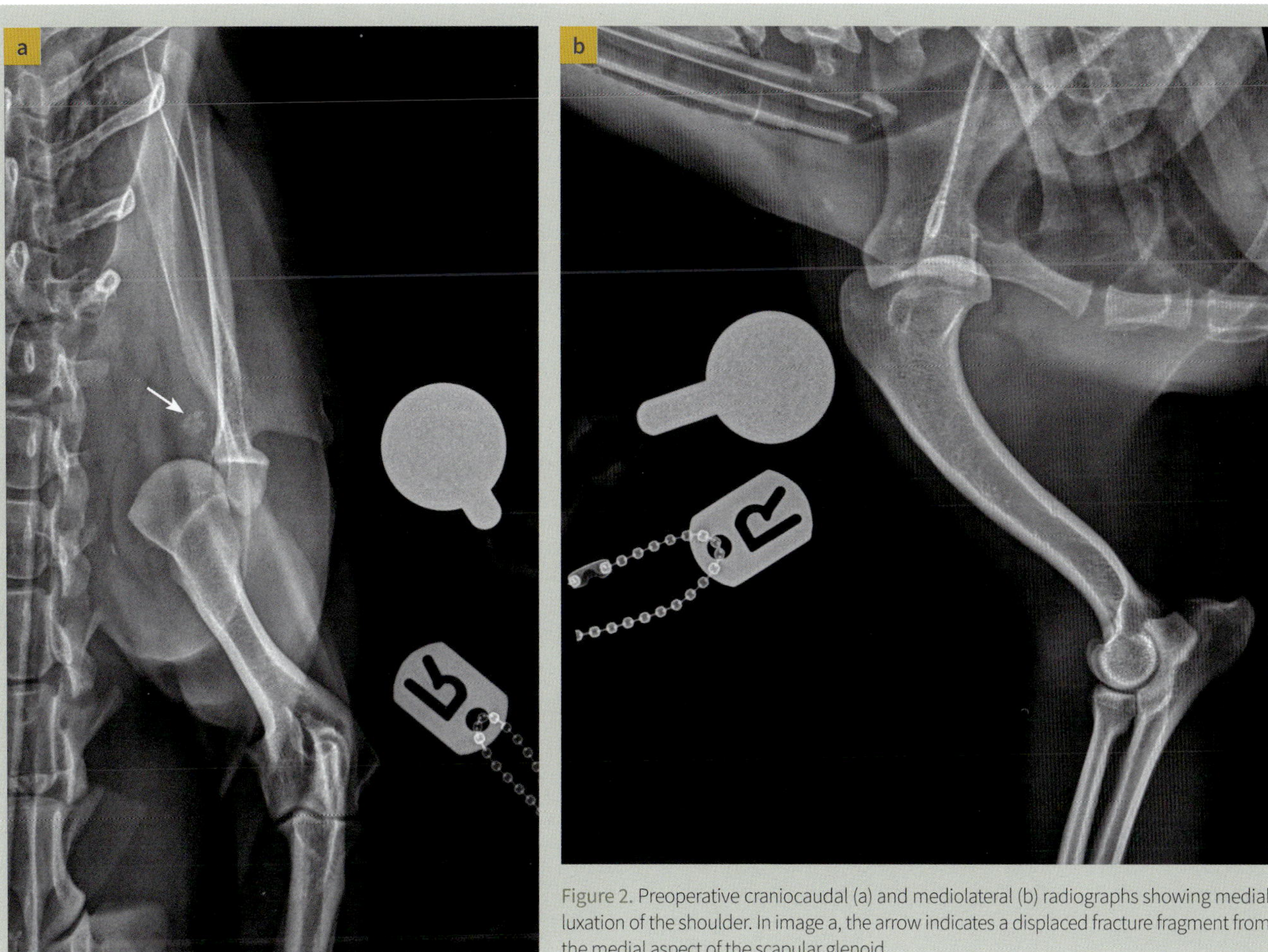

Figure 2. Preoperative craniocaudal (a) and mediolateral (b) radiographs showing medial luxation of the shoulder. In image a, the arrow indicates a displaced fracture fragment from the medial aspect of the scapular glenoid.

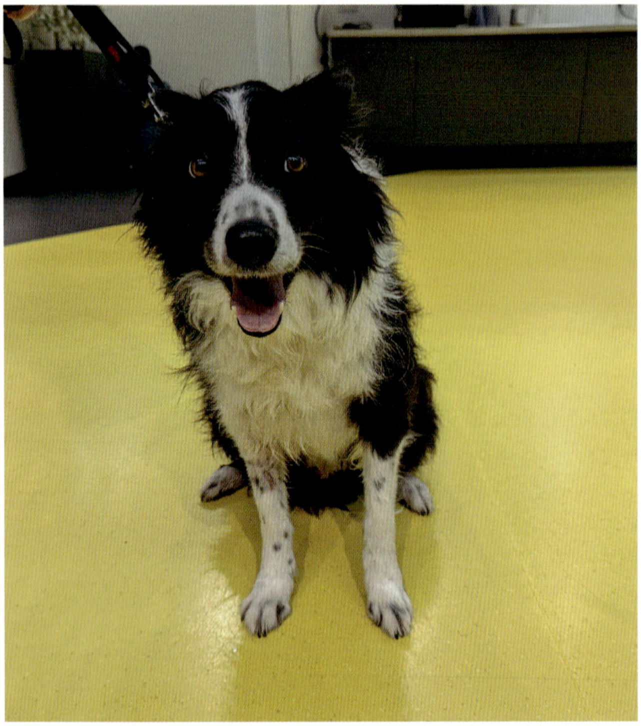

Figure 3. Abnormal loading of the left thoracic limb with abaxial displacement in the same dog as in Video 1.

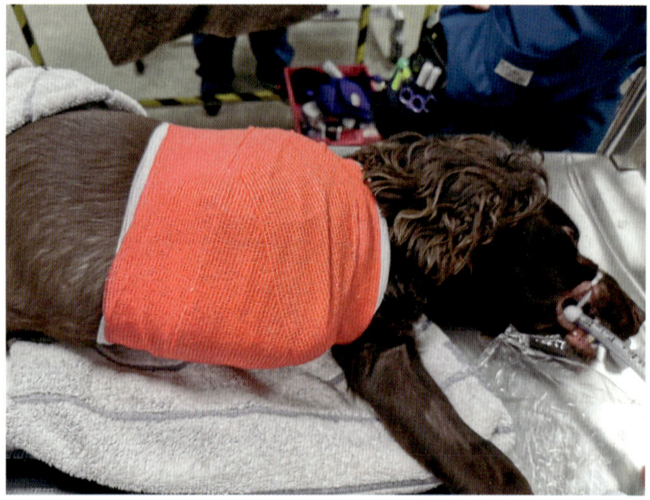

Figure 4. Dog with a non-weight-bearing Velpeau sling bandage.

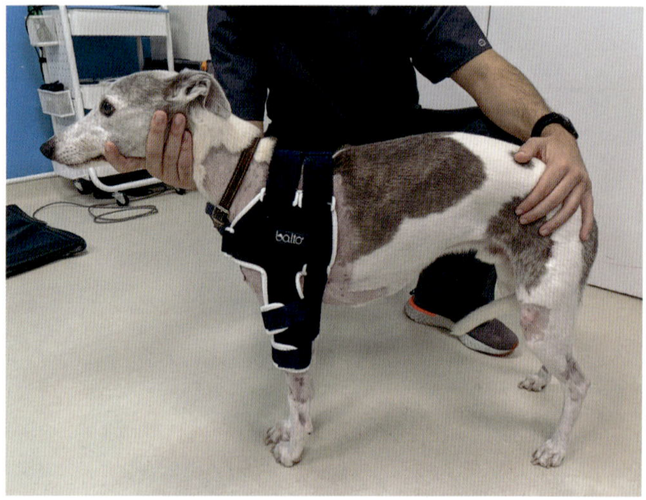

Figure 5. Shoulder stabilisation system to prevent shoulder abduction and extreme range of motion on the sagittal plane.

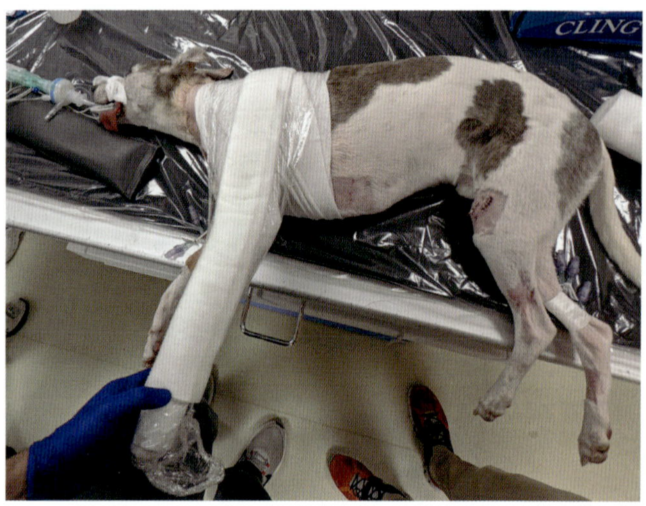

Figure 6. Spica splint using a casting material.

TREATMENT

CONSERVATIVE MANAGEMENT

In most cases conservative management is appropriate in the first instance. Closed reduction under sedation followed by immobilisation of the joint for 2–6 weeks is successful in many cases. The author prefers to immobilise for 4–6 weeks followed by 2–4 weeks of crate confinement before gradually returning to normal activity over the following 4 weeks.

A Velpeau sling (Fig. 4) is appropriate for medial luxations. Lateral luxations can be managed with a neutral sling (Fig. 5) that avoids adduction. Spica splints (Fig. 6) can be used in all cases, but given the difficulty for patients to tolerate this bandage, spica splints are usually reserved for cranial and caudal luxations.

SURGICAL MANAGEMENT

Surgical management is appropriate in shoulders that remain markedly unstable after closed reduction, in chronic cases, and in those cases in which conservative management has failed. Surgical options include biceps tendon transposition with or without supraspinatus tendon transposition, ligament reconstruction techniques and capsulorrhaphy.

Historically, biceps tendon transpositions (medial and lateral) were widely performed (Pucheu and Duhautois, 2008). Whilst generally good outcomes were reported, these techniques (particularly medial biceps tendon transposition) lead to alterations in joint biomechanics and congruity (Vasseur et al., 1982; Ringwood et al., 2001).

For medial luxations, the author prefers an adaptation of the medial glenohumeral ligament reconstruction technique described by Fitch et al. (2001) and Ringwood et al. (2001), which may provide more physiologically normal biomechanics than biceps tendon transposition.

Medial glenohumeral ligament reconstruction

The patient is positioned in lateral recumbency with the affected side up. The affected limb is hung and aseptically prepared. Four-quarter draping is performed to allow manipulation of the limb during surgery.

A craniomedial approach to the shoulder is performed, and the subscapularis muscle over the distal scapula is partially elevated to expose the medial aspect of the shoulder. The cranial and caudal origins in the scapula and the distal insertion of the medial glenohumeral ligament are identified, and suture anchors are placed in these locations. Two separate strands of monofilament nylon are used to allow reconstruction of the Y-shaped ligament (Fig. 8).

> The subscapularis muscle is often heavily damaged in patients with medial luxation.

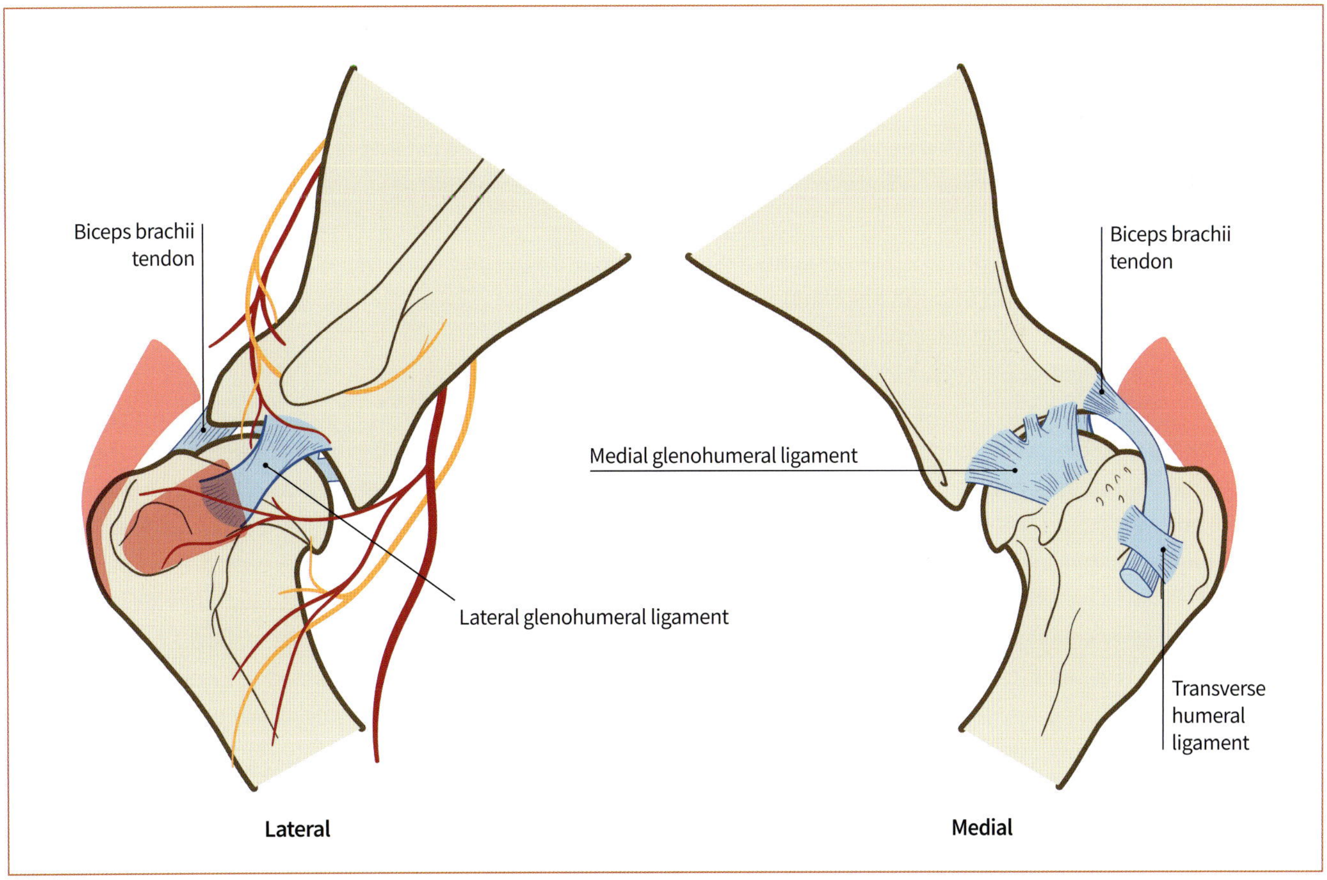

Figure 7. Schematic diagram of the anatomical location of the lateral and medial glenohumeral ligaments.

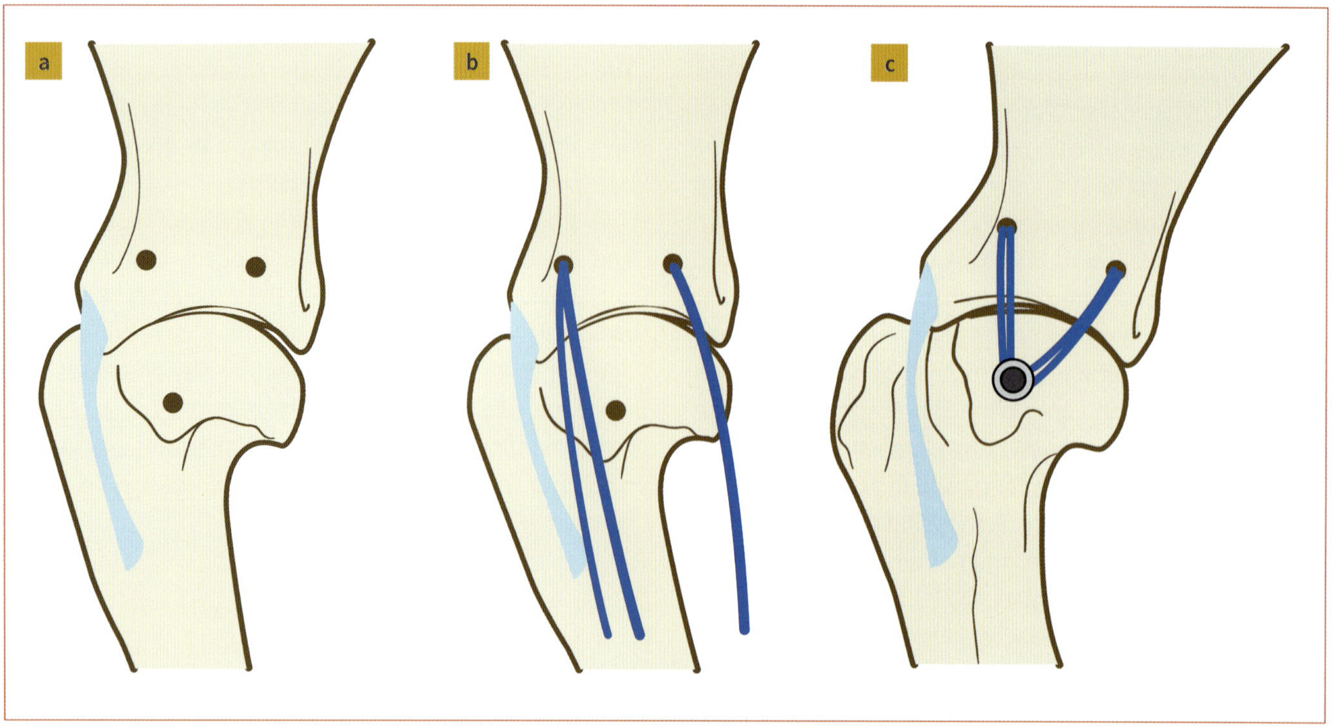

Figure 8. Medial aspect of the shoulder joint demonstrating the location of the humeral and glenoid suture anchors or bone tunnels.

Given the small amount of bone stock available for tissue anchors in this area, the author prefers an adaptation of this technique using bone tunnels.

There are two adaptations, both of which require an additional caudolateral approach to aid passage of the suture loops:

- Using scapular bone tunnels instead of bone anchors. One loop of nylon is passed through the humeral bone anchor and threaded through the cranial proximal bone tunnel and then passed underneath the infraspinatus and supraspinatus tendons directly against the lateral aspect of the scapula before being passed back medially through the caudal scapular tunnel. The loop is then tied off or crimped on the medial aspect of the joint. Other nonabsorbable suture materials such as FiberTape (Arthrex) can also be used.
- Using scapular and humeral bone tunnels. Two circumferential loops are used: one between the humeral and the cranial origin bone tunnels and the second through the humeral and caudal origin bone tunnels. This adaptation allows for reconstruction of the lateral support as well. This can be used as the primary approach in lateral luxations and in cases with gross instability due to multiligament disruptions.

Another technique is arthroscopic-assisted ligament reconstruction as described by O'Donnell et al. (2017). A full description of this technique is beyond the scope of this chapter, and the reader is referred to the "References and further reading" section at the end of this book for more information.

Capsulorrhaphy/capsular plication should be attempted in all cases. However, in the author's experience, the capsule is friable and often nonreconstructable.

POSTOPERATIVE MANAGEMENT

Postsurgical immobilisation (see Fig. 6 above) for 2–4 weeks followed by rehabilitation therapy (as described for conservative management) is recommended. For dogs with multiligament instability and reconstruction, the use of a spica splint for 2 weeks followed by a stabilisation brace for 2–4 additional weeks is recommended.

In multiligament disruptions and severely unstable joints, temporary immobilisation with a transarticular plate can be considered, as described by Post et al. (2008). In this study, the medial and lateral glenohumeral ligaments were repaired and a transarticular locking plate was applied laterally. After 25 days, the shoulder was functionally stable following plate removal.

> If medial shoulder luxation involves an avulsion fracture of the lesser tubercle, repair of the fracture with a lag screw may resolve any shoulder instability (Huck and Bergh, 2011).

OUTCOME AND COMPLICATIONS

In general, the outcomes reported following conservative and surgical management of shoulder luxations are good, although data is often mixed with shoulder instability syndromes (Pucheu and Duhautois, 2008; Post et al., 2008; Huck and Bergh, 2011; Fitch et al., 2001; Vasseur et al., 1982).

As with most joint injuries, some post-traumatic osteoarthritis is expected, although it may be more common in dogs that have undergone biceps tendon transposition.

Although biceps tendon transposition alters joint biomechanics and congruity, good outcomes have been reported; Pucheu and Duhautois (2008) reported around 85 % good to excellent function. However, cases with shoulder instability were also included in the outcome data, limiting the interpretation of this finding. Another study reported that 40 % of dogs had some degree of lameness at 2.5 years after surgery (Vasseur et al., 1982). Fitch et al. (2001) reported 9 out of 10 good to excellent outcomes, although only 1 case had a traumatic luxation.

O'Donnell et al. (2017) reported successful placement of the TightRope (Arthex) prosthetic ligament in 39 out of 39 dogs treated for management of medial glenohumeral instability. Complications were seen in 15 % of dogs. At the last follow-up (6–68 months), 77 % and 23 % of dogs were reported to have a full and acceptable function, respectively. It is noteworthy that only 4 out of 39 dogs in this case series had traumatic luxations of the shoulder.

Complications reported include persistent instability, infection, implant failure and, rarely, wound problems.

In cases with persistent shoulder luxation/instability, salvage procedures such as glenoid excision arthroplasty and shoulder arthrodesis can be considered.

OSTEOCHONDRITIS DISSECANS OF THE SHOULDER JOINT

Miguel Solano

INTRODUCTION

Osteochondrosis (OC) is a defect in endochondral ossification. Young, rapidly growing dogs of large and giant breeds are predisposed. When OC progresses forming a flap of cartilage, it is known as osteochondritis dissecans (OCD). The disease occurs mainly in large-breed dogs between 4 and 10 months of age (LaFond et al., 2002; Kuroki et al., 2005; Adamiak, 2007). The shoulder is the most common joint affected by OCD, followed by the elbow, the stifle and the hock. Males have a higher incidence than females, and dogs are likely (27–68 %) to have bilateral shoulder pathology. See chapter "Generalities of osteochondritis dissecans" for further general information on OC and OCD.

In the shoulder, OCD is generally localised in the caudocentral or caudomedial region of the humeral head (Fig. 1). Caudomedial OCD lesions are more commonly associated with positive outcomes compared with caudocentral lesions (Olivieri et al., 2007). Larger subchondral lesion size has also been associated with suboptimal clinical outcomes (Fitzpatrick et al., 2010).

CLINICAL PRESENTATION AND DIAGNOSIS

The degree of lameness at presentation is variable. Typically, it is more commonly reported in male dogs of large to giant breeds. Unilateral lameness is common despite the high incidence of bilateral shoulder OCD. Most dogs present with clinical signs of lameness before skeletal maturity, but some may present later in life with generalised

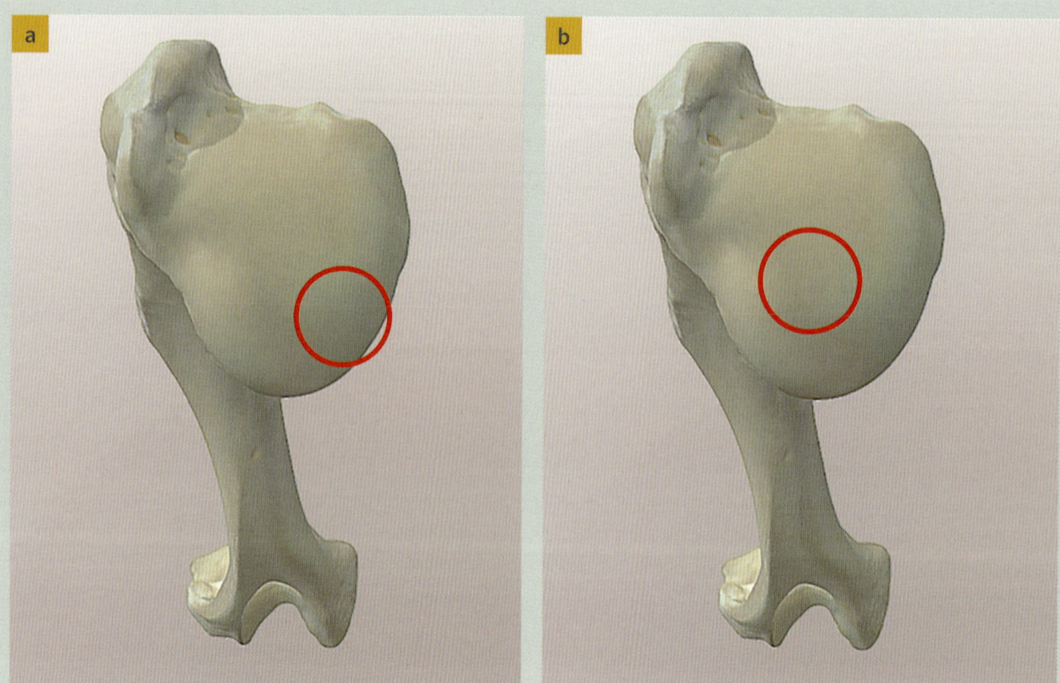

Figure 1. Representation of caudomedial (a) and caudocentral (b) OCD lesions on the humeral head.

degenerative joint disease in the affected shoulder. Some dogs may present with concurrent clinical signs of elbow and shoulder pathology. The author recommends elbow and shoulder imaging as standard workup for young dogs with thoracic limb lameness. Shoulder manipulation generally elicits pain. A definitive diagnosis can be established by radiography (with or without an arthrogram), CT or MRI (Figs. 2–4).

Mediolateral radiographs may evidence a subchondral defect on the caudal aspect of the humeral head, perilesional sclerosis and presence of a soft tissue opacity suggestive of shoulder effusion on the caudal pouch of the joint. Serial pronated and supinated mediolateral radiographs may help with the diagnosis.

> CT has become a more available imaging technique in veterinary practice. It allows evaluation of the location, size and depth of OCD lesions.

The diagnostic sensitivity, specificity and accuracy of radiography, ultrasonography and MRI were evaluated for detecting shoulder OC/OCD in dogs (Wall et al., 2015). The results were, respectively, 88.5 %, 90 % and 88.9 % for radiography; 92 %, 60 % and 82.6 % for ultrasonography, and 96 %, 88.9 % and 94.4 % for MRI. The odds of a correct diagnosis with MRI were 3.2 times more than with ultrasonography and 2 times more than with radiography.

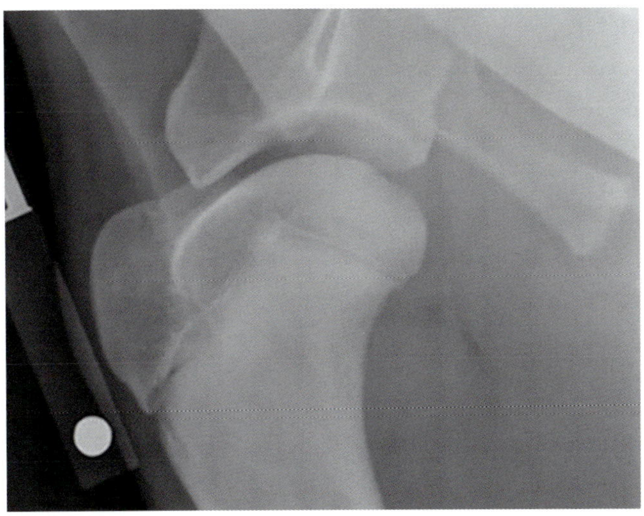

Figure 2. Mediolateral radiograph of the shoulder of a dog showing a subchondral defect on the humeral head.

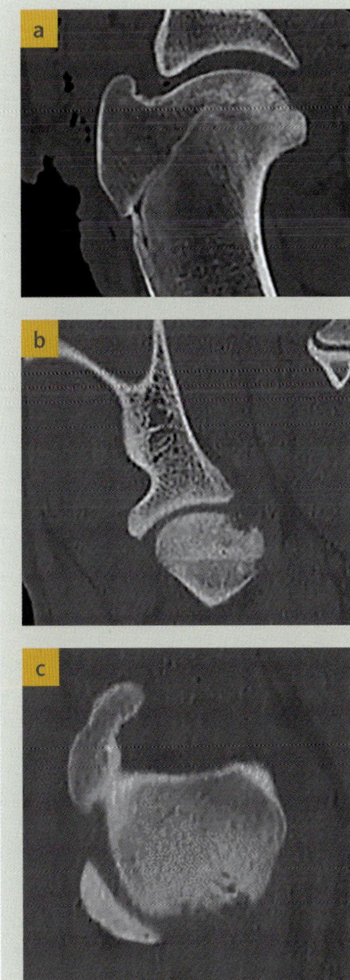

Figure 3. Sagittal (a), frontal (b) and transverse (c) plane CT images of a shoulder with a subchondral defect (OCD). Note the subchondral hyperattenuation.

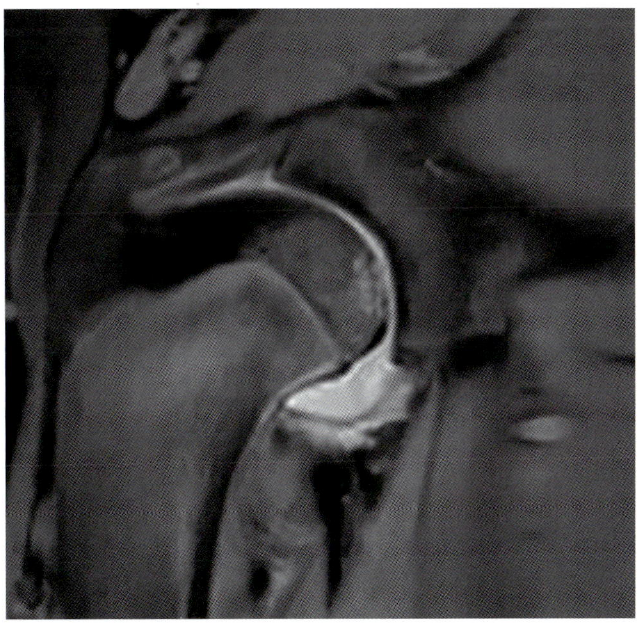

Figure 4. T2-weighted MRI sequence of a shoulder OCD lesion showing perilesional hyperintensity and increased signal suggestive of joint effusion.

TREATMENT

SURGICAL MANAGEMENT

Management of humeral OCD with arthrotomy/arthroscopy, debridement and curettage improves the outcome over nonsurgical management (Biezyński et al., 2012). Better short-term outcomes were reported in dogs of 6–10 months of age (Biezyński et al., 2012). The long-term outcome after surgical intervention has been reported frequently as favourable, but it may be poor for up to 25 % of cases managed by arthrotomy and debridement (Rudd et al., 1990). Previous studies have suggested that the poor outcomes after surgical debridement may be associated with the inferior biomechanical properties of replacement fibrocartilage compared with healthy hyaline cartilage and/or prolonged access of inflammatory mediators to exposed subchondral bone leading to degenerative joint disease. Taking this into consideration, some authors have explored the outcomes of management of large (>7 mm) caudocentral lesions with the use of osteochondral autograft transfer (OAT) and, more recently, synthetic osteochondral resurfacing (SOR) (Fitzpatrick et al., 2010; Murphy et al., 2019). Fitzpatrick et al. (2010) reported OAT as technically feasible, leading to amelioration or resolution of short-term lameness in 14 dogs. The same team reported the use of SOR as a viable implant to treat large caudocentral OCD lesions of the humeral head in 24 dogs (28 affected shoulders), with resolution of lameness at 1-year follow-up (Murphy et al., 2019).

> Based on the present evidence, it appears reasonable to recommend arthroscopic/modified Cheli approach debridement and curettage/microfracture for small clinical lesions and synthetic osteochondral resurfacing for large and centrally located lesions.

Arthroscopic debridement and curettage/microfracture

Shoulder arthroscopy is performed using a lateral approach (see chapter "Arthroscopy"). The joint is completely explored, taking pictures and videos to document the procedure. An instrument portal is created 2–4 cm caudal to the arthroscopic portal. The OCD flap is removed with grasping forceps, and the margins of the OCD lesion are probed. The subchondral bed is examined after flap removal and palpated with a probe. Lesions covered with apparently normal fibrocartilage do not require any further treatment. For partially covered lesions, microfracture is performed: subchondral tunnels are created until subchondral bone bleeding is seen. This can be performed with a small (6–8 mm) Kirschner wire driven with a motorised drill. The use of an arthroscopic sleeve may be beneficial to prevent skidding of the pin. Alternatively, a Chondro Pick (Arthrex Vet Systems) can be used to create the bone tunnels. Different angles of Chondro Pick are available (20, 40 and 60 degrees) to facilitate execution.

Video 1. Shoulder arthroscopy, OCD debridement and microfracture demonstrated by Ian Gordon Holsworth, with permission from Arthrex Vet Systems (©Arthrex GmbH).

Open approach and debridement/microfracture for shoulder OCD

Two surgical approaches to the humeral head are discussed below: the modified Cheli approach and the caudolateral approach. For central OCD lesions it is the author's preference to use the modified Cheli approach, whilst the caudolateral approach is only used for very caudomedial lesions.

Modified Cheli approach

This surgical approach was described in excellent detail by Vezzoni et al. (2021). The dog is positioned in lateral recumbency with the affected limb uppermost. The spine and acromion of the scapula and the greater tubercle of the humerus are identified. Forced hyperflexion of the shoulder with the elbow in extension is applied to the affected limb (Fig. 5). This, as proposed by Cheli in 1984, favours cranial displacement of the caudal surface of the humeral head. A longitudinal 1–1.5 cm skin incision is made in the craniolateral aspect of the shoulder, approximately midway between the cranial edge of the acromion process and the proximal greater tubercle. The joint capsule is located between the caudal aspect of the supraspinatus muscle and the cranial aspect of the acromial portion of the deltoideus muscle. Perpendicular Gelpi retractors are used to increase exposure of the joint capsule. The joint capsule is incised in a longitudinal fashion and cranial to the lateral collateral ligament. The Gelpi retractors can then be positioned retracting the joint capsule. The humeral head is rotated, and the OC/OCD lesion is inspected (Fig. 6).

The flap is carefully elevated and detached from its edges with the sharp end of a periosteal elevator or a number 11 scalpel blade (Fig. 7). Additional visualisation can be achieved by manipulation of the limb (forced adduction and internal rotation of the shoulder) and/or with the use of a Hohmann retractor to gently subluxate the humeral head.

Microfracture is then performed as with a Chondro Pick, with small (0.8–0.9 mm) Kirschner wires or a small drill bit (1.1 mm) (Fig. 8; Video 2). For large, centrally located lesions, a SOR procedure should ideally be performed (see below).

Caudolateral approach to the shoulder joint

This approach was classically described by Piermattei et al. (2006) (Figs. 9 and 10). The dog is positioned in lateral recumbency with the affected limb uppermost. The spine and acromion of the scapula and the greater tubercle of the humerus are identified. A skin incision is made from the distal aspect of the scapular spine to the proximal third of the humerus. The deep fascia is incised over the ventral border of the distal scapular spine to free the origin of the scapular part of the deltoideus muscle. This fascial incision is continued distally over the acromial part of the deltoideus muscle to the omobrachial vein. An incision is made on the ventral aspect of the scapular spine and continued distally to separate the acromial and scapular parts of the deltoideus muscle, which are divided by blunt dissection. A branch of the axillary nerve is identified and preserved. The joint capsule is incised distal to the teres minor muscle. Rotation of the shoulder helps visualise the OCD lesion.

Open approach and OCD lesion resurfacing with SynACART

Preoperative assessment of OCD lesion size is performed by CT in three planes (Fig. 11). SynACART implants (Arthrex Vet Systems) are 8 mm deep and are available in different diameter sizes (8, 10, 15, 20 and 25 mm).

A modified Cheli approach is performed (see above). The OCD lesion and any grossly diseased cartilage is debrided with a sharp number 11 scalpel blade and a curette.

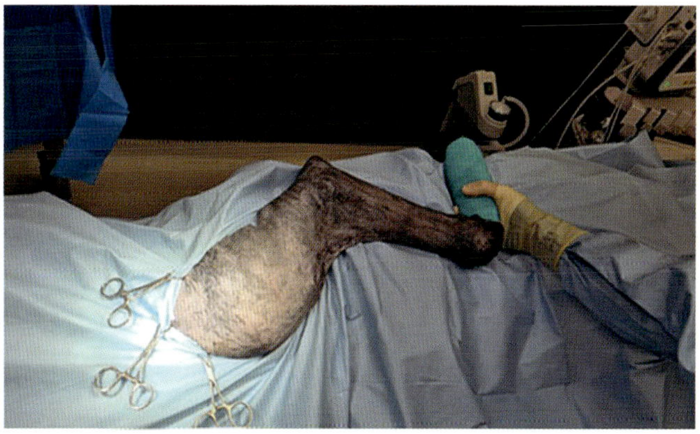

Figure 5. Patient positioning for a modified Cheli approach. Note the shoulder flexion with concurrent elbow extension.

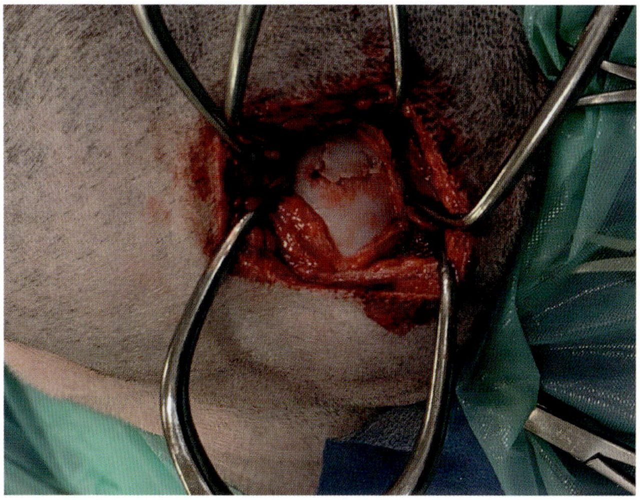

Figure 6. Intraoperative image of an OCD lesion on a canine humeral head.

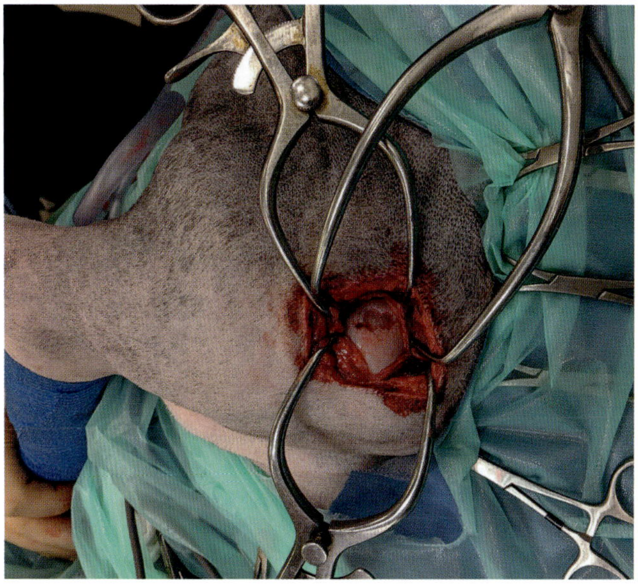

Figure 7. Intraoperative image of the same dog as in Figure 6 after OCD lesion debridement.

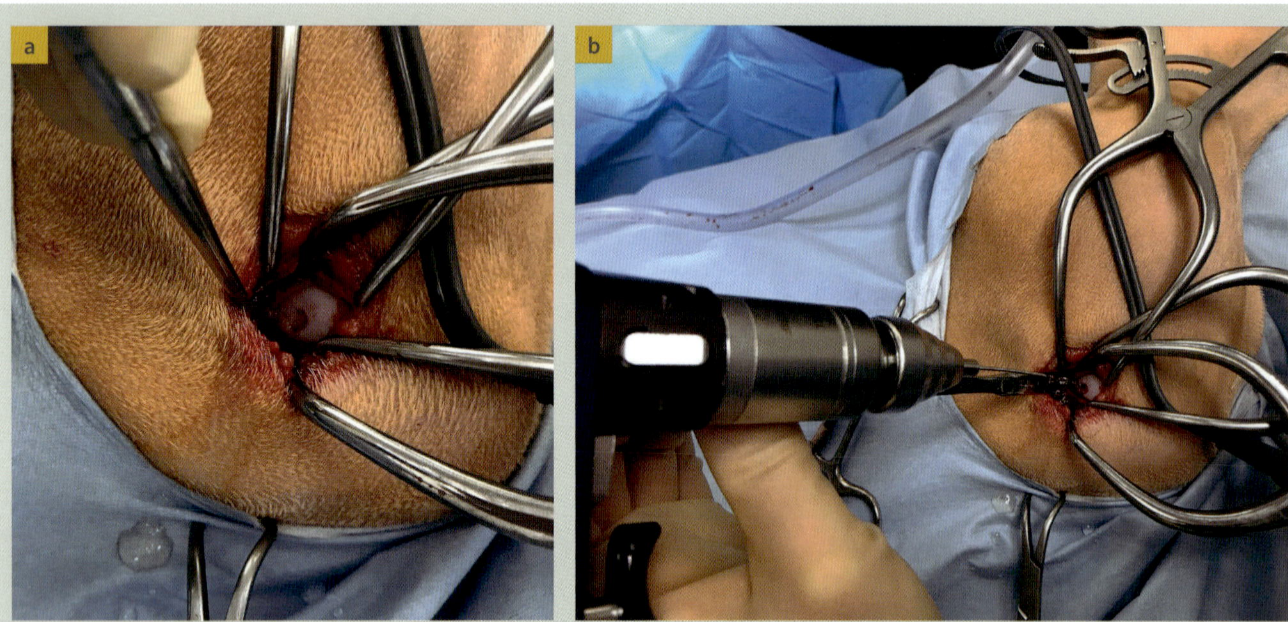

Figure 8. Intraoperative image of a canine shoulder with OCD (a). Drilling of the OCD lesion with a 1.1 mm drill bit after superficial debridement (b).

Video 2. Bleeding from the OCD lesion after drilling multiple small subchondral bone tunnels.

Video 3. Modified Cheli approach to the shoulder demonstrated by Ian Gordon Holsworth, with permission from Arthrex Vet Systems (©Arthrex GmbH).

The soft tissue retraction is maintained by Gelpi and Hohmann retractors. Sizing guides are used to determine the diameter of the chondral defect. This information is contrasted with preoperative planning data. The sizing guide is used as a drilling guide. The guide is positioned perpendicular to the defect, and a 2.4 mm pin is drilled through the centre. A motorised reamer of exactly the same diameter as the implant to be used is threaded over the pin to prepare the socket (Fig. 12). Care must be taken to ream the socket without bending the pin to avoid angulations in the execution. Abundant flushing should be applied during reaming. Ideally, reaming should be executed in a single go, without wobbling of the pin. This helps to create a perfect socket for implantation. The socket is then lavaged to remove any debris (Fig. 13).

The implant is inserted with a tamping tool and a mallet (Figs. 14 and 15). Care must be taken to avoid wedging the implant (i.e. mispositioning).

Ideally, the implant should be flush with the perilesional cartilage. Contouring of the implant has been reported using a fresh number 11 scalpel blade to enhance replication of the local articular topography (Murphy et al., 2019). The joint is then lavaged and closed as per routine. Postoperative radiographs and, when available, CT scans are taken to assess implant positioning (Figs. 16 and 17).

POSTOPERATIVE MANAGEMENT

Perioperative antibiotic therapy is given to all patients and discontinued at the end of the surgical procedure. A short course of oral nonsteroidal anti-inflammatory drugs is provided for 14 days. No bandage is generally needed, and it is recommended that cryotherapy is applied every 4–6 hours for the first 72 hours after surgery.

Strict rest is prescribed for 6 weeks (by confinement in a big cage or small room). No jumping, running, walking on slippery surfaces, off-lead exercise, steps or stairs are allowed. The patient can go outside on the lead

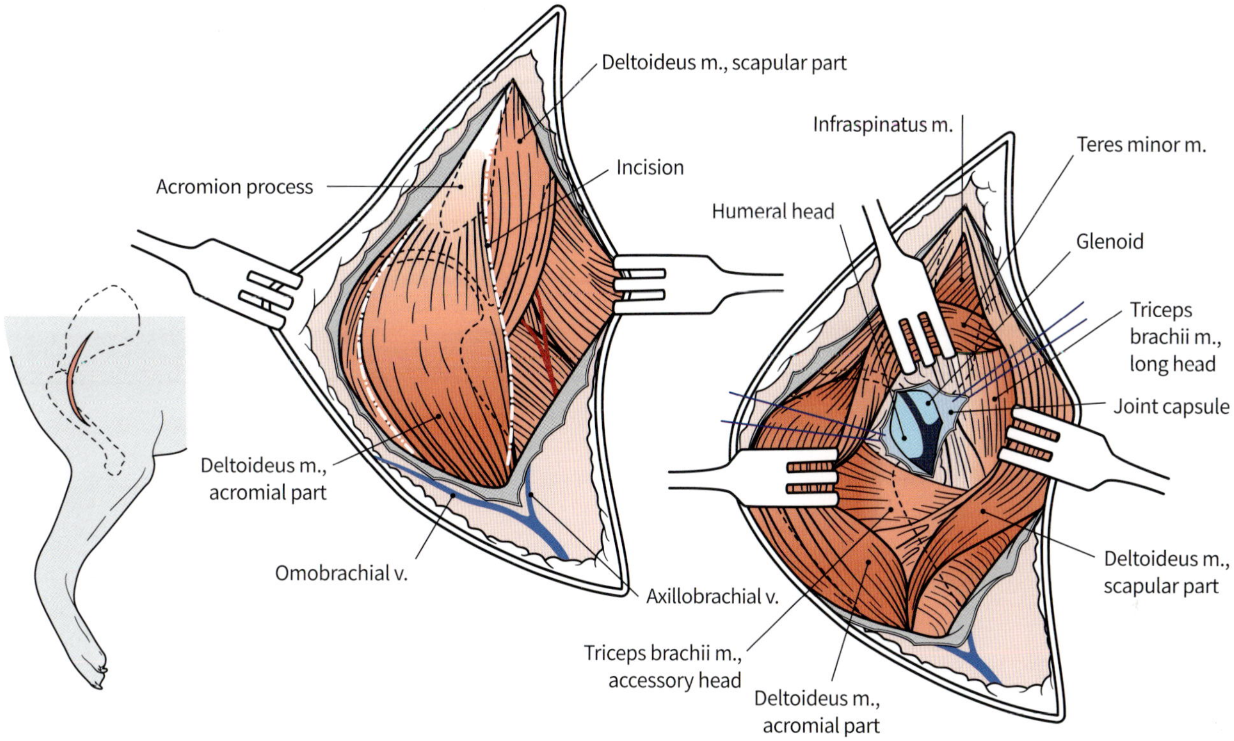

Figure 9. Caudolateral approach to the shoulder. Adapted from: Piermattei DL et al., *Brinker, Piermattei and Flo's Handbook of Small Animal Orthopedics and Fracture Repair*, 4th ed. (2006).

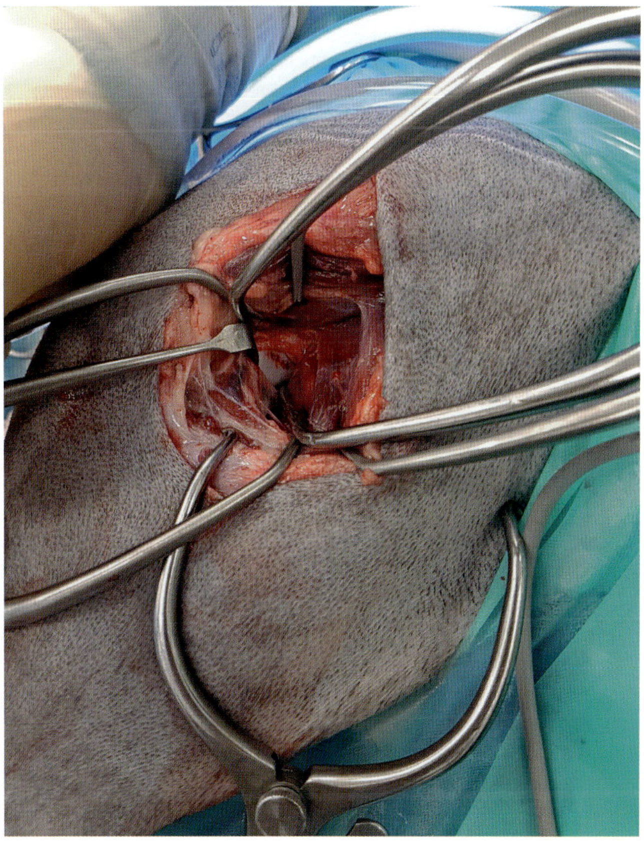

Figure 10. Intraoperative image of the caudolateral approach to a shoulder with an OCD lesion.

for 10 minutes 3–4 times a day for toilet purposes. The skin sutures or staples are removed after 12 days. Follow-up radiographs are taken under heavy sedation after 6 weeks.

Provided there is evidence of advanced healing and no implant-related issues, lead exercise can be increased by 5 minutes per walk on a weekly basis over a 4-week period, followed by slow reintroduction of off-lead exercise over an additional 4-week period. Physiotherapy and hydrotherapy can be considered after the 6-week follow-up visit.

Video 4. Synthetic osteochondral resurfacing with SynACART demonstrated by Ian Gordon Holsworth, with permission from Arthrex Vet Systems (©Arthrex GmbH).

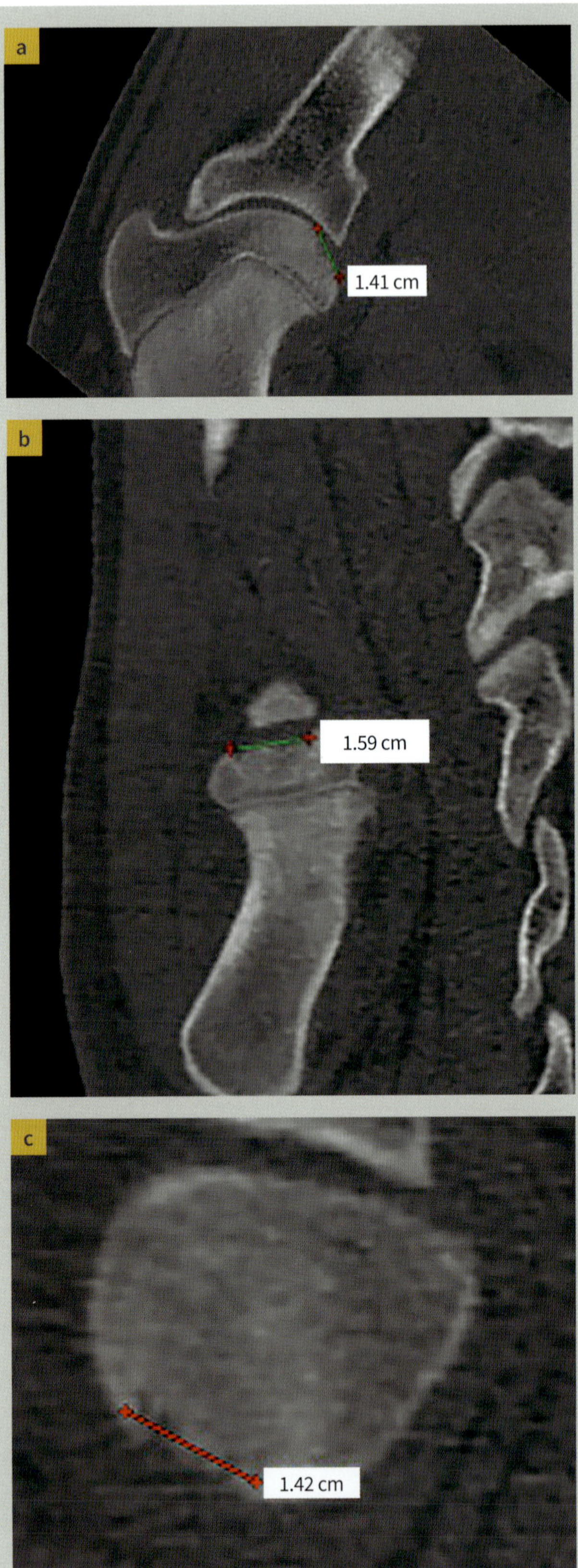

Figure 11. CT scan multiplanar reconstruction images (sagittal [a], frontal [b] and transverse [c] views) are used for selection of the SynACART implant. In this case, a 15 mm implant is likely to resurface most of the OCD defect.

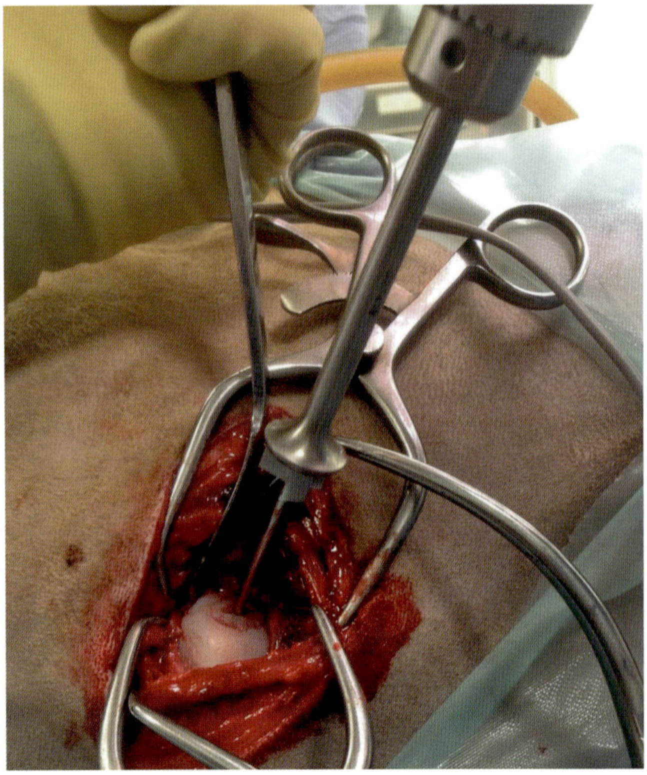

Figure 12. A reamer of appropriate size is put through the pin guiding the reaming.

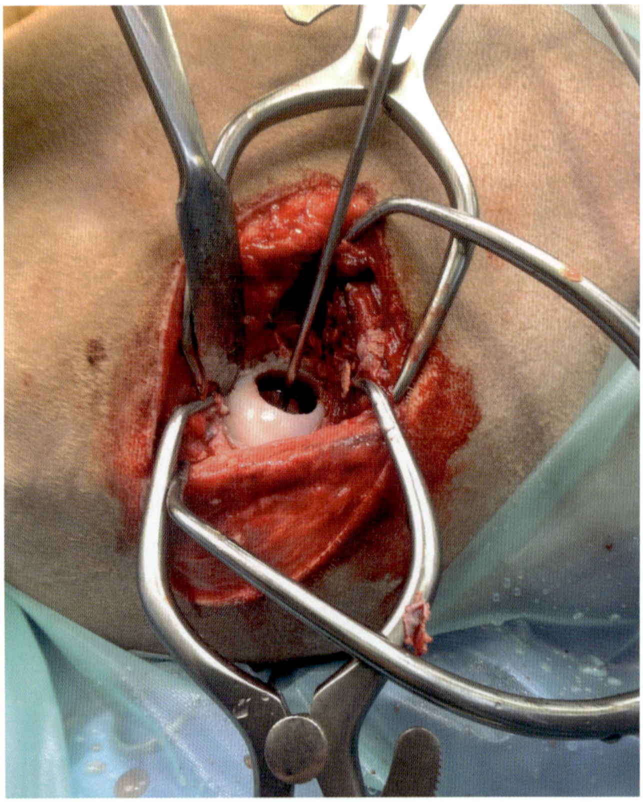

Figure 13. Intraoperative image of the socket created after reaming. The area is abundantly lavaged to remove any debris.

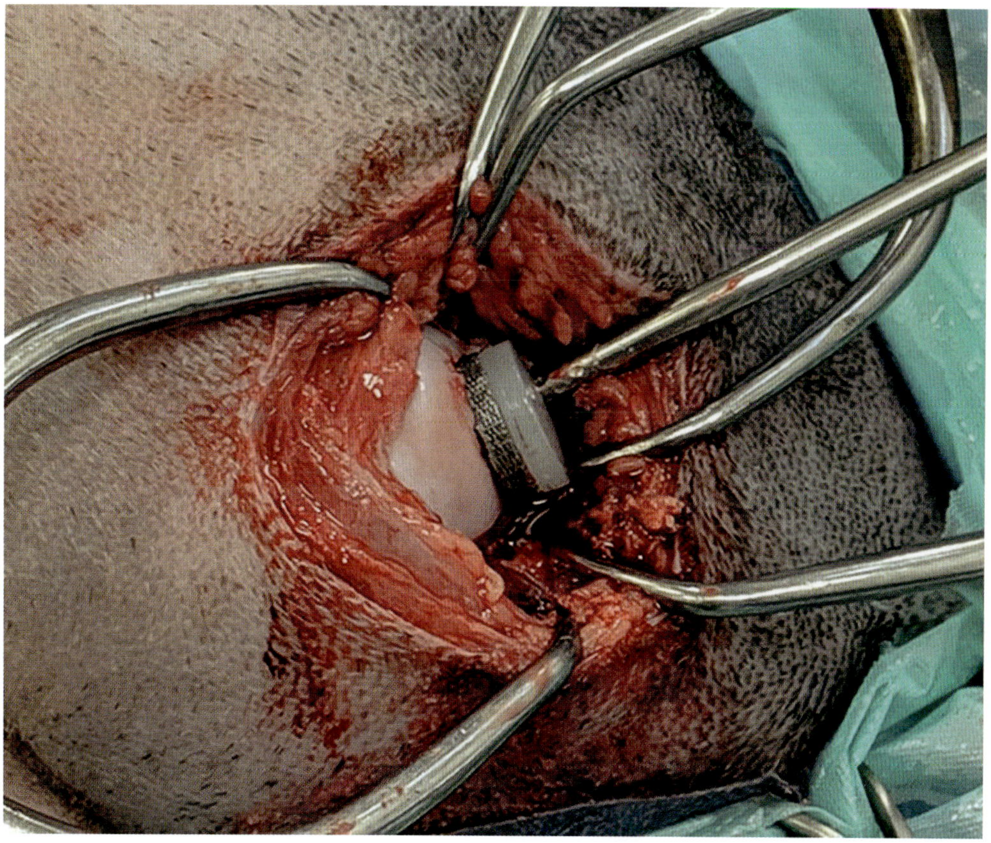

Figure 14. The SynACART implant is partially placed in the socket. Note the base of the implant, which favours osteointegration.

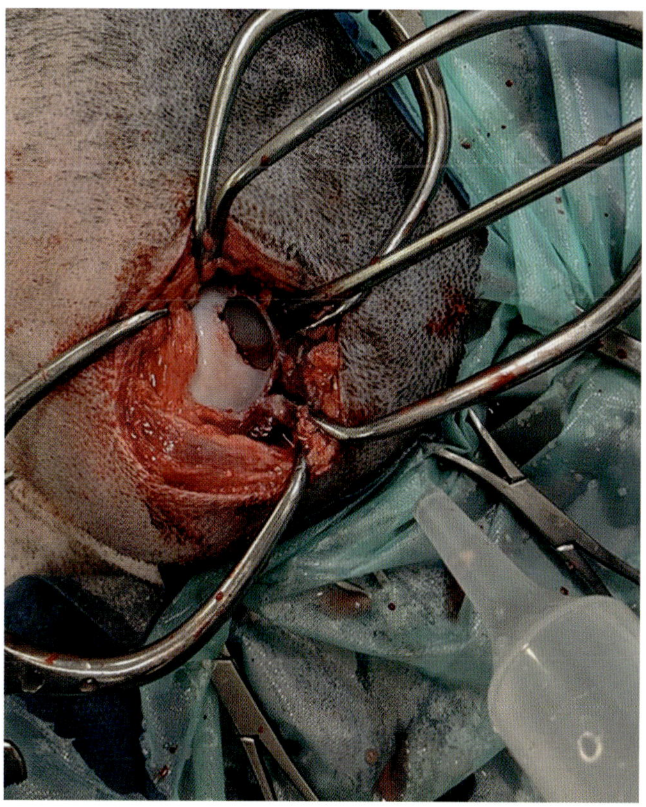

Figure 15. SynACART implant after implantation, providing appropriate resurfacing of the OCD lesion.

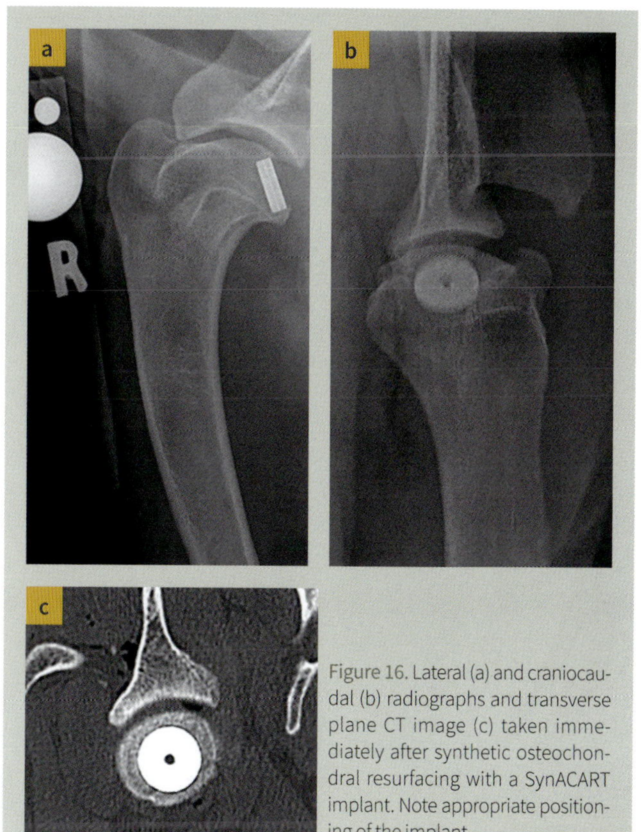

Figure 16. Lateral (a) and craniocaudal (b) radiographs and transverse plane CT image (c) taken immediately after synthetic osteochondral resurfacing with a SynACART implant. Note appropriate positioning of the implant.

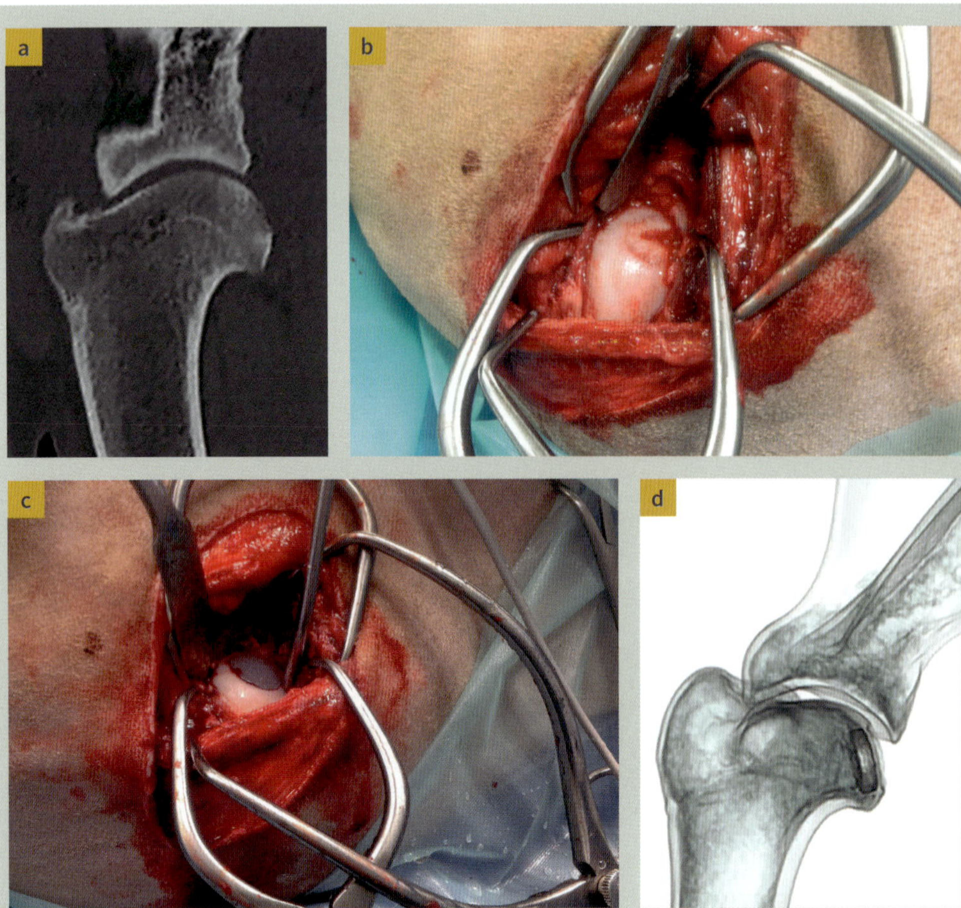

Figure 17. Preoperative sagittal plane CT image showing a subchondral defect on the humeral head (a). Intraoperative images showing the subchondral defect (b) and the implanted SynACART (c). Postoperative CT image for evaluation of implant positioning (d).

OUTCOME

The outcome after surgical management of shoulder OCD is generally good to excellent (Murphy et al., 2019; Vezzoni et al., 2021; Fitzpatrick et al., 2010; Olivieri et al., 2007). Dogs with caudomedial lesions appear to have a better outcome than those with caudocentral lesions (Olivieri et al., 2007). Management of a shoulder OCD lesion with a modified Cheli approach, arthrotomy and flap removal with or without microfracture was reported in 164 dogs (Vezzoni et al., 2021). Medium-term follow-up (6–12 months) was available for 70 cases and only one dog had intermittent lameness after exercise. For dogs with OCD lesions larger than 7 mm, excellent outcomes have been reported following SOR with SynACART (Murphy et al., 2019). All dogs were sound at long-term follow-up (>1 year).

COMPLICATIONS

Complications after the modified Cheli approach, arthrotomy and flap removal with or without microfracture were reported in 10 out of 164 (6 %) dogs, with surgical site seroma and persistent lameness being most common (Vezzoni et al., 2021). Complications after SOR with SynACART were reported in 9 out of 24 (37.5 %) dogs, with surgical site infection and seroma being most common (Murphy et al., 2019). The patients with superficial infection were successfully treated with antibiotic therapy. One dog with septic arthritis required implant explantation and revision 5 months after the original surgery (Fig. 18). None of the dogs with seroma required any additional intervention.

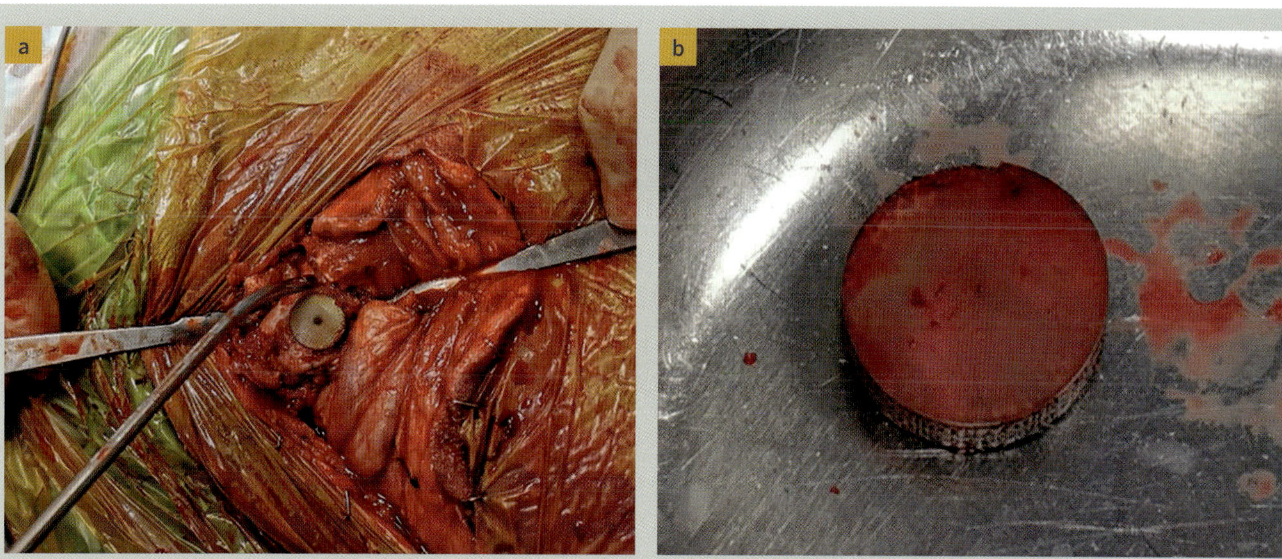

Figure 18. Intraoperative image of an infected SynACART (a). Explanted implant showing an irregular margin on the plastic component (b). This patient had subsequent shoulder arthrodesis.

INFRASPINATUS CONTRACTURE (FIBROTIC MYOPATHY)

Stephen Kalff

INTRODUCTION

Skeletal muscle heals through a combination of limited repair and replication of muscle cells and replacement of damaged tissue with fibrous connective tissue. Progressive fibrotic myopathy is a pathological process in which there is irreversible replacement of a myotendinous unit with fibrous connective tissue, leading to muscle contracture. This impedes normal joint movement, causing a mechanical, nonpainful gait abnormality that is characteristic for the muscle involved.

Fibrotic myopathy can theoretically affect any muscle. Whereas fibrotic myopathies of the infraspinatus, iliopsoas and supraspinatus muscles are commonly associated with myotendinous trauma, fibrotic myopathies of the gracilis, semitendinosus and sartorius muscles may have different aetiologies such as infection, ischaemic insults, immune-mediated disease and neoplasia.

Infraspinatus fibrotic myopathies are most frequently reported in highly active working-breed dogs. Patients often have a history of acute lameness which resolves, followed by a gradual progressive gait abnormality several weeks later. Once the muscle has completed the contracture process, the lameness typically remains static. The condition may occur bilaterally in some patients.

CLINICAL PRESENTATION AND DIAGNOSIS

Like most fibrotic myopathies, the gait alteration is pathognomonic. The limb circumducts and there is a distinct “carpal flip” into extension as the limb moves forwards (Video 1).

The shoulder exhibits a limited range of flexion, during which the elbow adducts and the antebrachium externally rotates and deviates laterally. There is marked focal atrophy of the infraspinatus muscle, which should be palpable.

Video 1. Dog with classic clinical signs of fibrotic myopathy of the left infraspinatus muscle.

> Palpation of the focal atrophy of the infraspinatus muscle may be difficult in overweight dogs.

Orthogonal radiographs are useful to exclude other pathologies but can appear unremarkable. Ultrasound, MRI or CT will confirm focal muscle atrophy; however, physical examination findings are generally sufficient for diagnosis.

TREATMENT

Failure to recognise the initial inciting injury and to initiate early treatment probably plays a significant role in the development of infraspinatus fibrotic myopathy. Early physiotherapy may prevent contracture development. However, once a contracture is present, treatment is release of the tendon of insertion of the infraspinatus muscle.

SURGICAL TREATMENT

The patient is positioned in lateral recumbency with the affected side up. The affected limb is hung and aseptically prepared. Four-quarter draping is performed to allow the surgeon and the assistant to manipulate the limb during surgery. A craniolateral approach to the shoulder is then performed (Fig. 1).

The infraspinatus tendon is isolated and released with a number 11 scalpel blade. Using a broad-based periosteal elevator over the incised tendon whilst flexing the shoulder

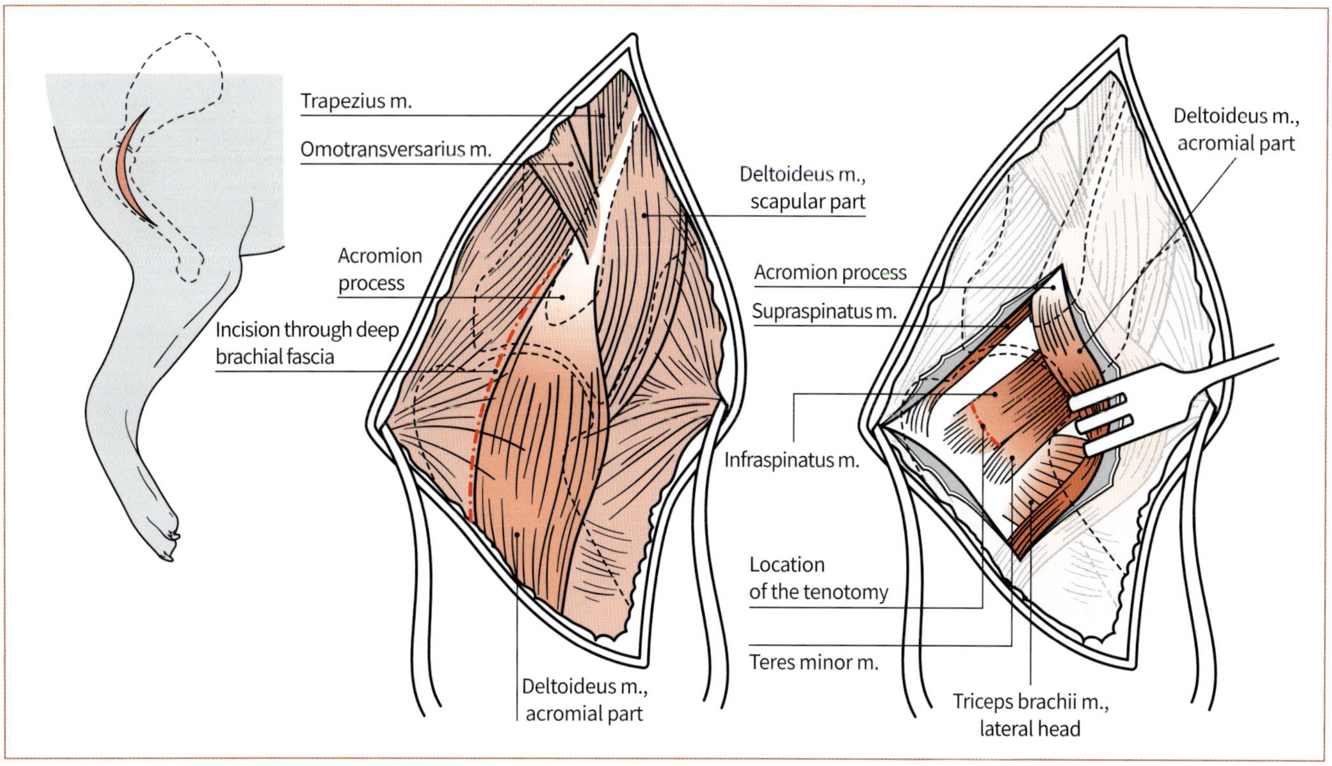

Figure 1. Craniolateral approach to the shoulder. Adapted from: Johnson KA, *Piermattei's Atlas of Surgical Approaches to the Bones and Joints of the Dog and Cat*, 5th ed. (2014).

can be helpful in completely releasing the tendon and any surrounding adhesions (Figs. 2–4). Once released, the shoulder range of motion should immediately return to normal. Often a distinct release point will be felt.

POSTOPERATIVE MANAGEMENT

The patient's activity should be restricted for 10–14 days, until sutures are removed, before reintroducing the dog to normal activity. Early return to activity may help prevent adhesion and recurrence.

OUTCOME

There are no reported recurrences in the literature and, in the author's experience, the prognosis for return to normal activity and work is excellent.

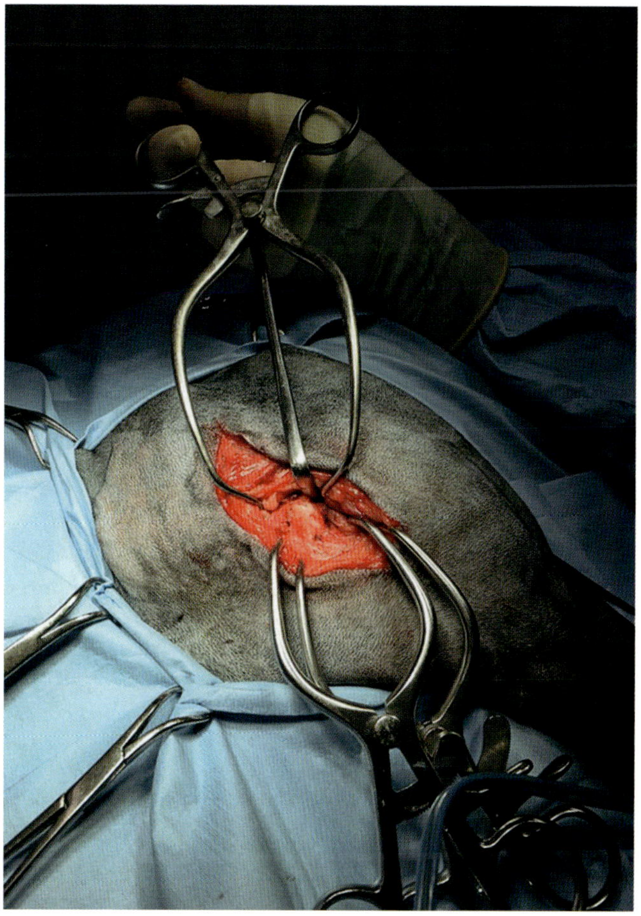

Figure 2. Intraoperative image of a surgical approach to the left infraspinatus tendon in a dog. Note the Langenbeck retractor displacing caudally the acromial part of the deltoideus muscle to expose the insertion of the infraspinatus tendon.

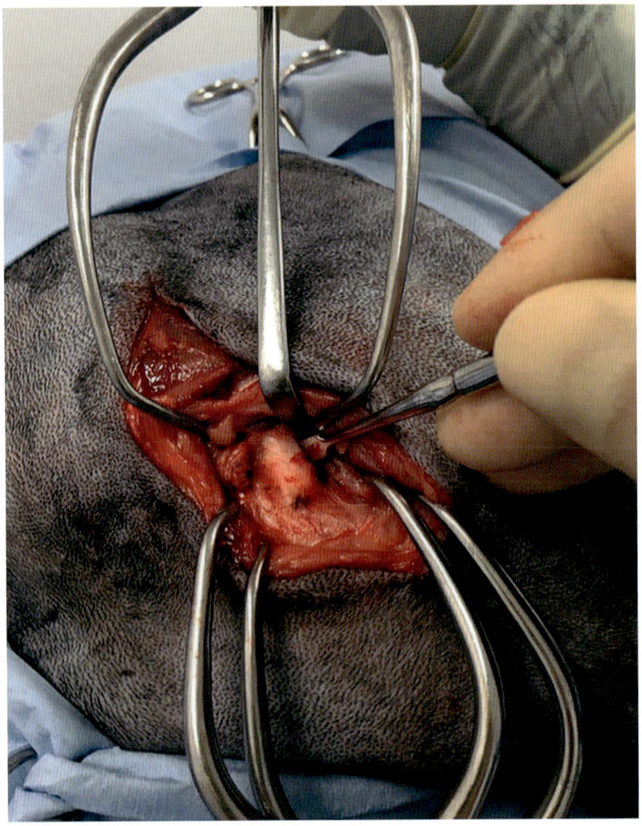

Figure 3. Intraoperative image of the same patient as in Figure 2. Note the periosteal elevator located at the caudal aspect of the tendon of insertion of the infraspinatus muscle.

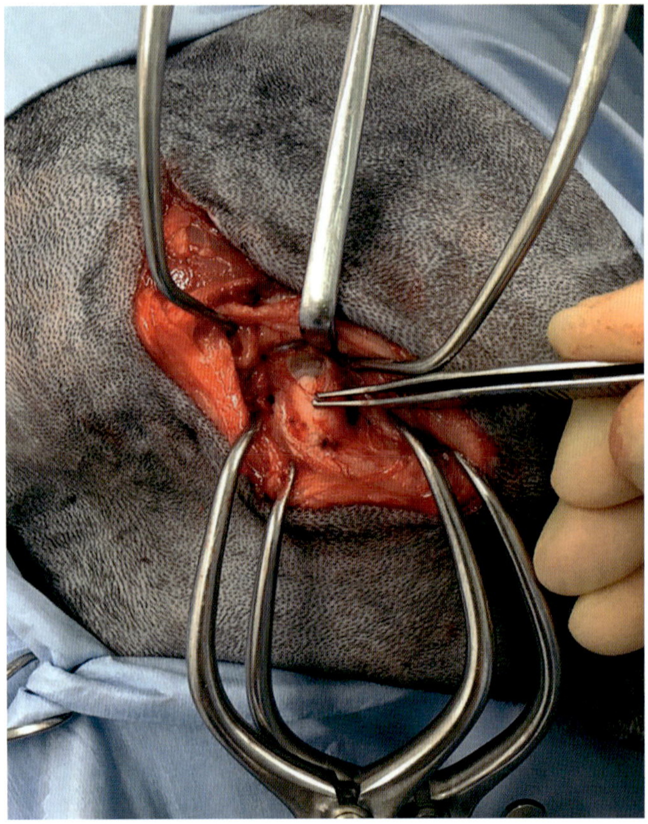

Figure 4. Intraoperative image of the same patient as in Figure 2. Note the transected insertion of the infraspinatus tendon.

BICEPS BRACHII TENDINOPATHY

Alan Danielski

INTRODUCTION

The biceps brachii tendon originates proximally from the supraglenoid tubercle and glenoid labrum and courses distally along the craniomedial aspect of the humeral head in the intertubercular groove, where it is held in place by the transverse humeral ligament. The tendon sheath extends to the level of the transverse ligament and is reflected over the tendon to form a visceral layer such that the intra-articular portion of the tendon is extrasynovial. The tendon sheath is filled with synovial fluid that is continuous with the synovial fluid in the shoulder joint (Bardet, 1999). The proportion of the tendon that is intra-articular changes when the joint is positioned in flexion or in extension.

Biceps brachii tendinopathy is considered one of the most common causes of shoulder lameness in dogs in conjunction with supraspinatus tendinopathy and osteochondritis dissecans lesions of the humeral head.

This tendinopathy is most commonly seen in middle-aged to older, medium- to large-breed dogs, and no breed or sex predisposition has been noted so far. It is particularly frequent in agility or working dogs, most likely as a result of the intense exercise levels they are subjected to, but it has also been described in sedentary or obese animals.

Affected dogs tend to exhibit chronic intermittent unilateral or bilateral lameness that deteriorates after intense exercise and is only partially and temporarily responsive to use of nonsteroidal anti-inflammatory drugs and exercise restriction.

Bicipital tendinopathy can be classified as primary or secondary (Gilley et al., 2002).

- Primary bicipital tendinopathy is the result of the inflammation of the tendon of origin of the biceps brachii muscle and is presumably a consequence of chronic overuse injury, similar to that described in humans (Kannus and Natri, 1997). Minor tendon injuries fail to heal appropriately due to the relative hypovascularity of the tendon near its origin on the supraglenoid tubercle, resulting in a nonhealing lesion which may predispose the tendon to mechanical failure (partial fraying or complete rupture). However, several studies have shown that histopathologic examination of the tendon of dogs diagnosed with bicipital tenosynovitis failed to support an inflammatory cause in every single case, and it is suggested that inflammation may not be the only cause of the disease (Gilley et al., 2002). A theory to explain tendon degeneration without inflammation is that the vascular supply to the tendon becomes impaired through aging, disease or trauma. Impaired blood supply to the tendon or tendon sheath could in fact lead to hypoxia and subsequent degeneration, such as has been reported in the Achilles tendon in humans (Slauson and Cooper, 1990; Averbukh et al., 1998; Handa et al., 1996).
- Secondary bicipital tendinopathy is usually the consequence of other intra-articular pathologies such as degeneration due to ageing or trauma, joint mice entrapment secondary to osteochondritis dissecans, or acute trauma to other tendons associated with the shoulder (Stobie et al., 1995).

Concomitant disease of the supraspinatus and biceps brachii tendons in the same joint has been reported and is believed to be due to the impingement of the biceps brachii tendon caused by the enlarged supraspinatus muscle tendon (Fransson et al., 2005).

CLINICAL PRESENTATION AND DIAGNOSIS

Diagnosis of bicipital tendinopathy can be made using a combination of physical examination and advanced imaging (e.g. radiography, arthroscopy, ultrasonography, CT, MRI).

PHYSICAL EXAMINATION

Dogs with biceps brachii tendinopathy usually show pain on focal pressure applied over the tendon in the intertubercular groove while flexing the shoulder joint and extending the elbow joint (Fig. 1). This manoeuvre is called the biceps tendon test. Dogs with an intact biceps brachii tendon should not be able to fully extend the elbow joint; therefore, hyperextension of the elbow joint with concomitant hyperflexion of the shoulder joint could indicate complete rupture of the biceps brachii tendon (Fig. 2). However, this rarely occurs, and it is strongly recommended to check the contralateral thoracic limb for comparison before diagnosing complete rupture of the tendon.

A significant pain response whilst performing the biceps tendon test and applying focal pressure to the biceps brachii tendon is commonly interpreted as diagnostic for bicipital tendinopathy by most veterinary surgeons, but it could also be interpreted as a sign of generalised shoulder pain.

A second test which is considered very useful to diagnose bicipital tendinopathy is the drawer test. The shoulder is partially flexed, the scapula is held still with one hand and the humerus is held with the other hand. By pushing the humerus cranially, pressure is applied to the biceps brachii tendon and, if this is diseased or inflamed, a painful response should be expected (Fig. 3).

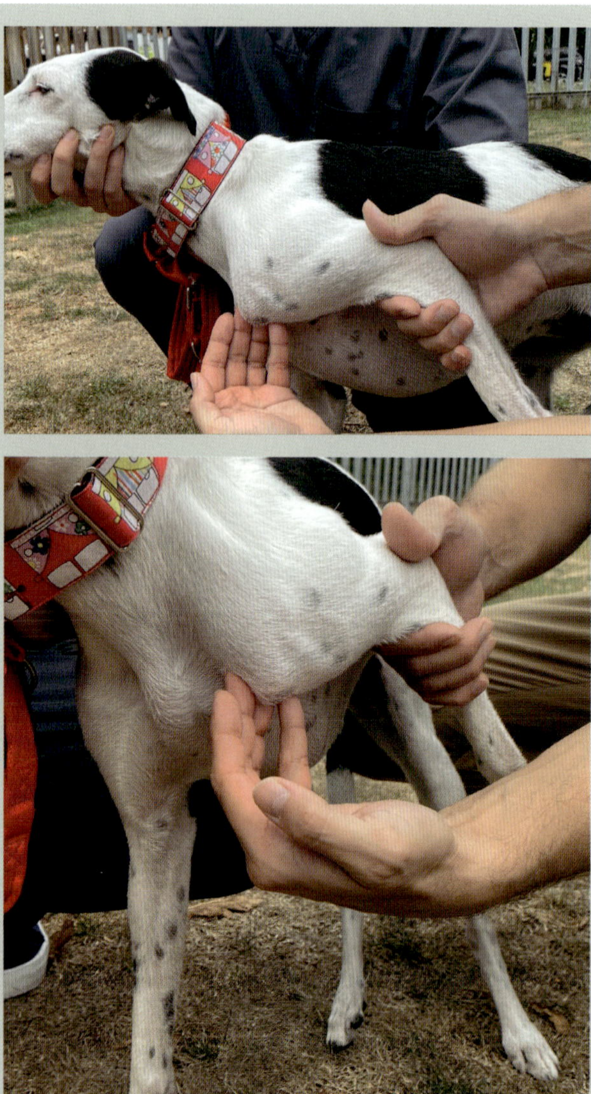

Figure 1. Biceps tendon test being performed in a dog. Focal pressure is applied to the proximal insertion of the biceps brachii tendon whilst the test is performed.

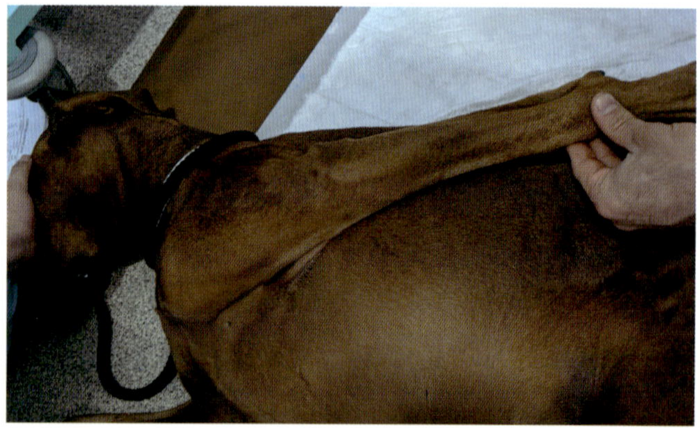

Figure 2. Positive biceps tendon test in a dog. If the biceps brachii tendon is intact, it should not be possible to fully extend the elbow joint.

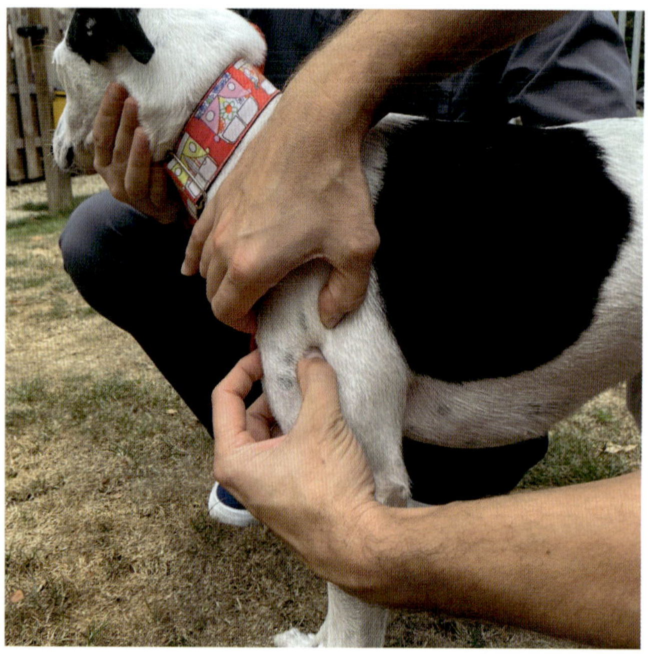

Figure 3. Drawer test being performed in the shoulder of a dog.

A third test usually used to diagnose biceps brachii muscle pain is called the biceps retraction test. With the dog in a weight-bearing position, the examiner's fingers are placed along the biceps brachii muscle close to the cranial aspect of the elbow, and pressure is applied by pulling the hand in a caudal direction (Fig. 4). A painful response would suggest biceps brachii tendinopathy.

RADIOGRAPHY

Orthogonal radiographs of the shoulder joint are usually useful only as a survey tool to look for secondary changes that could suggest bicipital tendinopathy and/or shoulder joint pathology. These changes consist of sclerosis of the intertubercular groove, increased periarticular osteophytosis at the level of the supraglenoid tuberosity, of the greater trochanter and at the caudal aspect of the shoulder joint, mineralisation of the biceps brachii and supraspinatus tendons and enthesophyte formation along the bicipital groove.

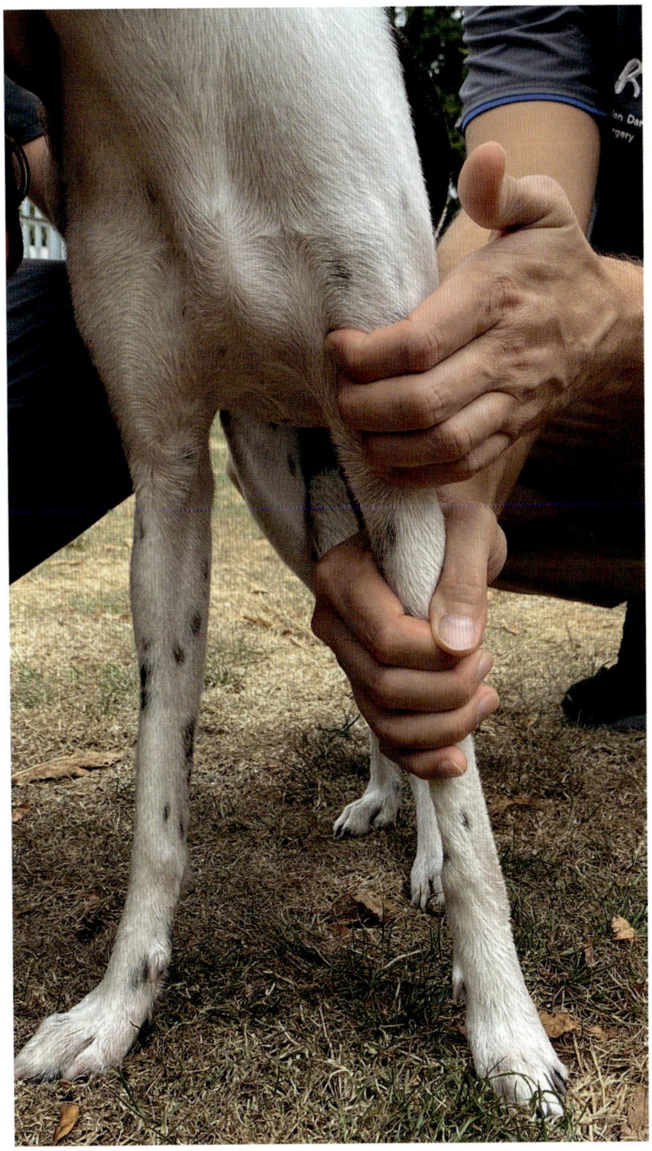

Figure 4. Biceps retraction test being performed in a dog. Note that the limb is maintained in a weight-bearing position whilst the test is performed.

A skyline view of the shoulder (i.e. a craniodistal–cranioproximal view of the humerus with the patient in sternal recumbency and the affected shoulder hyperflexed) may allow identification of irregularities within the intertubercular groove or areas of mineralisation of the tendon itself.

Positive-contrast arthrography can be performed to identify filling defects associated with the tendon and the surrounding synovium that could suggest a proliferative synovium, inflammation and adhesions between the tendon and the sheath or the presence of joint mice or enthesophytes (Fig. 5). In some cases, leakage of contrast material into the surrounding soft tissues can be noticed, and this should be interpreted as a rupture of the biceps brachii tendon sheath (Fig. 6). However, iatrogenic tendon sheath rupture caused by overdistension of the sheath during arthrography cannot be discarded.

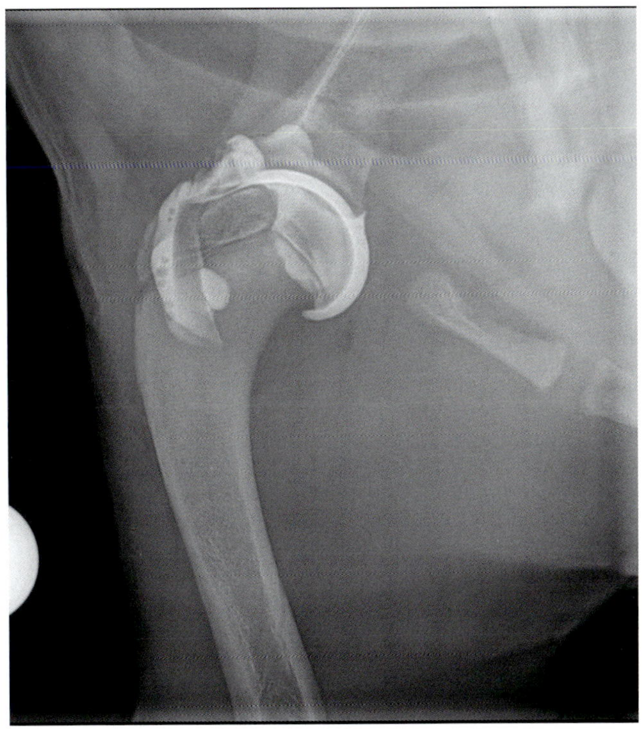

Figure 5. Positive-contrast arthrogram of the shoulder of a young dog. Note the filling defects looking like bubbles cranial to the biceps brachii tendon and the small synovial diverticulum at the caudal aspect of the tendon. A normal arthrogram should show good filling of the bicipital tendon sheath, with regular margins.

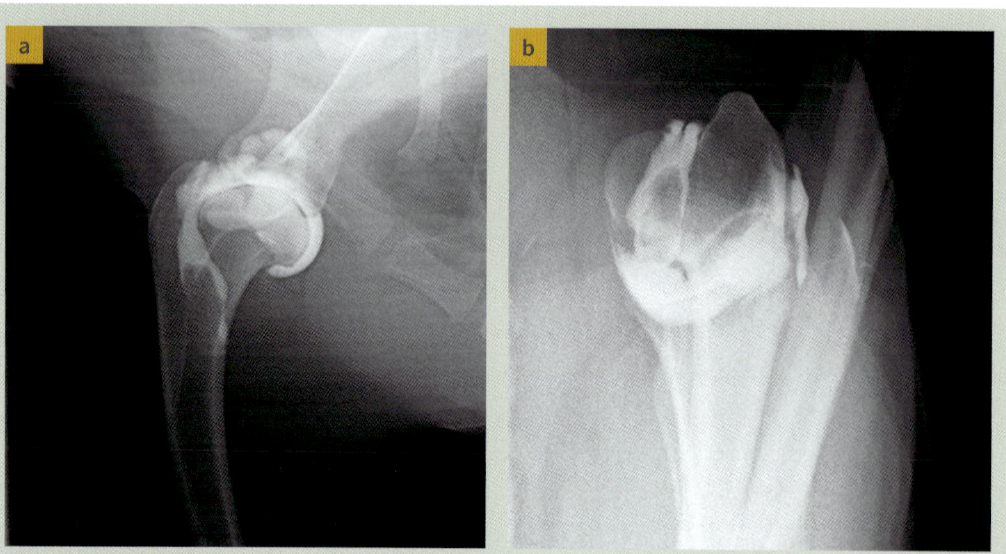

Figure 6. Positive-contrast arthrogram of the shoulder of an adult dog, mediolateral view (a) and skyline view (b). The contrast agent is filling the intertubercular groove, and it is not possible to evaluate the shape and contour of the biceps brachii tendon at the intertubercular groove, which is evident only at its very distal aspect. These findings are suggestive of rupture of the biceps brachii tendon.

ULTRASONOGRAPHY

Ultrasound imaging is the author's preferred method for investigation of biceps brachii tendinopathy because, if performed by an experienced ultrasonographer, it allows the identification of changes within the substance of the tendon that cannot be appreciated with radiography or arthroscopy.

Ultrasonographic examination of the shoulder joint has numerous benefits, as ultrasound is fast, noninvasive and more readily available, it has excellent tissue contrast, its cost is significantly less than that of MRI, it allows the ultrasonographer to perform a dynamic study (by placing the joint through its range of motion or in a position that helps delineating the lesion), and it guides diagnostic sampling (e.g. fine needle aspiration, biopsy). On the downside, it requires advanced expertise in imaging acquisition, it does not allow a complete 360-degree view of all the structures of the shoulder joint, and it has minimal ability to adequately image osseous structures.

Pathological findings in patients with bicipital tendinopathy usually include multiple hyperechogenic irregular structures with acoustic shadowing in the bicipital groove (enthesophytes), filling of the tendon sheath (adhesion formation or hypertrophic synovium), enlarged hypoechoic tendon with fibre pattern disruption or a sonolucent line around the tendon (fluid/effusion) (Figs. 7 and 8).

> Always remember to also assess the contralateral biceps brachii tendon as a comparison.

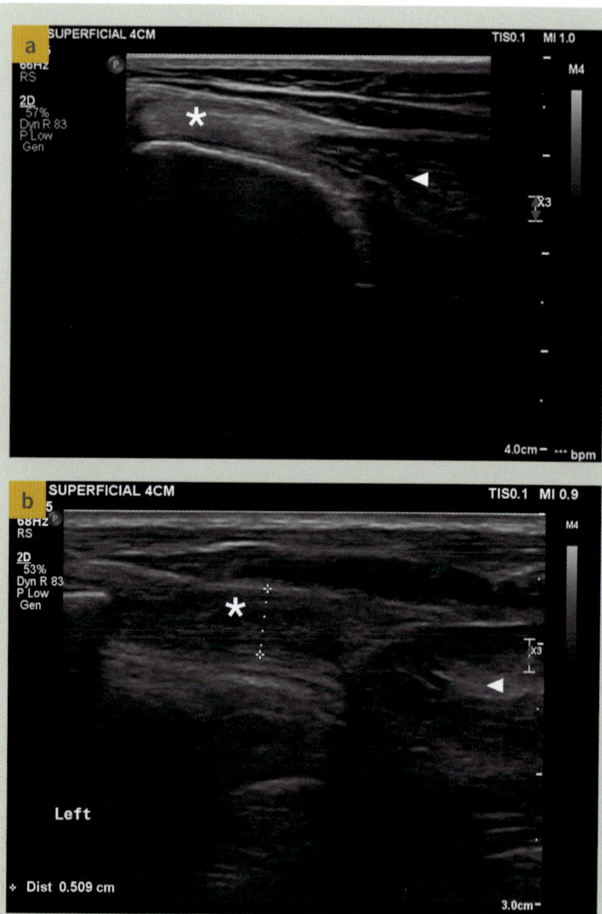

Figure 7. Sagittal ultrasound images of two different dogs showing the normal musculotendinous junction of the biceps brachii muscle (a) and a pathological biceps brachii tendon (b). In image b, note that, towards the musculotendinous junction, the tendon is swollen and has a heterogeneous appearance with small hypoechoic areas, and the normal pattern of muscle fibres cannot be recognised. The asterisk indicates the biceps brachii tendon, and the arrowhead points to the biceps brachii muscle.

MAGNETIC RESONANCE IMAGING

MRI has a remarkable soft tissue contrast resolution and allows easy identification of core lesions, tears, significant swelling and chronic changes (including mineralisation and fibrosis) of the tendon of the biceps brachii muscle (Fig. 9). It also allows a global view of the structures of the shoulder joint and permits evaluation of symmetry and secondary changes such as muscle atrophy or fibrosis. Impingement of the biceps brachii tendon secondary to supraspinatus tendon enlargement can also be assessed by MRI.

Disadvantages of using this imaging technique to assess biceps brachii tendinopathy include its high cost, the need for general anaesthesia and the much longer execution time.

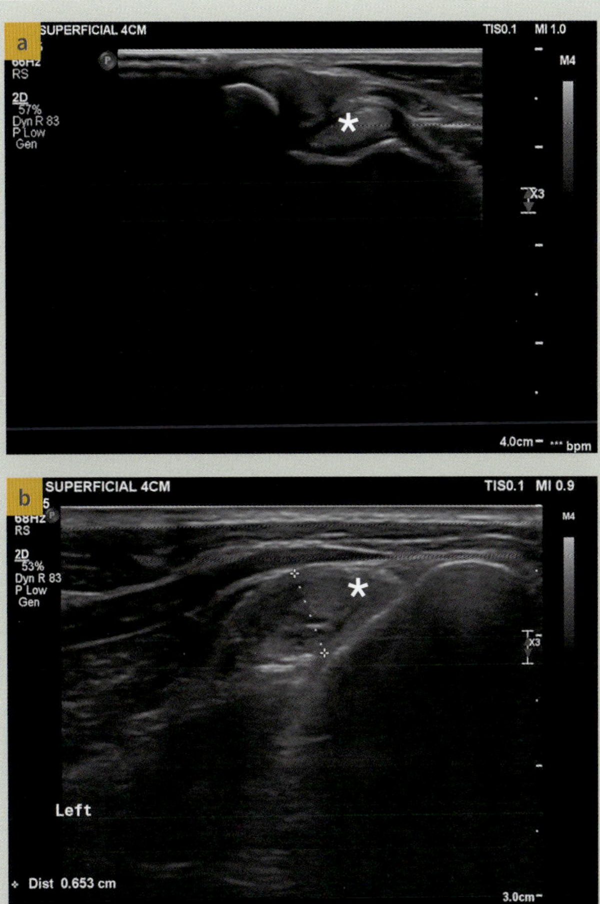

Figure 8. Transverse ultrasound images of the biceps brachii tendon (asterisk) of the same dogs as in Figure 7 showing a normal (a) and a pathological tendon (b). In image b, note the heterogeneous appearance of the enlarged tendon.

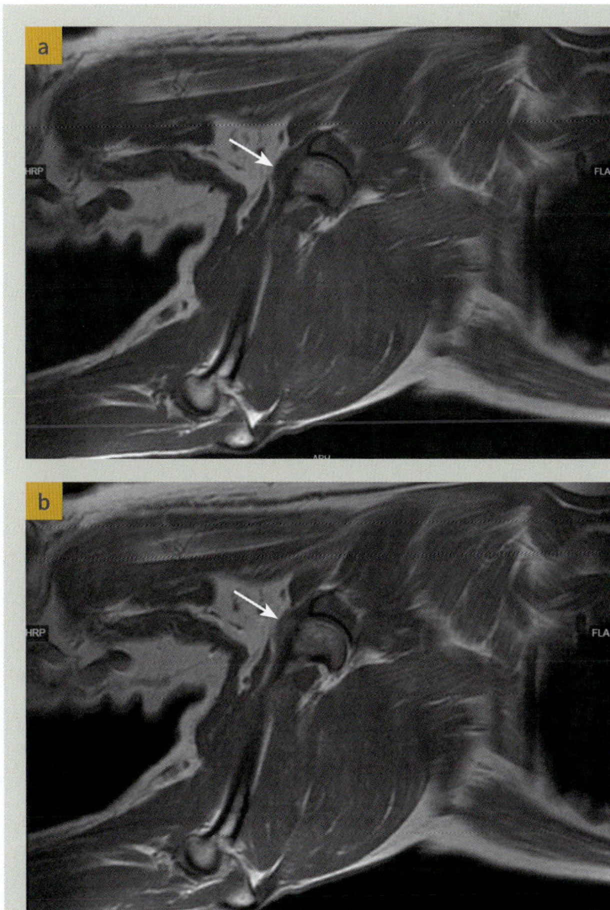

Figure 9. Sagittal view of T1-weighted magnetic resonance sequences of the shoulder region of a dog with bicipital tenosynovitis. The lesion (arrow) appears T1w isointense (a) and shows heterogeneous contrast enhancement in the postcontrast sequence (b).

TREATMENT

CONSERVATIVE TREATMENT

The primary objective of treatment is to reduce the degree of inflammation of the biceps brachii tendon and its synovial sheath. If the injury is acute and the pathological changes appear to be reversible, medical management using a long-acting corticosteroid (methylprednisolone acetate, 1 mg/kg) can be considered. The drug is injected intra-articularly using strict aseptic technique and, if necessary, it can be repeated once more 1–2 months later. This is followed by a period of strict cage rest and short lead walks for 6–8 weeks prior to a gradual return to normal activity.

> Whilst the use of corticosteroids is essential to reduce local inflammation and optimise the local environment for healing, exercise restriction is also considered critical to avoid continued injury to the tendon and to allow local inflammation to fully settle.

Continuous use of intra-articular long-acting steroids is not recommended, as it has been shown to negatively affect the articular cartilage by inducing chondrocyte apoptosis and accelerating osteoarthritis, which may already be present at the time of diagnosis (Fubini et al., 2001; Farkas et al., 2010).

Extracorporeal shock wave therapy (ESWT) has more recently been reported as an ancillary method to treat biceps brachii tendinopathy. The exact mechanism of action of ESWT is not completely understood, but it is thought that the release of energy caused by the sound waves emitted from the handheld trode can stimulate production and release of growth factors such as proliferating cell nuclear antigen (PCNA), transforming growth factor (TGF), insulin-like growth factor (IGF), platelet-derived growth factor (PDGF), vascular endothelial growth factor (VEGF) and fibroblast growth factor (FGF), which are responsible for tendon healing (Ogden et al., 2001; Notarnicola and Moretti, 2012).

A recent study reported good or excellent outcomes in 85 % of dogs with shoulder tendinopathy undergoing three treatment sessions with ESWT (over a 6-week period). There were no differences in outcomes between dogs that received ESWT with or without concomitant physiotherapy (Leeman et al., 2016).

Another study describing the use of ESWT in a dog following unsuccessful medical therapy reported that the patient demonstrated a substantial clinical improvement, having only minimal lameness during heavy exercise, 8 weeks after the first treatment session. Most importantly, diagnostic imaging revealed that the mineralised structures on the region of the intertubercular groove appeared less active after the first session, whilst additional treatment sessions did not demonstrate any further improvement in the radiographic appearance (Venzin et al., 2004).

SURGICAL TREATMENT

Although nonsurgical management of biceps brachii tendon pathology may be effective in some cases, surgical management often becomes necessary in a significant number of patients if a mechanical problem is found or when the animal does not respond to medical treatment.

The goal of surgery in all instances is to prevent the painful interaction between the diseased tendon and the inflamed tendon sheath as well as osteophyte formation in the intertubercular groove.

The most commonly reported surgical treatment options for biceps brachii tendon disease include tenodesis and tenotomy via an open or arthroscopic approach (Lincoln and Potter, 1984; Wall and Taylor, 2002; Cook et al., 2005).

Open tenodesis has traditionally been the preferred method to treat biceps brachii tendinopathy, especially in athletic dogs, based on recommendations extrapolated from human literature, and it provides good long-term outcomes in dogs (Adamiak and Szałecki, 2003; Stobie et al., 1995).

In these cases, the biceps brachii tendon is exposed by a cranial approach to the shoulder joint. The transverse humeral ligament and joint capsule are opened to expose the tendon and the intertubercular groove (Fig. 10). The tendon is then transected near the supraglenoid tubercle and is reattached to the humerus distal to the groove with a bone screw and a spiked washer (Fig. 11), with an interference screw or with a bone staple.

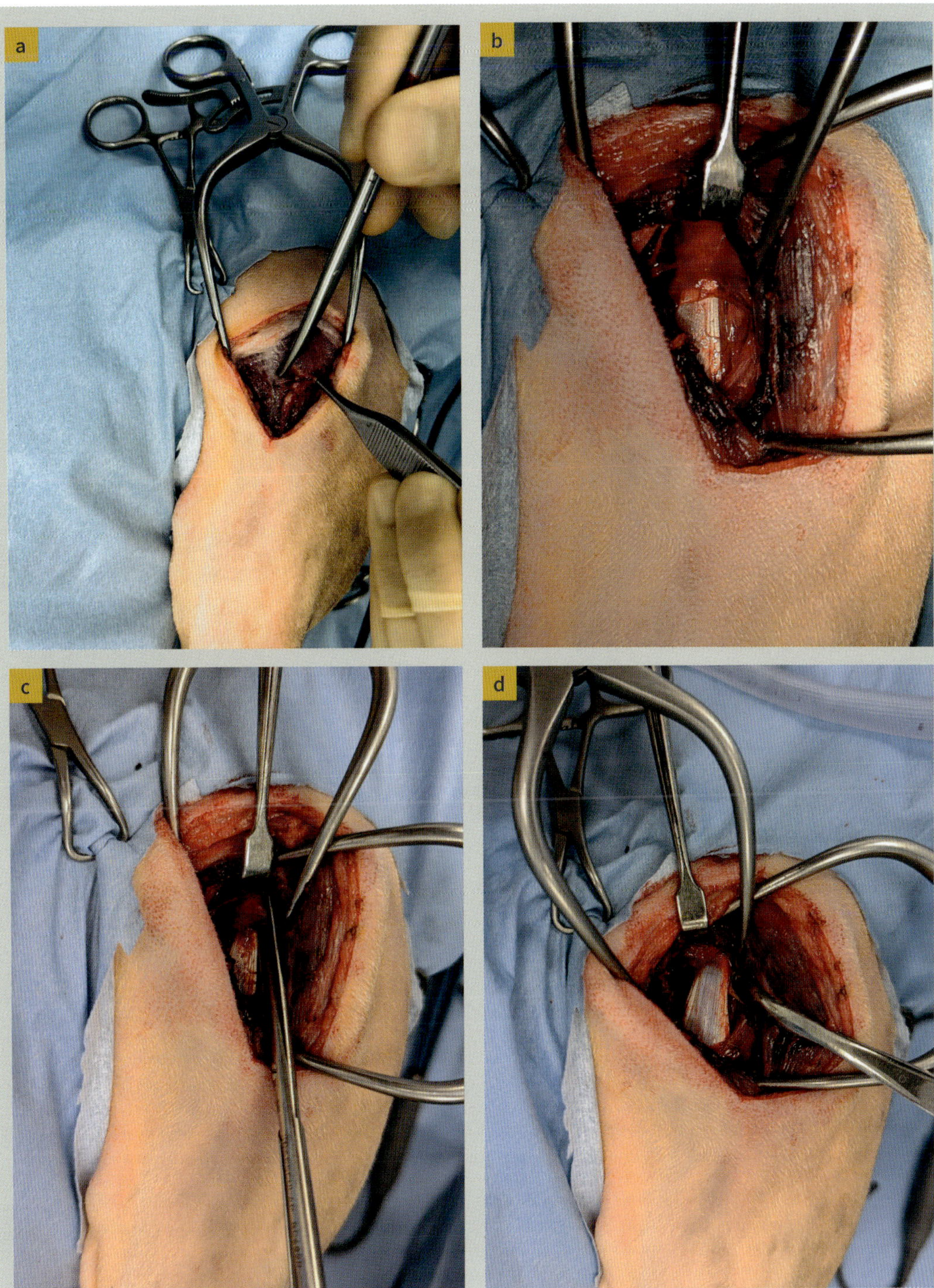

Figure 10. After incision and retraction of the subcutaneous tissues, the brachiocephalicus muscle is identified (a) and retracted medially following a fascial incision along its lateral border. With the limb externally rotated, the insertions of the superficial and deep pectoral muscles are freed from the humerus and retracted medially. The transverse humeral ligament and the musculotendinous portion of the biceps brachii muscle are exposed (b) and transected (c) to gain access to the tendon of the biceps brachii muscle (d).

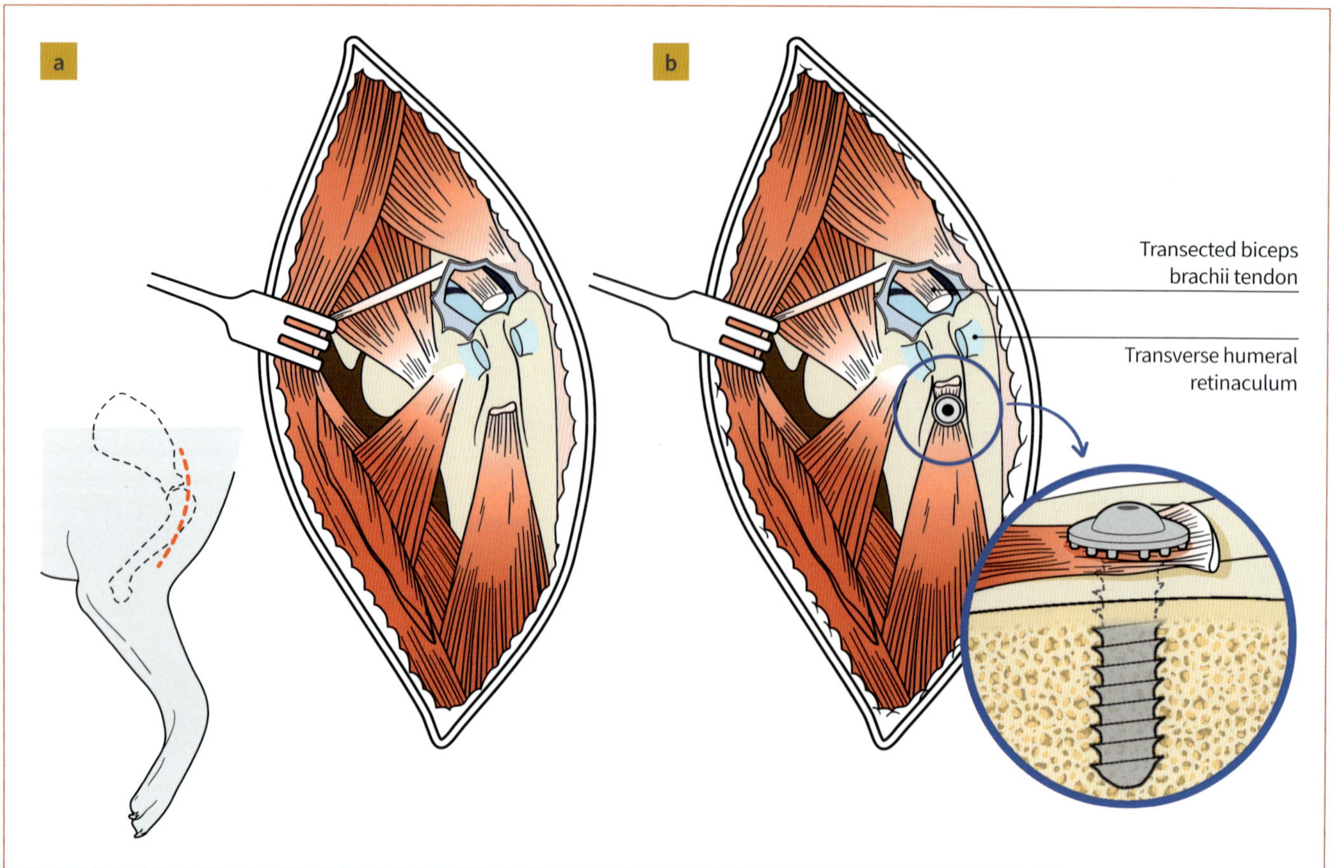

Figure 11. Medial approach to the left biceps brachii tendon. After cutting the transverse humeral retinaculum and exposing the biceps brachii tendon, the tendon is cut close to the supraglenoid tubercle (a) and fixed to the humerus further distally with a bone screw and a spiked washer (b). Adapted from: DeCamp CE et al., *Brinker, Piermattei, and Flo's Handbook of Small Animal Orthopedics and Fracture Repair*, 5th ed. (2015).

Arthroscopic biceps brachii tenodesis has also been reported as an option for the surgical management of biceps brachii tendon pathology (Cook et al., 2005). The proposed advantages over open tenodesis and open or arthroscopic tenotomy are decreased morbidity and improved function. This kind of tenodesis can be performed by using bone staples, cannulated interference screws, or screws and spiked washers.

The tendon of origin of the biceps brachii muscle is an important stabiliser of the shoulder joint and, theoretically, its role should not be underestimated. However, due to the fact that dogs do not need to lift objects with their limbs and no adverse biomechanical sequelae have been reported in the literature, tenotomy alone appears to be a completely acceptable alternative to tenodesis, with the advantages of being quicker, cheaper and with less risk of complications. Tenotomy can be performed via an open or arthroscopic approach. The latter approach has the advantage of being minimally invasive and the treatment procedure can be carried out at the time of performing diagnostic arthroscopy.

The tendon of insertion of the biceps brachii muscle is visualised and inspected with a 2.7 mm arthroscope inserted from a lateral portal. In case of tendinopathy, synovial hyperaemia and proliferation, partial tearing of tendon fibres, mineralisation and hypertrophy of the tendon, and osteophyte production within the intertubercular groove are evident. Most cases of bicipital tendinopathy occur at the origin and at the midsubstance level of the tendon. However, careful evaluation of the entire intra-articular portion of the tendon by use of a blunt instrument is recommended to fully evaluate the integrity of the tendon and avoid diagnostic error (Figs. 12 and 13).

An instrument portal is then created at the craniomedial aspect of the shoulder joint. An arthroscopic knife or a large needle inserted through the instrument portal is used to cut the tendon at its insertion on the supraglenoid tubercle. Once the tendon is fully released, it should retract distally

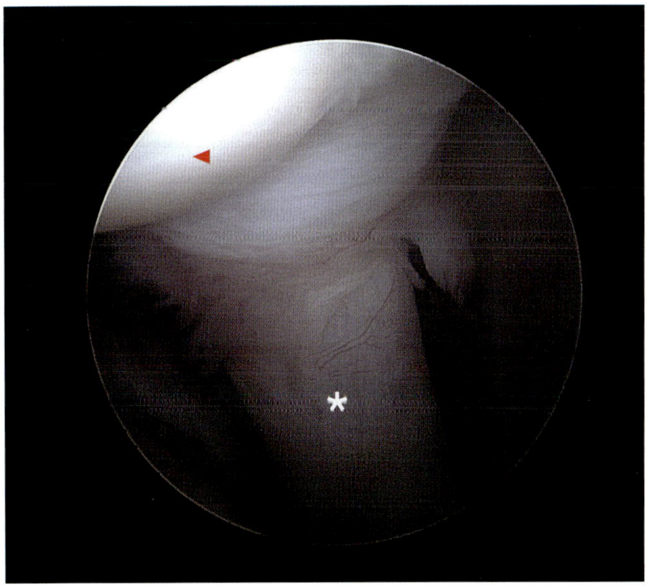

Figure 12. Arthroscopic image of a normal biceps brachii tendon (asterisk) and its attachment to the supraglenoid tubercle (arrowhead).

within the intertubercular groove and disappear from the field of view of the arthroscope (Video 1). Manipulation of the shoulder in extension and flexion immediately after cutting the tendon facilitates its distal displacement and guarantees complete transection of the tendon.

Video 1. Arthroscopic release of the biceps brachii tendon demonstrated by Ian Gordon Holsworth, with permission from Arthrex Vet Systems (©Arthrex GmbH).

POSTOPERATIVE MANAGEMENT

Cold or warm packing, use of nonsteroidal anti-inflammatory drugs for 3–4 weeks, physiotherapy, cage rest for 6 weeks and lead-only walks for 12 weeks are recommended in the postoperative period.

OUTCOME AND COMPLICATIONS

Conventional open tenodesis carries good to excellent long-term results. However, this technique is associated with several noted complications, such as seroma formation, infection and implant migration (Stobie et al., 1995).

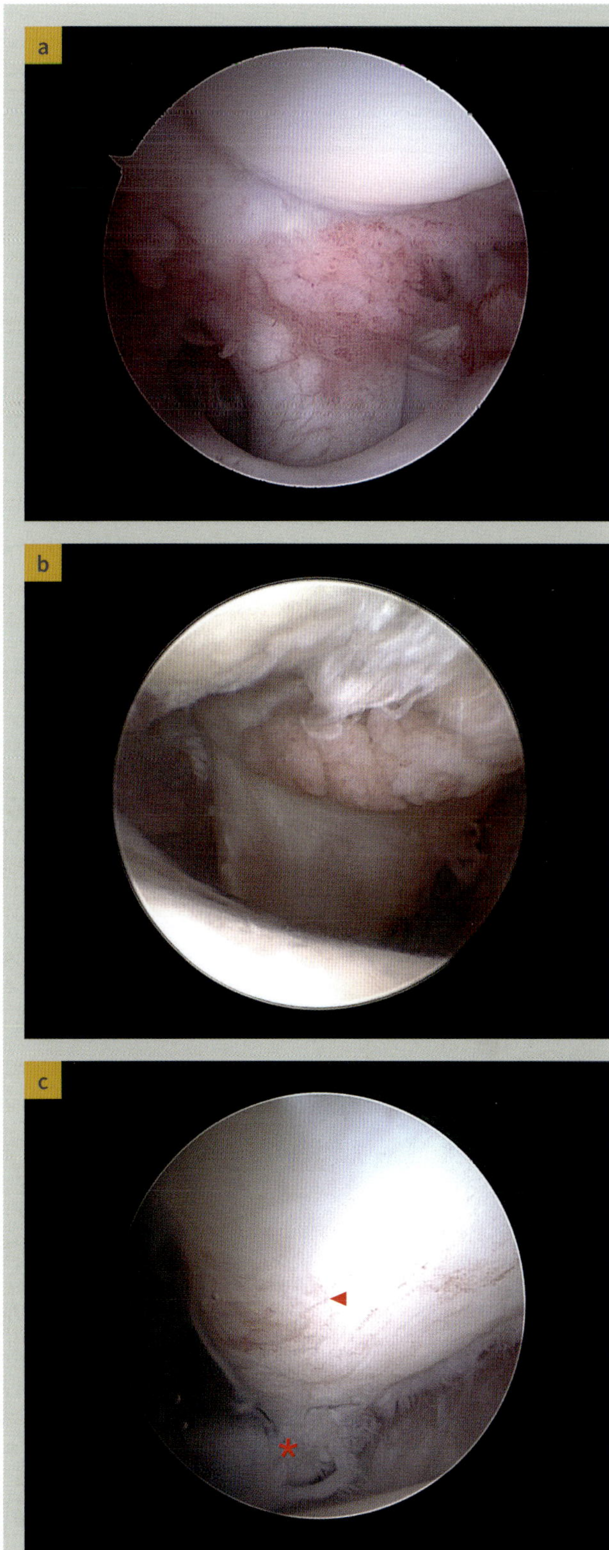

Figure 13. Arthroscopic images showing examples of biceps brachii tendon pathologies in dogs. Severely inflamed tendon (a). Note the severe synovitis affecting the tendon and the surrounding joint capsule. Partial rupture of the tendon associated with chronic synovitis and cartilage fibrillation (b). Complete rupture of the tendon (asterisk) at its attachment to the supraglenoid tubercle (arrowhead) (c). Image b courtesy of Dr Andreoni, DipECVS, Switzerland.

A case series of six dogs treated with arthroscopic tenodesis confirmed resolution of lameness in all cases, with full return to function in all patients by 12–18 weeks (Cook et al., 2005). The only complication reported in this study was seroma formation. Whilst arthroscopic tenodesis offers the advantages of decreased morbidity and improved function, it is important to note that it is technically more demanding, the surgeon has to be very proficient in performing arthroscopy and the learning curve to carry out this procedure is steep.

Arthroscopic tenotomy performed with radiofrequency in five dogs produced good to excellent long-term results (Stobie et al., 1995). In one case, the owner reported a mild, intermittent lameness after intense exercise 6 months after surgery.

Another study of 25 shoulder joints treated with arthroscopic tenotomy performed by using hook scissors reported excellent clinical outcomes and no complications in 22 shoulders, with relief of clinical signs at a mean time of 3 weeks. The remaining two dogs (3 shoulders) showed, respectively, a low and a moderate degree of lameness at the follow-up appointment. The authors of the study believe that this was the result of incomplete tenotomy of the biceps brachii tendon at the time of initial surgery (Bergenhuyzen et al., 2010).

SUPRASPINATUS TENDINOPATHY

Miguel Solano

INTRODUCTION

Supraspinatus tendinopathy is a common cause of thoracic limb lameness in the dog. The aetiology of this pathology is unknown, but it is thought to be associated with repetitive strain activity and overuse, with a failure of adequate remodelling. Supraspinatus tendinopathy occurs more frequently in young to middle-aged large-breed dogs, with no sex predilection. Labrador Retrievers and Rottweilers appear to be overrepresented (Lafuente et al., 2009).

CLINICAL PRESENTATION AND DIAGNOSIS

Clinical signs, when present, involve intermittent weight-bearing lameness that worsens after exercise and is typically refractory to rest and conservative management.

PHYSICAL EXAMINATION

The most common findings on orthopaedic examination are a moderate weight-bearing lameness and pain associated with the palpation of the affected shoulder. Although most dogs have unilateral supraspinatus pathology, dogs with bilateral pathology have also been reported (Lafuente et al., 2009). Nonspecific signs of muscle atrophy may be seen in the supraspinatus and infraspinatus muscles of the affected limb (Fransson et al., 2005). Affected shoulders are typically stable in the abduction and drawer tests. Pain can be seen associated with shoulder extension or flexion or when digital pressure is applied on the tendon of insertion of the supraspinatus muscle. Dogs can have concurrent bicipital tendon impingement and respond to direct palpation over the tendon of origin of the biceps brachii muscle and/or to a biceps stretch test.

IMAGING

Radiographic evaluation of the affected limb generally involves mediolateral, craniocaudal and skyline (cranioproximal–craniodistal) projections. Diagnosis of calcified supraspinatus tendinopathy is readily confirmed by radiographic imaging. The skyline projection allows for better observation of the intertubercular groove and localisation of the abnormal calcification adjacent to the greater tubercle in mineralised tendinopathies (Figs. 1 and 2). Other common causes of thoracic lameness (e.g. developmental elbow disease, shoulder OCD, concurrent bicipital tenosynovitis) should be excluded by careful orthopaedic and imaging examination. The author recommends including the elbow (mediolateral and craniocaudal projections) and, when pertinent, considering distal limb radiographs as part of the initial workup.

Typically, radiographs reveal an egg-shaped, rounded or irregularly delineated mineralisation near the greater tubercle of the humerus.

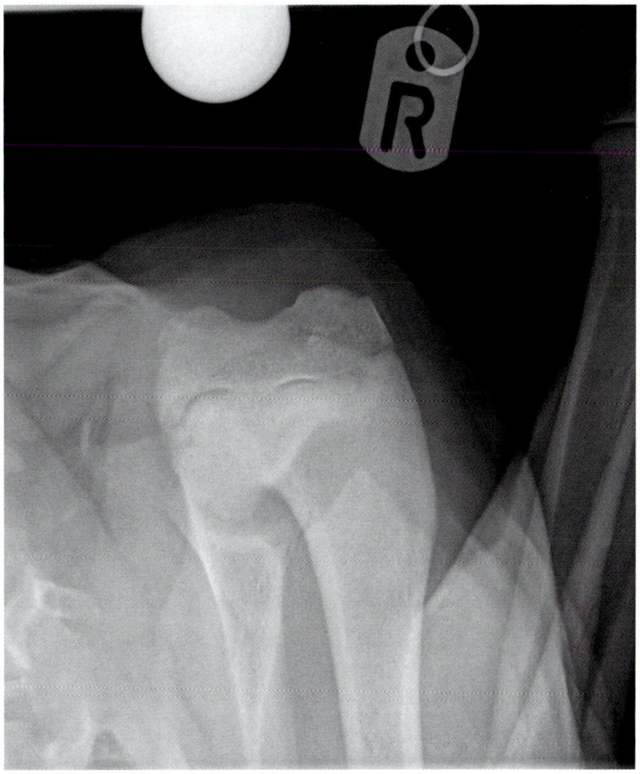

Figure 1. Skyline radiograph of a normal shoulder. This view is ideal to locate mineralisation associated to the greater tubercle (supraspinatus tendon) or the intertubercular groove (biceps brachii tendon).

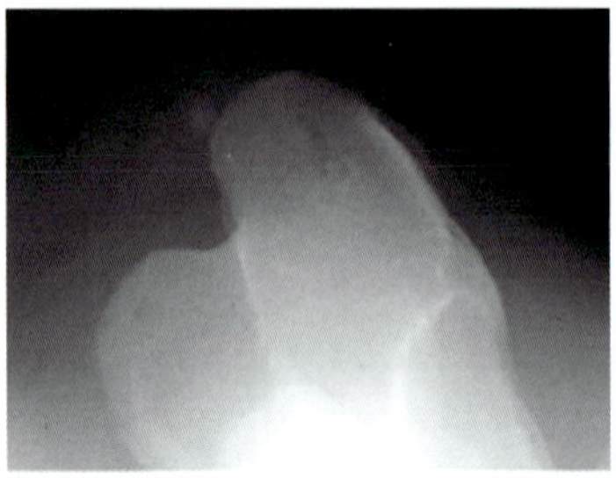

Figure 2. Skyline radiograph of a shoulder showing mineralisation of the tendon of insertion of the supraspinatus muscle.

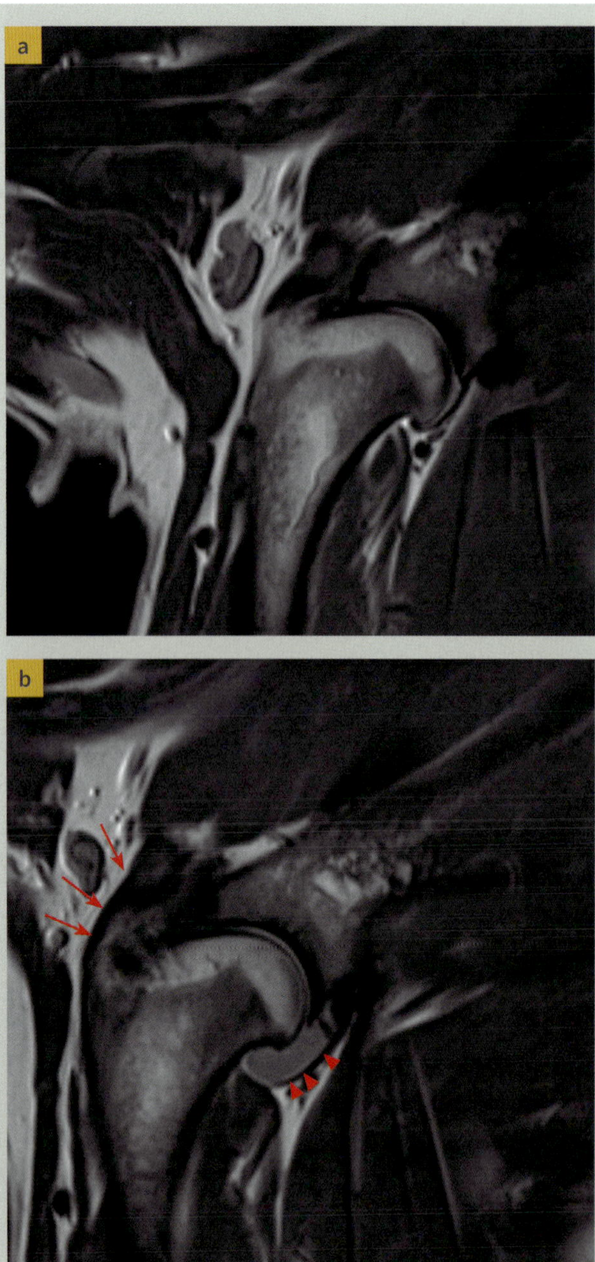

Figure 3. Sagittal view of an MRI sequence of a dog with a normal left (a) and an abnormal right shoulder (b). Note the presence of joint effusion on the caudal aspect of the humeral head (arrowheads) and the presence of a heterogeneous tendon of insertion of the supraspinatus muscle on the greater tubercle (arrows).

Tendon ultrasonography is a simple, noninvasive and cost-effective tool for the diagnosis of mineralised supraspinatus tendinopathy (Mistieri et al., 2012). The most common ultrasonographic finding in mineralised supraspinatus tendinosis is a heterogeneous tendinous pattern in combination with mineralised hyperechoic deposits (Mistieri et al., 2012).

The clinical relevance of calcifications of the supraspinatus tendon is uncertain, as was demonstrated in a study examining 89 dogs with thoracic limb lameness that underwent CT scan (Maddox et al., 2013). In this study, 24.7 % of dogs had supraspinatus mineralisation, but this was not a significant source of shoulder pain for the majority of affected dogs.

> A presumptive diagnosis of supraspinatus mineralisation can only be made by a combination of signalment, history, physical examination and imaging supportive of such a diagnosis.

In contrast, noncalcified supraspinatus tendinopathy has been more recently reported and investigated with advanced imaging (Spall et al., 2016). Common findings with presumptive nonmineralised supraspinatus tendinopathy reported a subjective impression of enlarged, heterogeneous and hyperintense lesions. Final diagnosis requires histological examination; however, the invasive nature of the procedure makes this diagnosis modality impractical. Research performed by Spall et al. (2016) documented an absolute and normalised larger supraspinatus tendon volume in dogs with histologically confirmed supraspinatus tendinopathy when compared to controls. This makes supraspinatus MRI scan volume determination a helpful aid in the diagnosis of suspected nonmineralised supraspinatus tendinopathy (Fig. 3; Videos 1 and 2).

> Supraspinatus tendinopathy can present as mineralised or nonmineralised changes in the supraspinatus tendon.

Other more common causes of thoracic lameness (e.g. developmental elbow disease) should be excluded by careful orthopaedic and imaging examination (radiographs, CT scan and/or MRI scan). The author recommends a systematic screening of the thoracic limbs.

Video 1. MRI scan of the normal shoulder of the same dog as in Figure 3.

Video 2. MRI scan of the abnormal shoulder of the same dog as in Figure 3. Bicipital tendinopathy, supraspinatus tendinopathy, joint effusion, periarticular osteophytes and signs of glenoid and humeral head degeneration can be seen.

Supraspinatus tendinopathy can be challenging to diagnose. Other causes of lameness should be excluded.

TREATMENT

Management of supraspinatus tendinopathy includes rest, analgesia, physical therapy, steroid injections, biologic injections, extracorporeal shock wave therapy, and surgery.

Nonsurgical management should be trialled first for 3 months. Surgery should be recommended when a nonsurgical approach has failed to alleviate the lameness and other causes of lameness have been ruled out.

CONSERVATIVE TREATMENT

A previous study including 327 dogs suggested that supraspinatus tendinopathies are difficult to treat, with 75 % of dogs failing to respond to nonsteroidal anti-inflammatory drugs (NSAIDs) and rest, and 40 % failing to respond to a dedicated physiotherapy programme (Canapp et al., 2016a).

Local therapies such as intratendinous injections and extracorporeal shock wave therapy, in combination with therapeutic exercises (physiotherapy), have been reported for the nonsurgical management of supraspinatus tendinopathy (Canapp et al., 2016a; Ho et al., 2015; McDougall et al., 2018; Leeman et al., 2016).

Short-term (90 days) outcomes after ultrasound-guided injections of adipose-derived stem cells and platelet-rich plasma showed promising results, with resolution of lameness in 88 % of dogs and reduction in supraspinatus tendon size based on ultrasonographic assessment (Canapp et al., 2016b). All patients received weekly physiotherapy including laser therapy for 8 weeks and underwent a twice-daily at-home physiotherapy programme. The authors of the study recommended considering this programme for dogs that had failed to respond to conservative management and physiotherapy alone.

Similar positive ultrasonographic results were reported by McDougall et al. (2018) using intralesional ultrasound-guided injections of bone marrow aspirate in combination with platelet-rich plasma.

These results suggest a promising role for the use of ultrasound-guided injections of biological products for the management of supraspinatus tendinopathies unresponsive to a simpler approach consisting of NSAIDs, rest and physiotherapy.

Extracorporeal shock wave therapy has been reported for the management of supraspinatus tendinopathy in combination with biceps tendinopathy (Leeman et al., 2016) (Fig. 4). Short-term results showed good to excellent outcomes in 85 % of dogs. The availability of an extracorporeal shock wave therapy machine is a limitation for widespread clinical use.

An initial nonsurgical management is strongly recommended for 3 months before considering surgery. The role of intralesional biological products in combination with therapeutic exercises is very promising.

SURGICAL TREATMENT

In dogs not responding to a classic approach (i.e. NSAIDs, rest and physiotherapy), nor to biological therapies consisting of intralesional injections of platelet-rich plasma and stem cells, surgical resection of the mineralised and inflamed sections of the supraspinatus tendon can be considered.

The patient is positioned in lateral recumbency with the affected limb uppermost. The affected limb is aseptically prepared and draped.

Arthroscopy can be considered for screening and management of concurrent intra-articular pathology (OCD, biceps tenosynovitis) (see chapter "Biceps brachii tendinopathy"). Shoulder arthroscopy may not be indicated in dogs that had a preoperative MRI scan without obvious

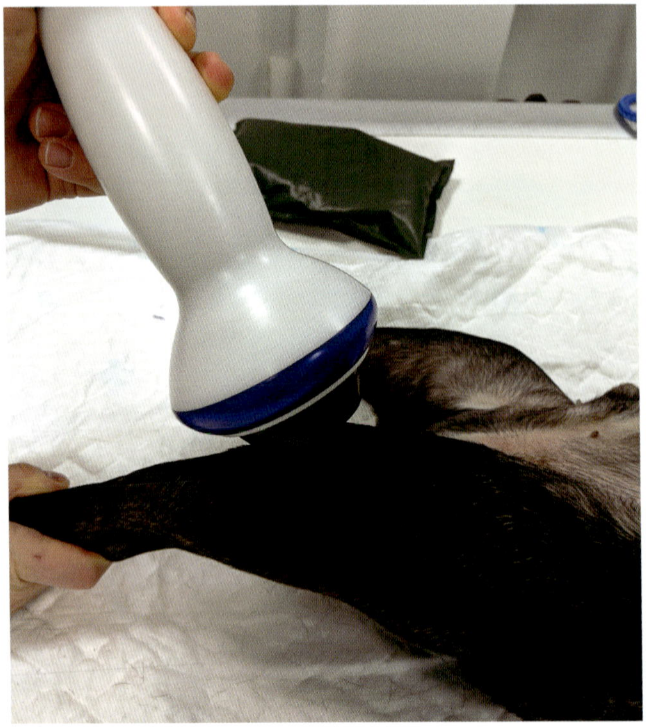

Figure 4. Extracorporeal shock wave therapy being applied to the patellar tendon.

signs of intra-articular pathology nor biceps pathology. The indication for shoulder arthroscopy must be assessed case by case. Lafuente et al. (2009) reported 3 out of 20 dogs with concurrent biceps pathology on arthroscopy that was not diagnosed on preoperative MRI. These three dogs had increased fluid content observed with ultrasound and MRI at the time of supraspinatus tendinopathy diagnosis.

A craniomedial approach to the greater tubercle of the humerus is performed. A skin incision of adequate size is made. The fibres of the brachiocephalicus muscle are retracted medially, revealing the supraspinatus tendon. A cranial incision to the tendon is made to elevate the pectoralis muscle. For mineralised cases, reviewing lesion location on radiographs is recommended. Longitudinal incisions are made in the tendon until calcified material is observed and removed. Usually, small longitudinal elliptical portions of the tendon are debrided as well. Closure is performed as per routine in three layers, with polydioxanone sutures for the tendon and muscles.

POSTOPERATIVE MANAGEMENT

Perioperative antibiotic therapy is given to all patients and discontinued at the end of the surgical procedure. A short course of oral NSAIDs is provided for 7–14 days. Generally, no bandage is used. It is recommended that cryotherapy is applied every 4–6 hours for the first 72 hours after surgery.

The skin sutures or staples are removed after 12 days. Follow-up assessment is performed at 2 (suture removal) and 6 weeks after surgery.

Physiotherapy is recommended for 8–12 weeks. Daily therapeutic exercises and lead-only walks are advised for 6 weeks.

OUTCOME

Lafuente et al. (2009) reported good to excellent outcomes in 21 out of 24 dogs after surgical management of supraspinatus tendinopathy. There was no difference in outcome for patients with mineralised and nonmineralised lesions. Three dogs had concurrent bicipital pathology and had biceps release performed.

> Surgical outcomes after surgical resection of the supraspinatus tendon are good to excellent in the majority of dogs with supraspinatus tendinopathy.

DORSAL SCAPULAR LUXATION

Miguel Solano

INTRODUCTION

Dorsal scapular luxation is an uncommon cause of thoracic limb lameness in dogs and cats.

CLINICAL PRESENTATION AND DIAGNOSIS

Traumatic rupture of the extrinsic muscles of the thoracic limb inserting on the cranial angle and dorsal aspect of the scapula allows displacement of the scapula when the affected limb is loaded. Disruption of the serratus ventralis, rhomboideus and trapezius muscles is commonly seen (Jones et al., 2017). Patients tend to present with an obvious severe weight-bearing lameness. The dorsal scapular border protrudes dorsal to the vertebral column when the limb is loaded but returns to its normal position when the limb is unloaded (Jones et al., 2017). Scapular manipulation can elicit dorsal displacement of the scapula (Video 1) but is not usually associated with pain.

Neurological injury is not common (Jones et al., 2017). Dogs may present with oedematous swelling of the ventral thorax and axillary region (Jones et al., 2017).

Radiographic examination should be performed to confirm dorsal displacement of the scapula and to rule out other concurrent conditions (Fig. 2).

> Radiographic examination is particularly important in patients with a history of trauma.

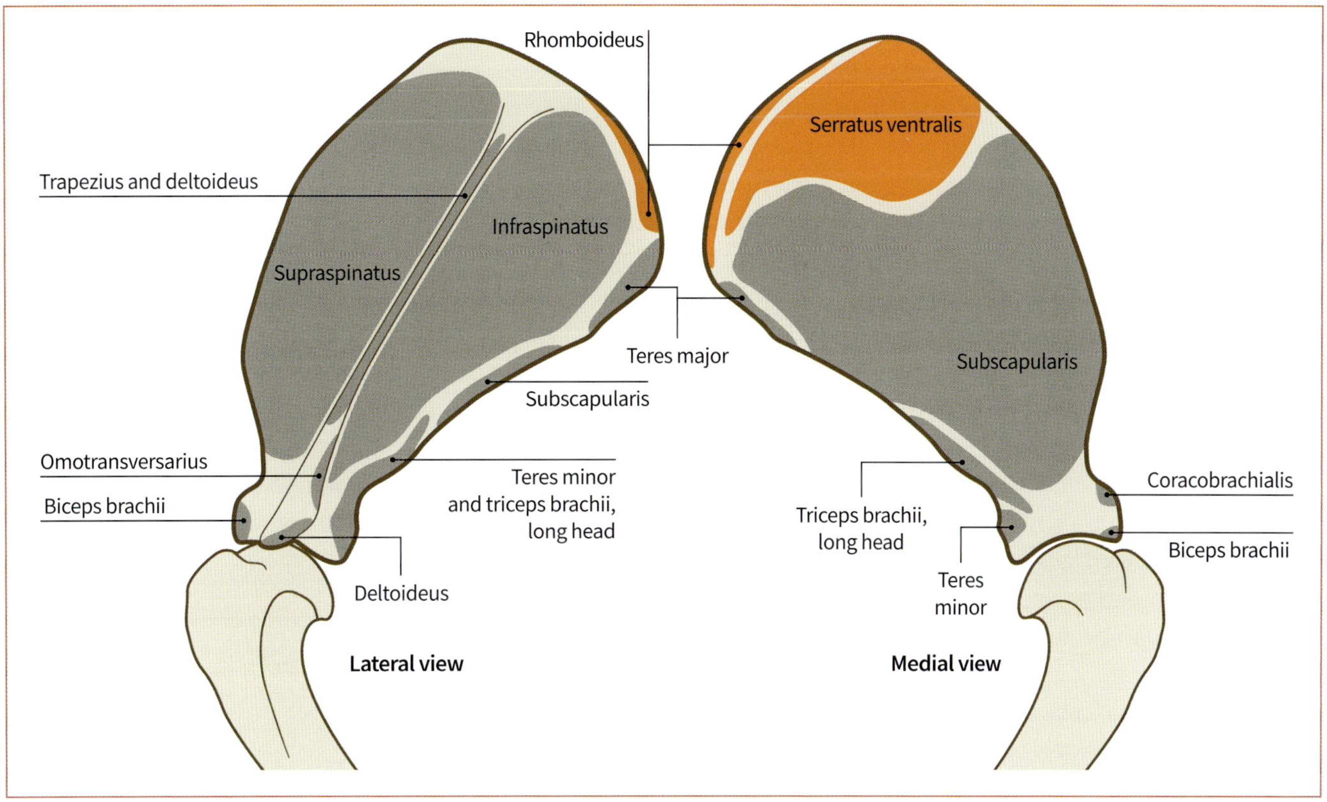

Figure 1. Insertion of extrinsic and intrinsic muscles on the canine scapula. Note the area of insertion of the serratus ventralis and rhomboideus muscles.

Video 1. Intraoperative video of a feline patient in lateral recumbency with dorsal luxation of the right scapula. Dorsal displacement of the scapula is clearly seen beyond the spine when pressure is applied.

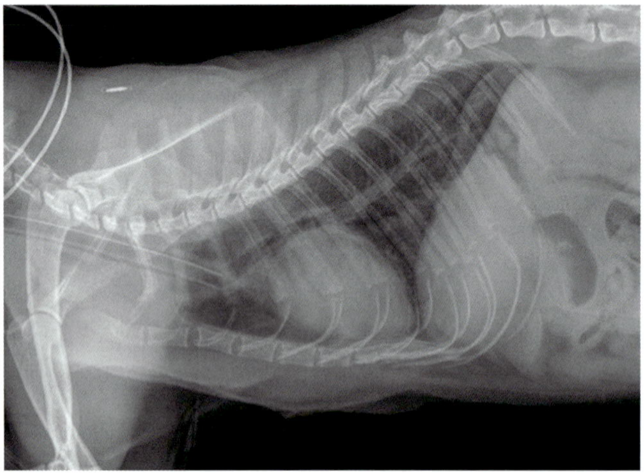

Figure 2. Laterolateral radiograph of the same patient as in Video 1 showing dorsal displacement of the right scapula.

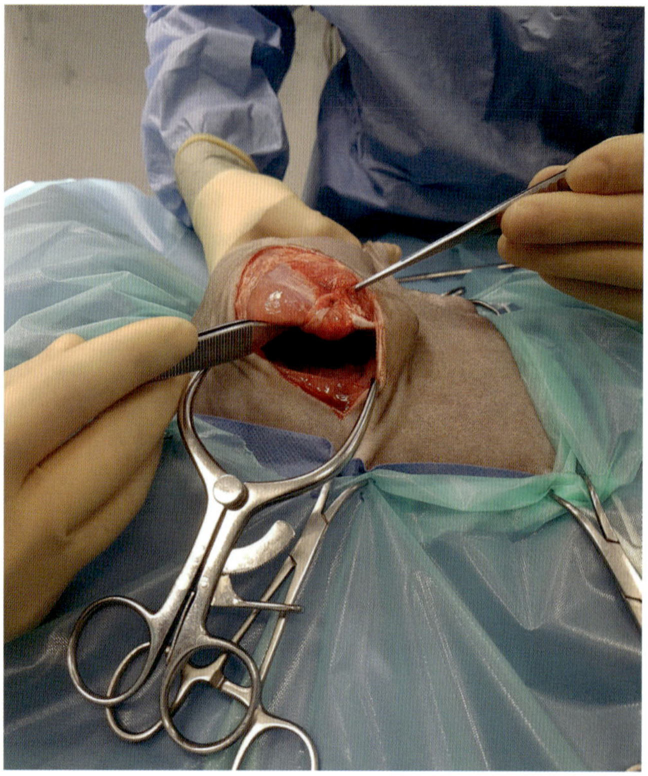

Figure 3. Intraoperative image of the same patient as in Video 1 showing partial tearing of the rhomboideus and serratus ventralis muscles.

TREATMENT

SURGICAL TREATMENT

The patient is positioned in lateral recumbency with the affected limb uppermost. Following surgical preparation of the limb, a surgical approach to the scapula is made from proximal to distal and centred caudal to the scapular spine. The integrity of the rhomboideus, trapezius and deltoideus muscles is examined (Fig. 3).

For patients with a clear dorsal scapular luxation and intact rhomboideus and trapezius, these muscles may need transection for appropriate exploration and repair of the serratus ventralis muscle. Stay sutures are placed on the edge of the transected muscles to facilitate closure.

For patients with an obvious tear of the rhomboideus–trapezius, the serrated face of the scapula can be inspected by gently lifting and/or rotating the scapula (see Fig. 3). Primary repair can be achieved by different methods. For cats and small dogs, it is the author's preference to repair the musculotendinous attachments of the serratus ventralis, trapezius and rhomboideus muscles by drilling small holes with a 1.1–1.5 mm drill bit to create anchoring tunnels in the dorsal and caudal angles of the scapula (Fig. 4).

A large (3 in cats, 3.5 metric in small dogs) polydioxanone suture thread is then used to anchor the serratus ventralis and rhomboideus muscles to the scapula in an interrupted pattern. Sutures are preplaced before tightening (Fig. 5).

The trapezius and deltoideus muscles can be sutured to the fascia immediately dorsal to the proximal aspect of the scapular spine. If needed, bone tunnels can be drilled in the proximal aspect of the scapular spine for appropriate anchorage. Similar size suture material is used.

For medium- to large-breed dogs, the use of additional sutures (nylon, FiberTape [Arthrex], etc.) around the second

Video 2. Intraoperative video demonstrating resolution of the dorsal scapular luxation after repair.

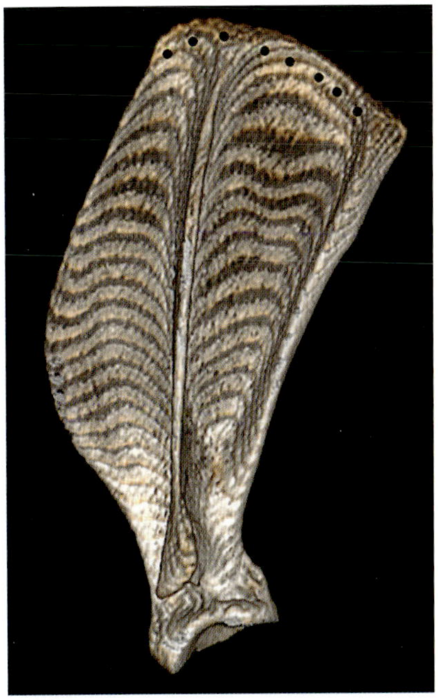

Figure 4. Three-dimensional volume of a canine scapula. Note the holes drilled in the dorsal and caudal aspect of the scapula. These holes are used for anchoring the musculotendinous attachments of the torn muscles.

rib and to the supraspinatus and infraspinatus fossae has been reported (Jones et al., 2017). The supraspinatus and infraspinatus muscles are elevated along the proximal half of the scapular spine to expose the junction between the body and the spine. After identifying the second rib, a double strand of suture material is passed around it using a blunt hernia needle. Four holes are drilled through the scapular body: two holes separated by 1 cm immediately cranial to the scapular spine (in the supraspinatus fossa) and two holes separated by 1 cm immediately caudal to the scapular spine (in the infraspinatus fossa). The two ends of the suture material are passed from medial to lateral through either cranial or caudal holes, and the ends of the sutures are clamped using haemostat forceps in preparation for tightening. The sutures for reattachment of the serratus ventralis, rhomboideus and trapezius muscles are preplaced through the holes in the dorsal and caudal aspect

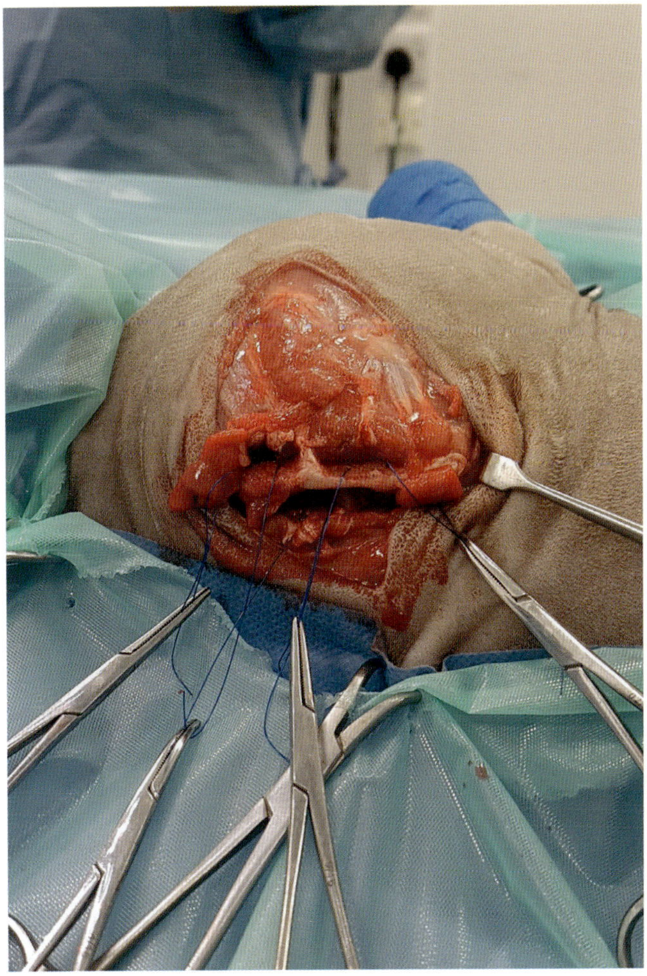

Figure 5. Intraoperative image of the same patient as in Video 1 after preplacement of polydioxanone sutures through the drill holes and the musculotendinous portion of the torn muscles.

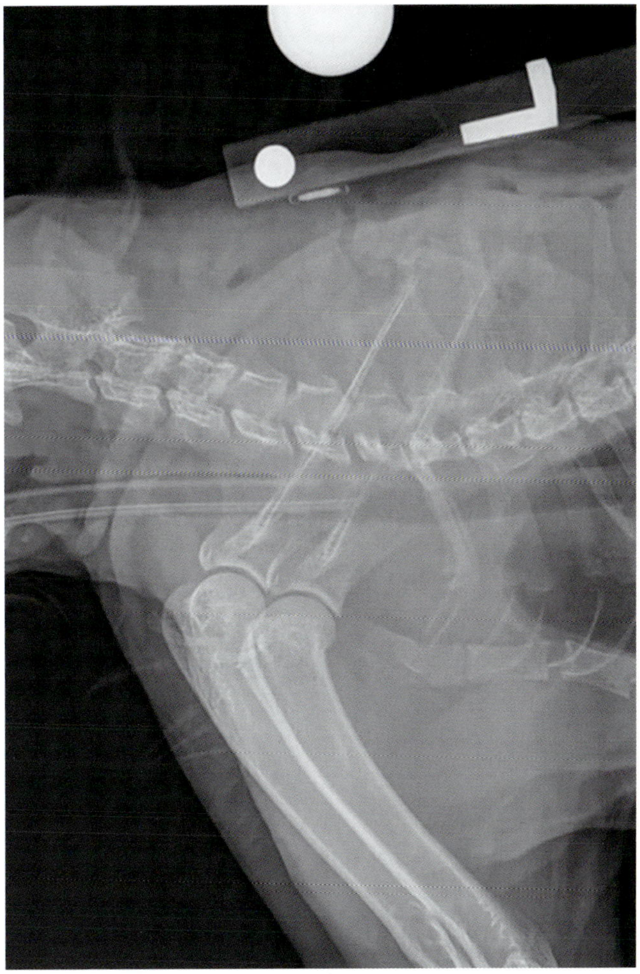

Figure 6. Laterolateral radiograph of the same patient as in Video 1. Note the reduction of the right scapula to its normal anatomical position after repair (compare with Figure 2).

of the scapula (see above). For these larger patients, a 3.5 or 4 metric polydioxanone suture thread is recommended. The sutures around the second rib (cranial and caudal) are tightened (Fig. 7), followed by the sutures on the dorsal and caudal aspect of the scapula. The supraspinatus and infraspinatus muscles are closed as per routine. The surgical wound is closed in two layers.

POSTOPERATIVE MANAGEMENT

Perioperative antibiotic therapy is given to all patients and discontinued at the end of the surgical procedure. A short course of oral nonsteroidal anti-inflammatory drugs is provided for 14 days. Bandages are generally not necessary, and it is recommended that cryotherapy is applied every 4–6 hours for the first 72 hours after surgery. The use of a non-weight-bearing Velpeau sling for 2 weeks can be considered for heavy or boisterous patients.

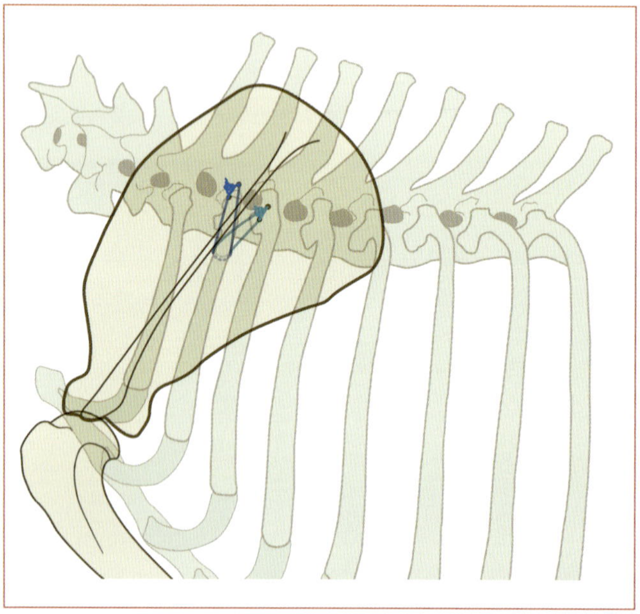

Figure 7. Schematic drawing illustrating scapular reduction with the use of synthetic suture material around the second rib and secured in the infraspinatus and supraspinatus fossae. Adapted from: Jones SC et al., Surgical management of dorsal scapular luxation in three dogs, *Vet Comp Orthop Traumatol* (2017).

Strict rest is prescribed for 6 weeks (confinement in a big cage or small room). No jumping, running, walking on slippery surfaces, off-lead exercise, steps or stairs are allowed. The patient can go outside on the lead for 10 minutes 3–4 times a day for toilet purposes. The skin sutures or staples are removed after 12 days. Follow-up examination is performed at 6 weeks after surgery.

Provided there is good clinical progression, lead exercise can be increased by 5 minutes per walk on a weekly basis over a 4-week period, followed by slow reintroduction of off-lead exercise over an additional 4-week period. Physiotherapy can be considered 2 weeks after surgery.

OUTCOME AND COMPLICATIONS

The current literature on dorsal scapular luxation is very sparse; therefore, further research is warranted to provide more robust guidelines on outcomes and complications.

Clinical outcomes have been described as excellent for a small number of dogs with long-term telephone follow-up (Jones et al., 2017). In the author's experience, cats and small dogs have an excellent long-term outcome.

Anticipated complications are reluxation (failure of the repair) and surgical site infection (as with any other clean orthopaedic procedure). Revision strategies may include the use of larger suture material and the use of a postoperative non-weight-bearing sling/bandage for longer periods of time.

SHOULDER ARTHRODESIS

Miguel Solano

INTRODUCTION

Arthrodesis has been reported as a salvage procedure for the management of a number of conditions including shoulder dysplasia, nonreconstructable articular fractures, chronic shoulder instability, acute or chronic shoulder luxation, and severe shoulder osteoarthritis (OA) unresponsive to medical therapy (Fitzpatrick et al., 2012; Oxley, 2017) (Fig. 1).

The surgical procedure is performed following the classic principles of arthrodesis (see chapter "General concepts about arthrodesis"), including removal of articular cartilage, use of graft (ideally cancellous bone graft) and rigid fixation with a functional angle of arthrodesis (Fitzpatrick et al., 2012).

SURGICAL PLANNING

The contralateral shoulder angle in standing position should serve as a guide for choosing the appropriate angle for arthrodesis; this angle is commonly 110 degrees. Although plates and screws are the implants of choice for shoulder arthrodesis, the use of crossed pins, tension bands and single compression screws has been reported in several studies in small and toy dog breeds (Vasseur, 1990; Herron, 1989).

Implant selection is based on the standard AO guidelines (Johnson et al., 2005). The use of locking implants can provide some advantage for shoulder arthrodesis (Fitzpatrick et al., 2012). Considering the particular biomechanical properties of the scapula and the extremely challenging plate contouring for non-locking plates, the use of reconstruction plates seems to be more suitable for aggressive contouring to match the local anatomy (Piermattei et al., 2006; Fitzpatrick et al., 2012). Plates that are specifically designed to be bent on a lateral plane, like the string of pearl in titanium or stainless steel, the advanced locking plates or other type of reconstruction plates, may facilitate plate contouring and, thus, surgical execution. Recently, it has been described that the use of preoperative plate contouring based on three-dimensional (3D) printed shoulder

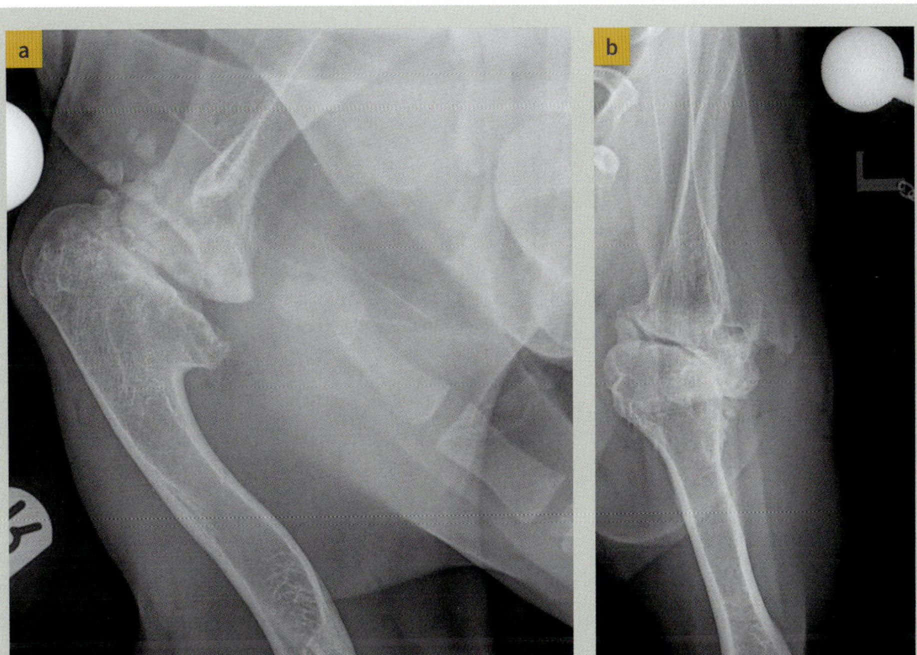

Figure 1. Lateral and craniocaudal radiographs of a canine shoulder with severe humeral head and glenoid remodelling. Note the presence of subchondral sclerosis and periarticular osteophytes.

models reduced operative time and helped enhance arthrodesis (Oxley, 2017). This author reported consistent excellent outcomes with the use of locking compression plates (LCPs) despite their limitation for lateral bending. In addition, custom plates may be a suitable alternative to simplify this surgery in the future.

> The plates should be of sufficient length to allow at least three screws to be placed both proximally and distally to the arthrodesis site.

Autogenous cancellous bone is harvested from the osteotomised humeral head or from the lateral aspect of the proximal metaphyseal region of the humerus. Bone graft harvesting is commonly performed with rongeurs. The graft material is then placed around the arthrodesis site.

SURGICAL TECHNIQUE

The dog is positioned in lateral recumbency with the affected limb uppermost. The surgical approach is performed through a modified craniolateral approach to the shoulder joint (Piermattei and Johnson, 2004). A skin incision is made over the midpoint of the scapular spine to the mid-shaft humerus (Fig. 2). The omotransversarius muscle is transected at its insertion along the scapular spine, revealing the supraspinatus muscle (Fig. 3).

At this stage, further approach to the shoulder joint can be performed through tenotomies and/or osteotomies; the author's preference is to proceed with tenotomies. Tenotomy of the origin of the acromial part of the deltoideus muscle is performed close to the acromion of the scapula. The attachment of the supra- and infraspinatus muscles to the scapular spine is dissected from proximal to distal towards the acromion. Great care must be taken to avoid suprascapular nerve injury, as this nerve enters the supraspinatus fossa and continues its course to the infraspinatus fossa underneath the acromion.

Retraction of the acromial portion of the deltoideus muscle allows direct visualisation of the infraspinatus tendon insertion and the teres minor tendon on the lateral aspect of the proximal humerus, and both tendons are transected (Fig. 4). The shoulder is externally rotated and the supraspinatus tendon is transected at the level of its insertion in the greater tubercle (Fig. 5). The joint capsule is then visible and an arthrotomy is performed (Fig. 6).

The articular cartilage is completely removed with a high-speed burr (Fig. 7; Video 1) or by femoral head and glenoid ostectomy. Compared to articular cartilage burring, ostectomy yields a larger surface area of cancellous bone and greater inherent angular stability. However, an improperly executed ostectomy could lead to potentially serious drawbacks (e.g. malalignment on the frontal plane and/or suboptimal angle of arthrodesis). Malalignment and undesirable loss of bone stock could be prevented by the use of computer-aided design and 3D printed guides (Oxley, 2017).

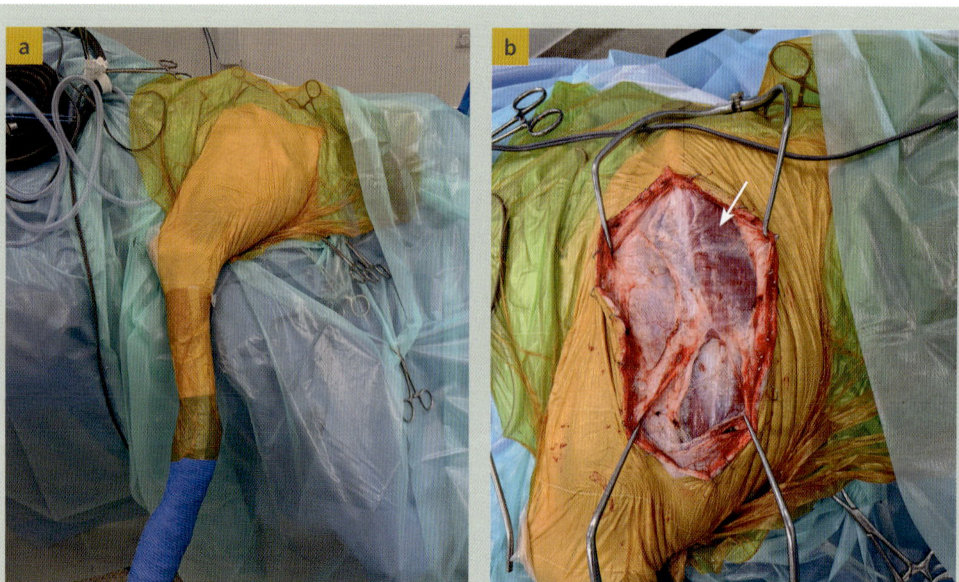

Figure 2. Patient positioning in lateral recumbency with iodine-impregnated sticky drape to avoid touching the dog's skin. Initial approach to the shoulder joint (a). The omotransversarius muscle is visible (arrow) (b).

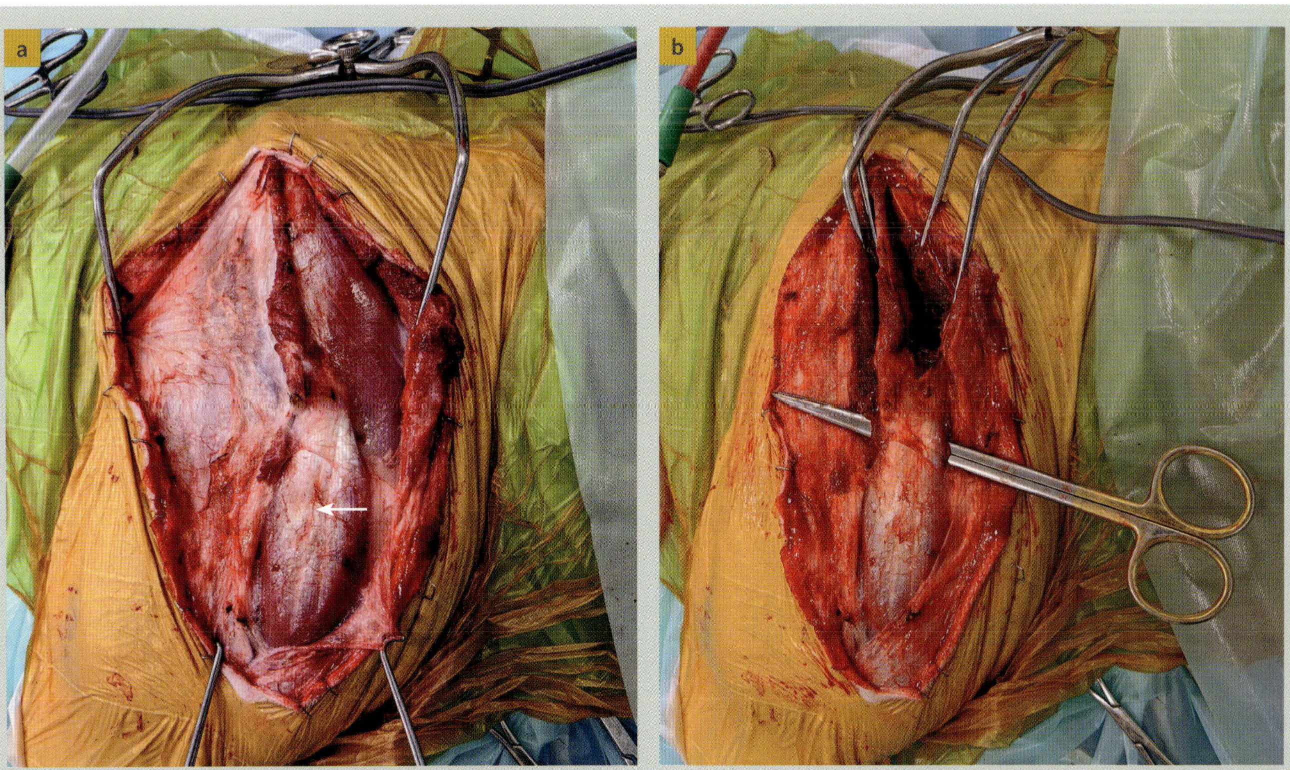

Figure 3. The omotransversarius muscle is transected at its insertion along the scapular spine. The supraspinatus muscle is visible. The arrow indicates the acromial portion of the deltoideus muscle (a). Metzenbaum scissors are placed under the tendon of origin of the acromial part of the deltoideus muscle prior to tenotomy (b).

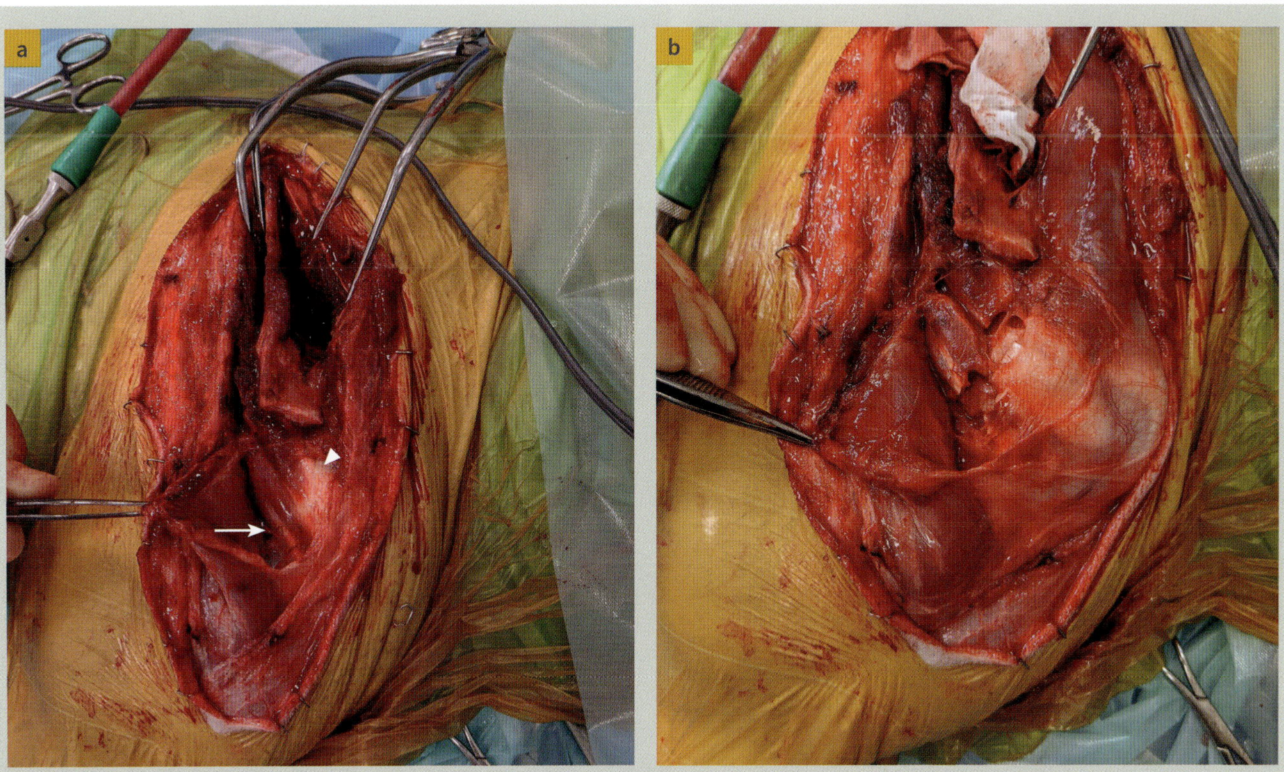

Figure 4. Caudal retraction of the acromial portion of the deltoideus muscle (a). The infraspinatus tendon insertion (arrowhead) and teres minor tendon (arrow) are seen. Intraoperative image after transection of the tendons of the infraspinatus and teres minor muscles (b).

Video 1. Cartilage debridement with a high-speed burr.

The shoulder with subluxation of the humeral head is externally and internally rotated by using a Hohmann retractor in order to make cartilage debridement easier. A small (proportionately small compared to the size of the humeral head in dogs) burr is used to create channels to promote arthrodesis in the surface of the humeral head and glenoid (Fig. 8; Video 2). At this stage, cancellous bone graft can be obtained from the lateral aspect of the proximal metaphyseal region of the humerus; in cases in which articular ostectomies have been previously performed, it can be obtained by morselising the ostectomised bone fragments.

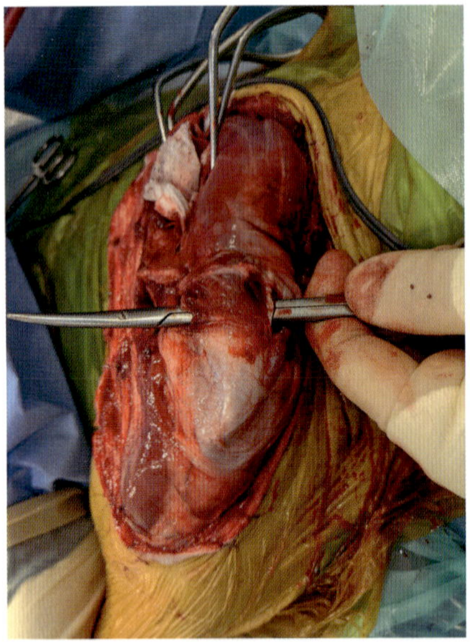

Figure 5. Metzenbaum scissors under the supraspinatus tendon at its insertion in the greater tubercle of the humerus prior to tenotomy.

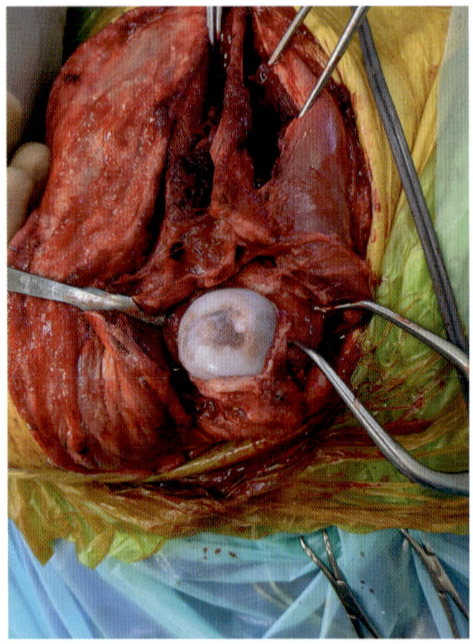

Figure 6. Image after arthrotomy of the joint capsule showing extensive signs of full-thickness cartilage erosion in this dog's humeral head.

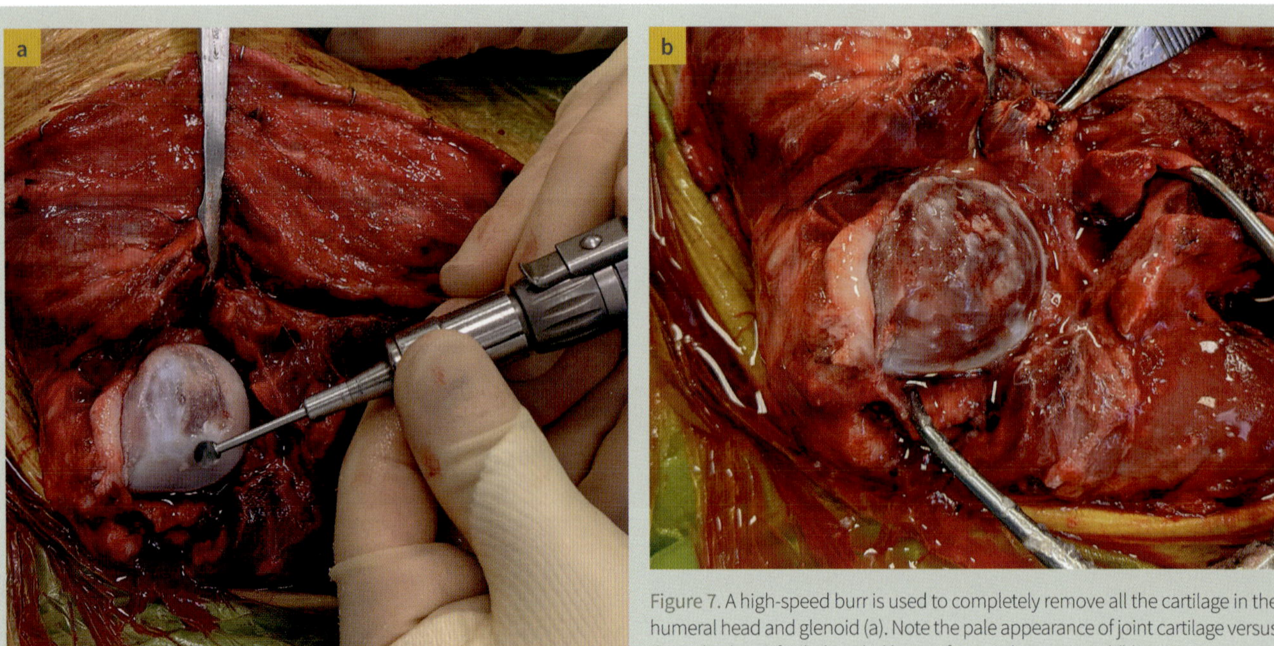

Figure 7. A high-speed burr is used to completely remove all the cartilage in the humeral head and glenoid (a). Note the pale appearance of joint cartilage versus the red colour of subchondral bone after cartilage removal (b).

Video 2. Humeral head after cartilage debridement and creation of bone tunnels. Note the bleeding from the highly vascularised subchondral bone.

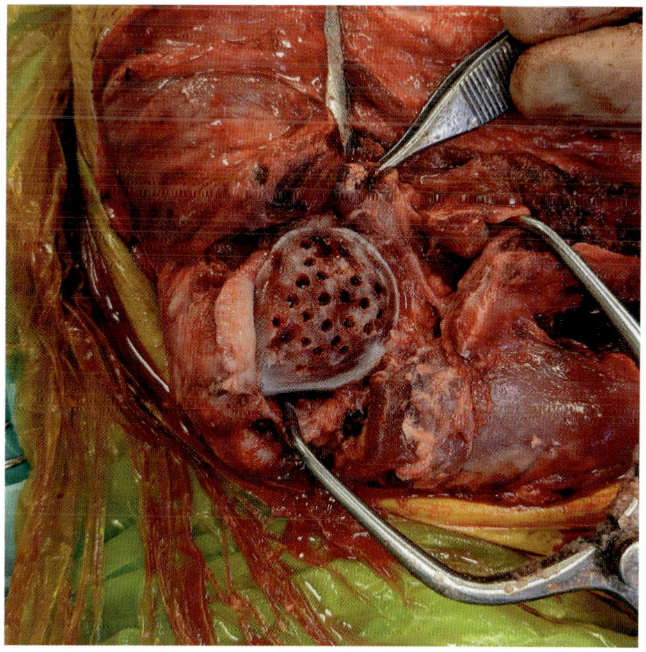

Figure 8. Intraoperative image of the humeral head after cartilage debridement and creating multiple bone tunnels with a small high-speed burr.

Crossed Kirschner wires (K-wires) are used to stabilise the joint at the intended angle of arthrodesis (i.e. 110 degrees). K-wires are inserted from the cranial aspect of the humeral head to the caudal aspect of the glenoid, and from the cranial aspect of the glenoid to the caudal aspect of the humeral head. Manual scapulohumeral compression prior to K-wire placement is recommended. Following the AO principles, further compression at the arthrodesis site can be achieved with plates and screw application. Placement of the K-wires can be achieved with an inside–out technique.

Both the angle of arthrodesis on the sagittal plane and the scapulohumeral alignment on the frontal plane are carefully evaluated and verified. A sterile goniometer is used to evaluate the angle of arthrodesis (Fig. 9).

A plate of sufficient size and length is selected as discussed above. According to the author's preference, the application of the plate starts from the most dorsal aspect of the infraspinatus fossa to the lateroproximal aspect of the humerus (Piermattei at al., 2006). The screws are ideally driven at a 45-degree angle between the scapular spine and each fossa (see Fig. 14) to maximise bone purchase at the level of the scapular spine (Fig. 10). The locking plate may require twisting and bending. At least three screws per segment are used. Interfragmentary compression is desirable.

At this stage, both K-wires can be replaced with transarticular screws. Screw head countersinking of the transarticular screws can be considered to avoid potential interference with additional plating.

A second plate is placed from the supraspinatus fossa to the cranial proximal third of the humerus (Figs. 11–13). This plate contouring may be very time-consuming compared to the first one, thus becoming a greater challenge. Bending (lateral and craniocaudal) and twisting is likely to be necessary. Contouring of reconstruction and preoperative plates

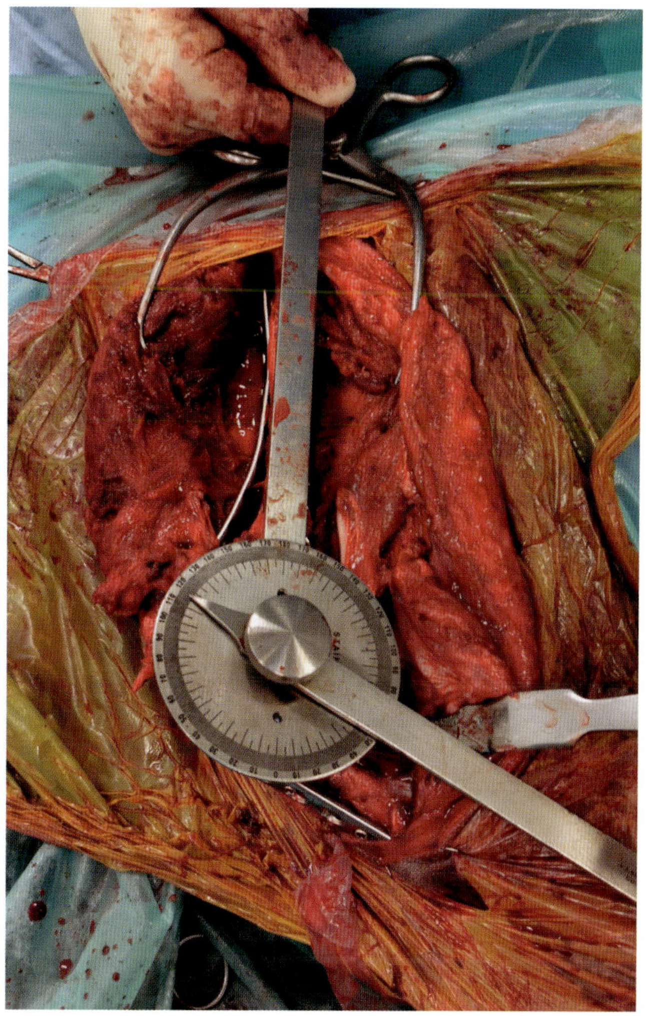

Figure 9. A sterile goniometer is used to verify the angle of arthrodesis. The scapular spine and the longitudinal axis of the humerus (between the supraspinatus tendon insertion and the lateral epicondyle of the humerus) are used. ▶

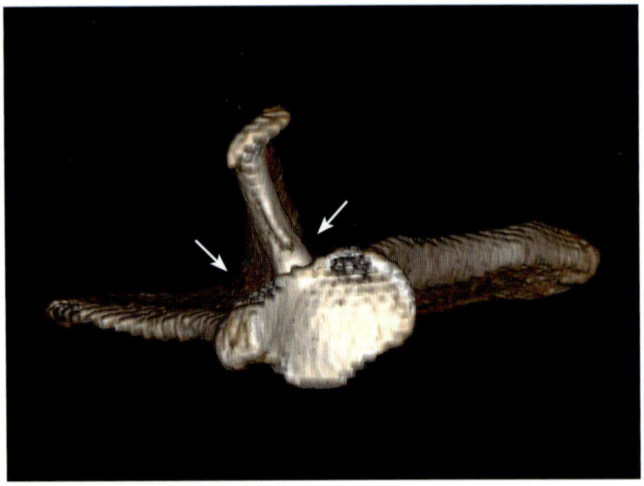

Figure 10. Computerised axial scan of a canine scapula showing the optimal screw angulation (45 degrees) for maximising bone purchase during plating in the infra- and supraspinatus fossa.

on a 3D printed model may simplify and shorten the time taken for this process (Oxley, 2017).

Closure is performed by apposition of the excised tendons to its origin/insertion when possible; tendon suture patterns (locking loop, three-loop pulley) or mattress sutures with polydioxanone are used. Subcutaneous tissue and skin are closed as per routine (Fig. 14). A protective spray dressing is applied to the skin wound and an adhesive wound dressing is positioned on it.

Postoperative radiographs of the shoulder are taken under anaesthesia in the lateral and caudocranial/craniocaudal plane (Fig. 15). The images are reviewed for apposition, apparatus (screw length, plate positioning, screws per segment, etc.) and alignment (particularly in the frontal plane). The angle of arthrodesis is also verified.

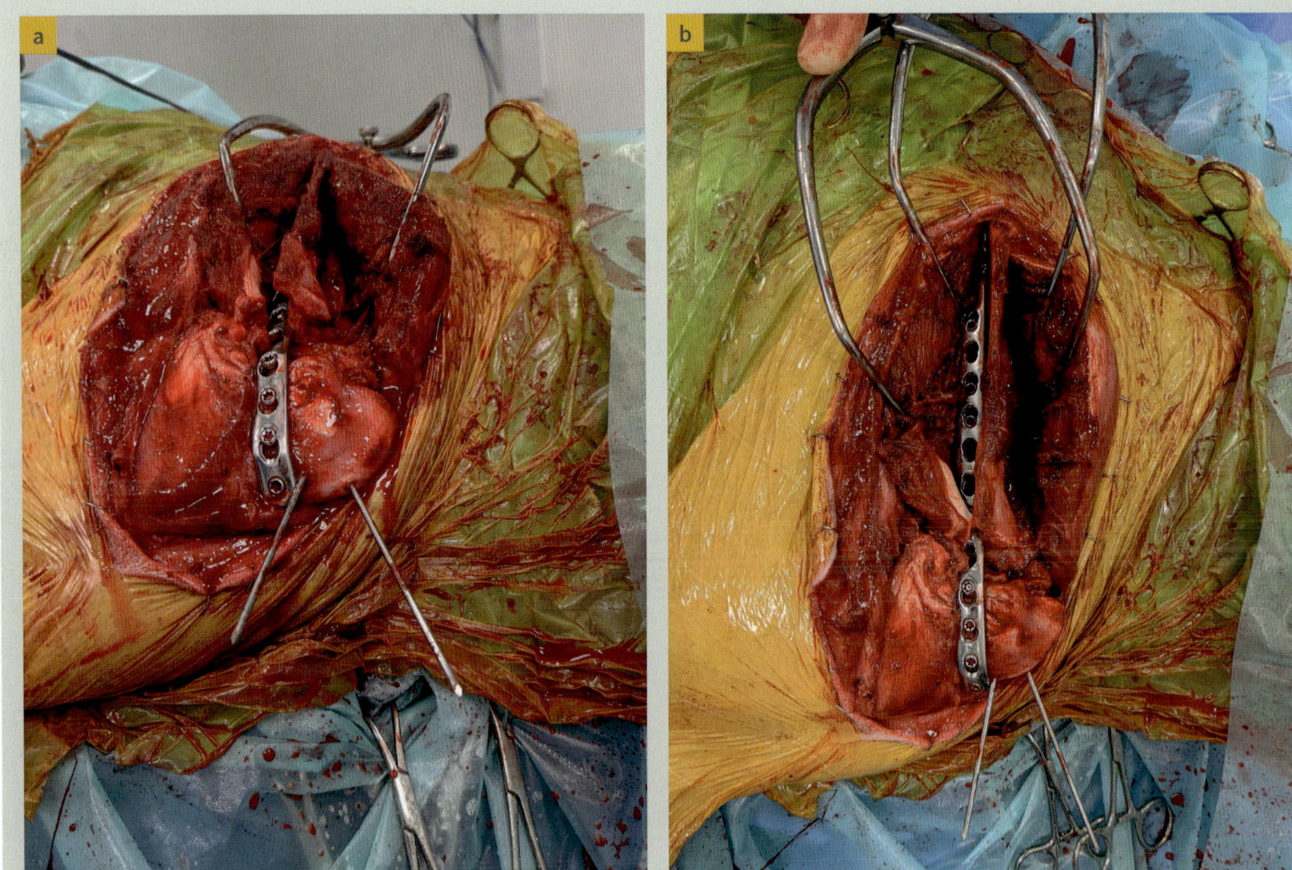

Figure 11. Intraoperative images showing positioning of a 3.5 mm locking compression plate (LCP) in the infraspinatus fossa at the lateral aspect of the proximal humerus.

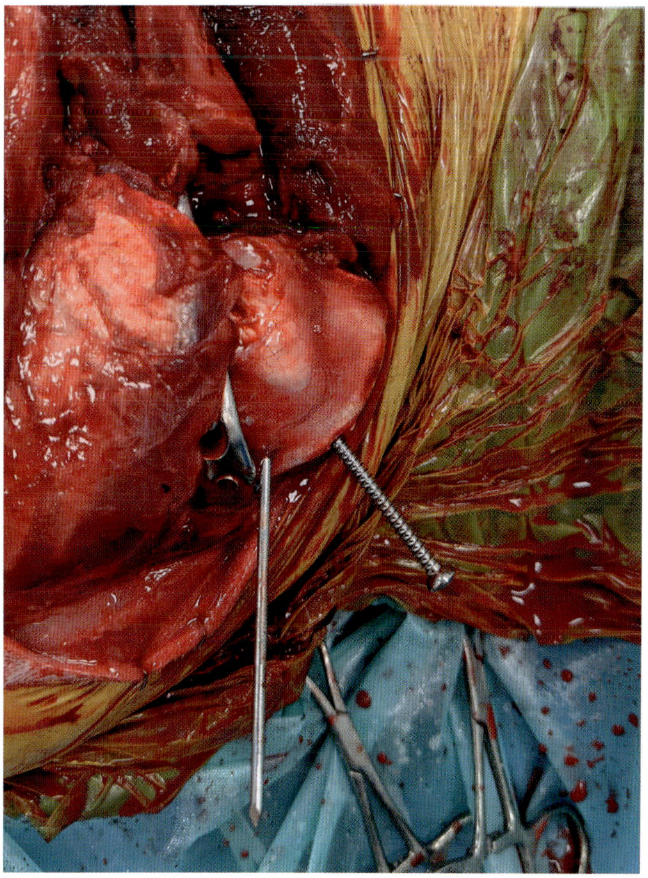

Figure 12. The transarticular K-wires are replaced with 3.5 mm cortical screws.

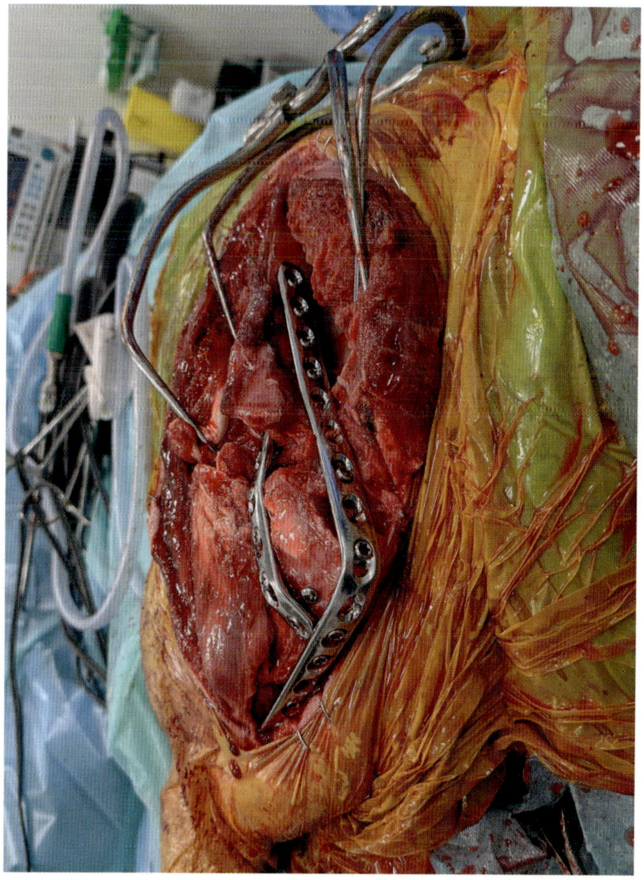

Figure 13. Plate positioning. Note that the plate extends from the supraspinatus fossa to the cranial aspect of the proximal third of the humerus.

POSTOPERATIVE MANAGEMENT

Perioperative antibiotic therapy is given to all patients and discontinued at the end of the surgical procedure. A short course of oral nonsteroidal anti-inflammatory drugs (NSAIDs) is provided for 14 days. Generally, no bandage is used. It is recommended that cryotherapy be applied every 4–6 hours for the first 72 hours after surgery.

Video 3. Dog walking 72 hours after left shoulder arthrodesis. Partial weight bearing is typically seen very shortly after surgery.

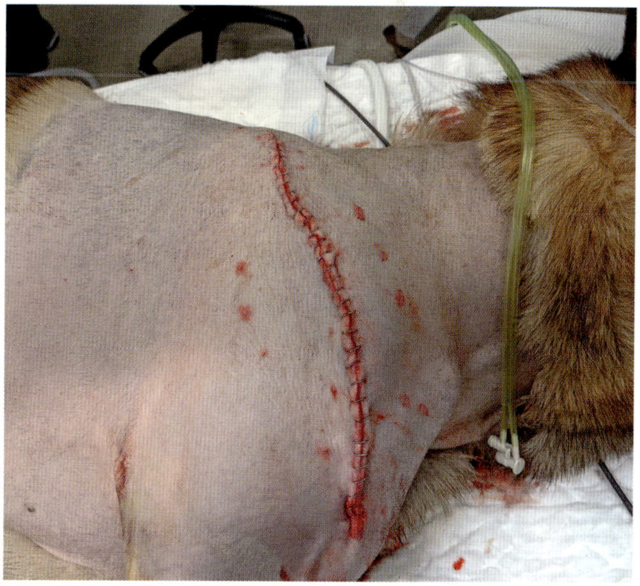

Figure 14. Surgical wound after closure with skin staples prior to final cleaning and application of a wound dressing.

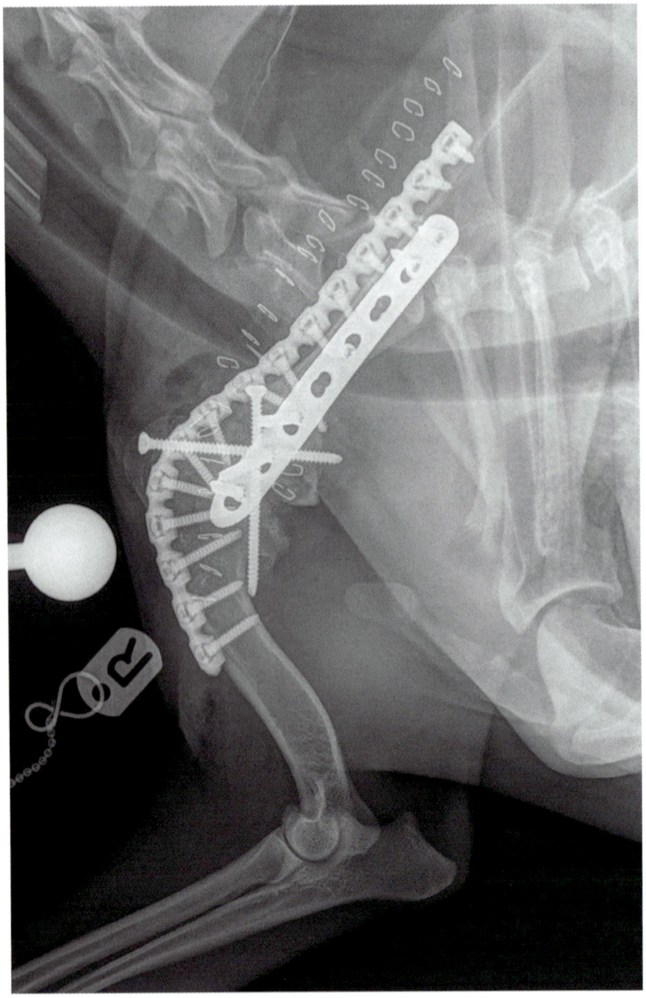

Figure 15. Postoperative lateral radiograph of a dog after being submitted to shoulder arthrodesis. A 3.5 mm locking compression plate (LCP) was used in the infraspinatus fossa at the lateral aspect of the proximal humerus and a titanium plate on the supraspinatus fossa at the cranial aspect of the proximal humerus.

Strict rest is prescribed for 6 weeks (by confinement in a big cage or small room). No jumping, running, off-lead exercise, walking on slippery surfaces or up and down steps or stairs is allowed. The patient can go outside for 10 minutes 3–4 times a day for toilet purposes. The skin sutures or staples are removed after 12 days. Follow-up radiographs are taken after 6 weeks under heavy sedation (Fig. 16).

Provided that there is evidence of advanced healing and no implant-related issues, lead exercise can be increased by 5 minutes per walk each week over a 4-week period, followed by slow reintroduction of off-lead exercise over an additional 4-week period. Physiotherapy and hydrotherapy can be considered after the 6-week follow-up visit.

OUTCOME

The clinical outcome after shoulder arthrodesis has been found to be good or excellent in over 85 % of the reported cases (Oxley, 2017). In a case series study carried out by Fitzpatrick et al. (2012), dogs were likely to bear weight within 5 days after surgery, and most of them were described to be free of pain at the 5–8-week clinical follow-up visit, with a moderate degree of thoracic limb lameness. An improvement in lameness was recorded in most of the evaluated dogs 11–16 weeks after surgery, with 71 % of them being sound or showing functional rather than painful lameness. In the same study, a mid- to long-term (range 6–20 months) telephonic questionnaire follow-up was conducted and showed promising positive results: minor difficulties to do specific tasks, such as rising from a prone position, ascending or descending stairs or jumping in or out of a car, were reported. Most of the evaluated dogs (72 %) had no pain to mild ongoing pain and ranged from sound to mildly lame (81 %).

COMPLICATIONS

The present literature on shoulder arthrodesis is rather sparse. The study conducted by Fitzpatrick et al. (2012) documented the outcome of the largest number (14) of dogs undergoing this surgical procedure. Complications were recorded in seven dogs (nine complications in total); two of them were considered catastrophic (14 %), leading to amputation in one case and to euthanasia in the other. Complications occurred in the perioperative period and were resolved with medical and/or surgical management in five out of the seven dogs (71 %).

> Due to the high rate of reported complications, shoulder arthrodesis should be considered a last resort when managing shoulder pathology.

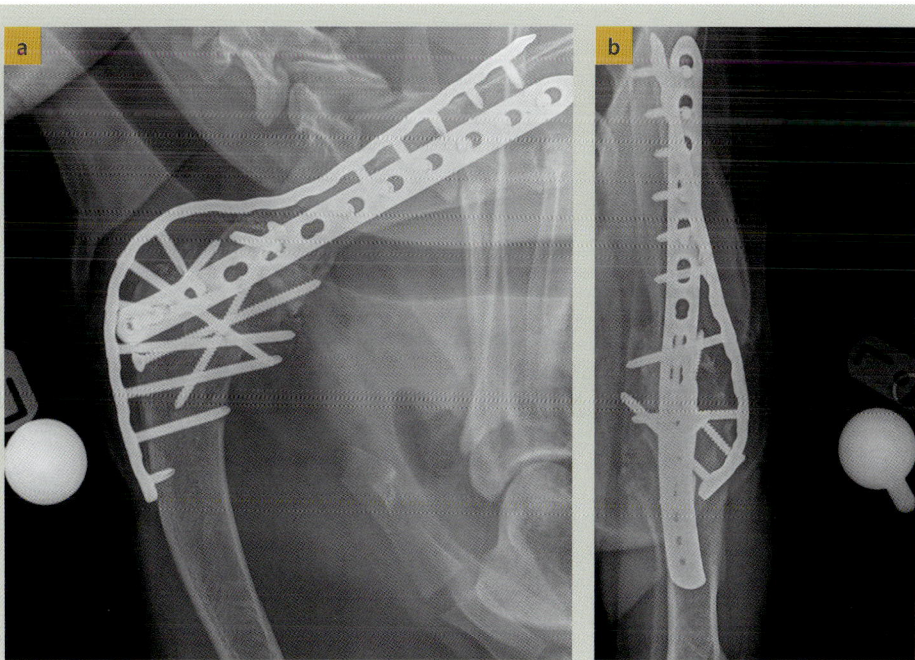

Figure 16. Mediolateral (a) and craniocaudal (b) radiographs of a dog 6 weeks after left shoulder arthrodesis. Note the signs of bone bridging across the humeral head and scapular glenoid.

03

ELBOW

TRAUMATIC ELBOW LUXATION

Stephen Kalff

INTRODUCTION

The elbow is a semiconstrained hinge joint. Although the elbow relies on the integrity of the collateral ligaments, there are several additional anatomical features that provide a degree of inherent stability. The anconeal process interlocks with the olecranon fossa of the humerus within the range of 45 degrees of flexion to full extension, and the larger and steeper articular surface of the medial condyle (relative to the lateral condyle) also helps prevent medial translation of the radius and ulna (Fig. 1). As a result, traumatic elbow luxations are uncommon compared with fractures in the same location, and lateral luxations account for over 90 % of cases in most reports (Campbell, 1971; O'Brien et al., 1992; Sajik et al., 2016; Schaeffer et al., 1999; Mitchell, 2011).

CLINICAL PRESENTATION AND DIAGNOSIS

Patients with traumatic elbow luxation typically present non-weight-bearing on the affected limb. In the case of lateral luxation, the antebrachium is usually abducted and externally rotated (Fig. 2). Pain and crepitus are noted on physical examination. The affected elbow is swollen, and the anatomical landmarks are difficult to palpate.

Definitive diagnosis requires orthogonal radiographs (Fig. 3), which should be performed under heavy sedation.

> If closed reduction is to be attempted, the patient should be anaesthetised and additional articular trauma/fractures ruled out.

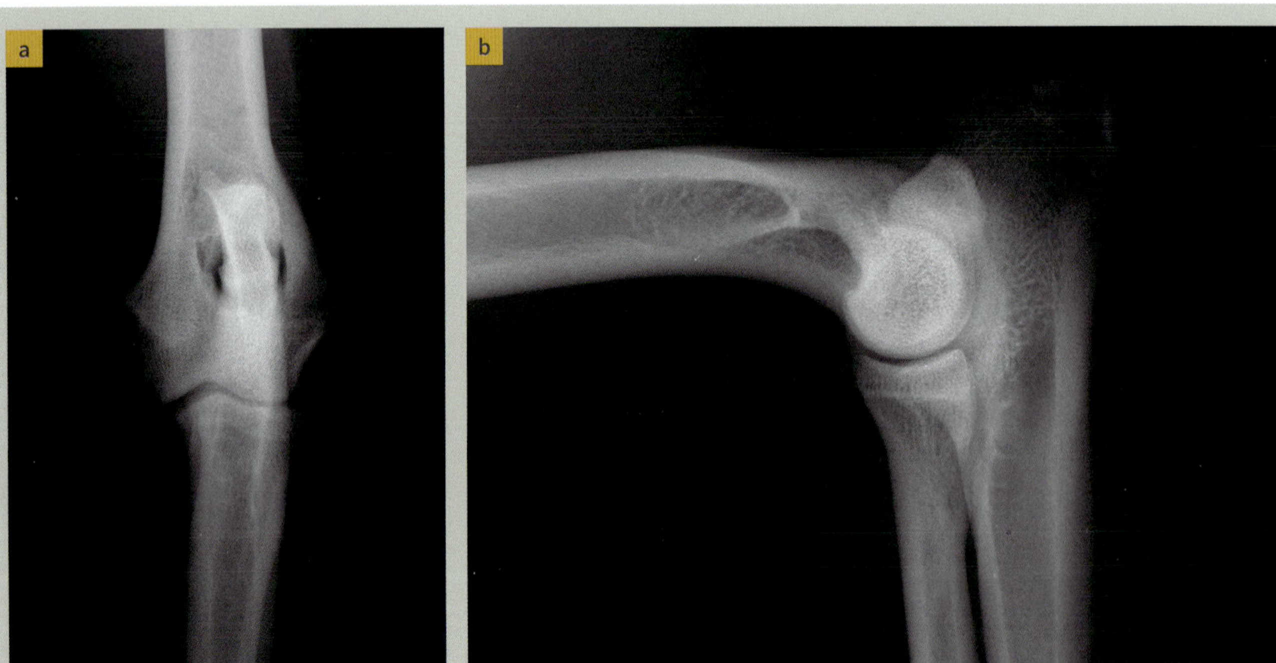

Figure 1. Craniocaudal radiograph of an elbow showing the steep articular surface of the medial condyle relative to lateral condyle (a). Mediolateral radiograph of an elbow showing the anconeal process in the olecranon fossa (b).

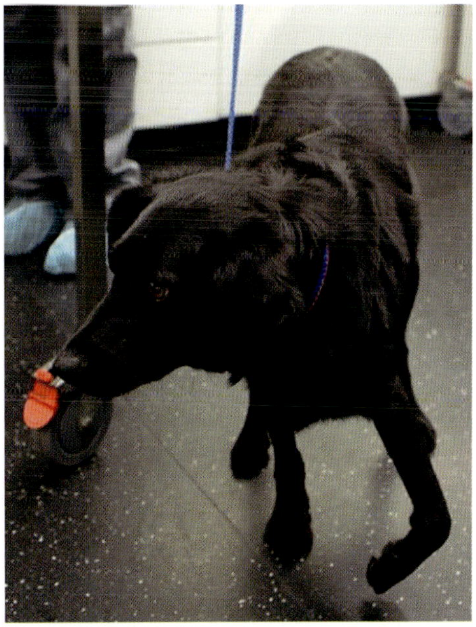

Figure 2. Dog with left lateral elbow luxation. Image courtesy of M. Farrell.

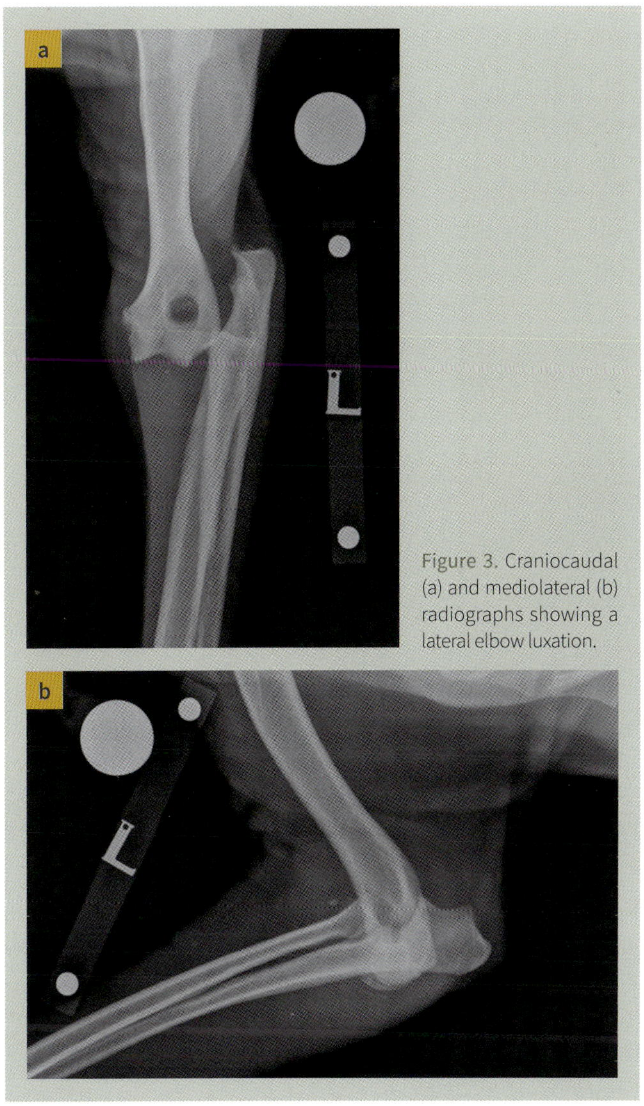

Figure 3. Craniocaudal (a) and mediolateral (b) radiographs showing a lateral elbow luxation.

TREATMENT

JOINT REDUCTION

Closed reduction should be attempted within the first few days following trauma. The technique ultimately depends on the direction of the luxation. It should only be attempted with the patient anaesthetised and once imaging has been performed to confirm the direction of the luxation and to document any additional joint trauma.

Significant force may be required to reduce the luxated elbow. To reduce the risk of iatrogenic injuries, care should be taken to understand the anatomy prior to any attempt.

Contraindications for closed reduction of the elbow may include concurrent articular and periarticular fractures.

Closed reduction of lateral luxations

The patient is anaesthetised and then positioned in lateral recumbency with the affected side up. Hanging the luxated limb or fully flexing the elbow for 5–10 minutes prior may relax periarticular soft tissues enough to help reduction.

With the elbow flexed to 90–100 degrees, and holding the distal limb with one hand, the carpus is flexed to 90 degrees and pronated. Using the thumb of the other hand, medial pressure is applied to the olecranon to force the tip of the anconeal process over the lateral condyle. Once the tip of the anconeal process hooks over the lateral condyle, the elbow is slightly extended whilst maintaining medial pressure on the olecranon. Medial pressure is then applied to the radial head, and distal limb pronation is slightly increased to force the radial head into reduction (Fig. 4).

Orthogonal radiographs should be performed to confirm the reduction of the luxation and document any other joint pathology.

> If closed reduction is not possible, open reduction and stabilisation is indicated.

Assessment of elbow stability

The integrity of the collateral ligaments following reduction can be reliably assessed with the Campbell's test. This test measures the degrees of pronation and supination possible with both the elbow and carpus at 90 degrees of flexion (Fig. 5). In normal canine cadaveric elbows, 60–70 degrees of supination and 40–50 degrees of pronation have been

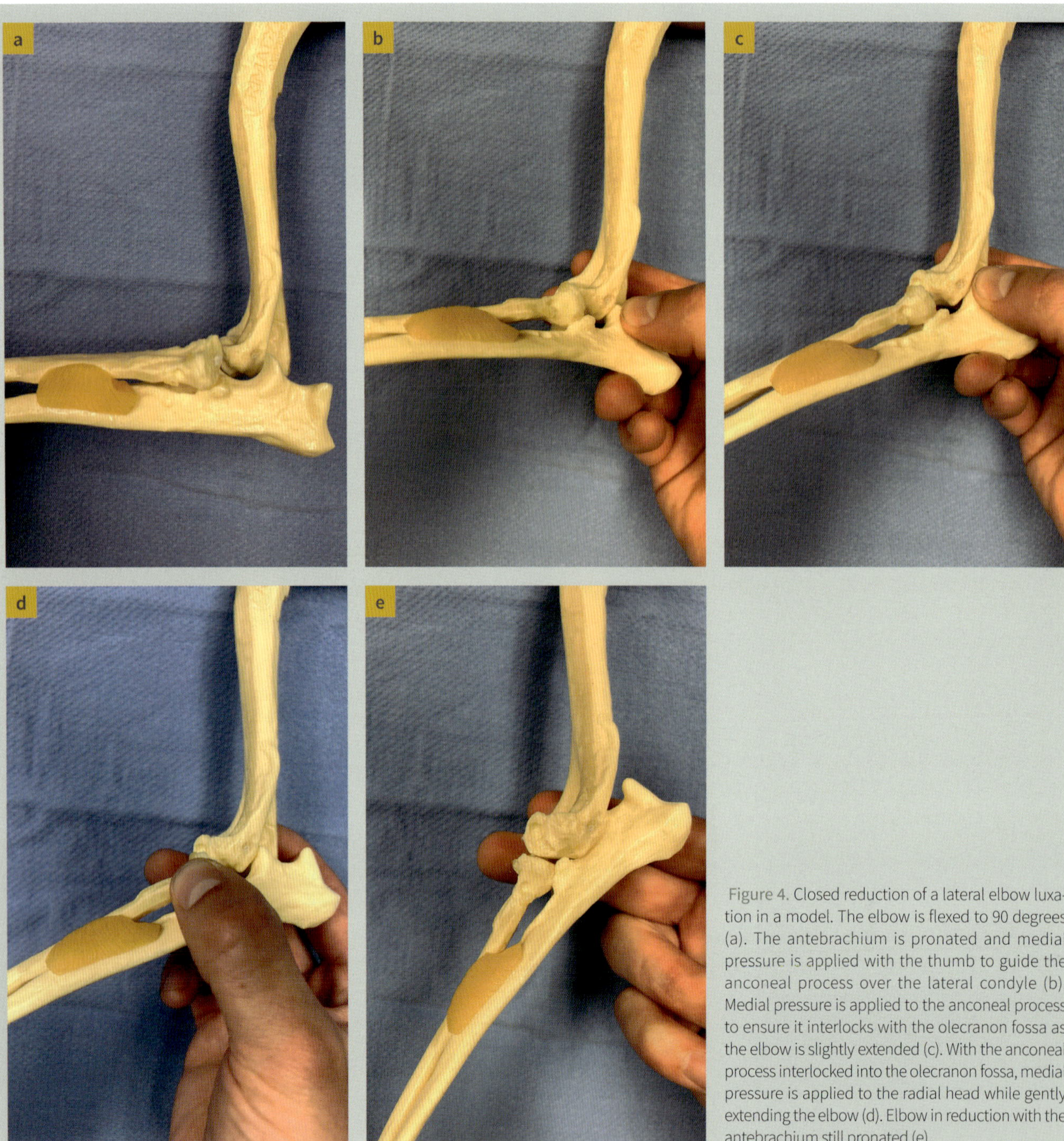

Figure 4. Closed reduction of a lateral elbow luxation in a model. The elbow is flexed to 90 degrees (a). The antebrachium is pronated and medial pressure is applied with the thumb to guide the anconeal process over the lateral condyle (b). Medial pressure is applied to the anconeal process to ensure it interlocks with the olecranon fossa as the elbow is slightly extended (c). With the anconeal process interlocked into the olecranon fossa, medial pressure is applied to the radial head while gently extending the elbow (d). Elbow in reduction with the antebrachium still pronated (e).

reported (Campbell, 1969). This study showed that transection of the lateral collateral ligament increased supination to 120–140 degrees and transection of the medial collateral ligament allowed 90–100 degrees of pronation.

Campbell's test was validated by Farrell et al. (2007), who also demonstrated that elbow luxation was not possible without transection of at least the lateral collateral ligament. This study also showed that significant variability exists between dogs. As such, the contralateral limb should ideally be used as a comparison, when possible.

Ultimately, assessment of elbow stability is subjective. In the author's experience, elbows that remain reduced during the normal range of the Campbell's test can usually be managed conservatively, whereas those that luxate or feel "loose" require surgical stabilisation.

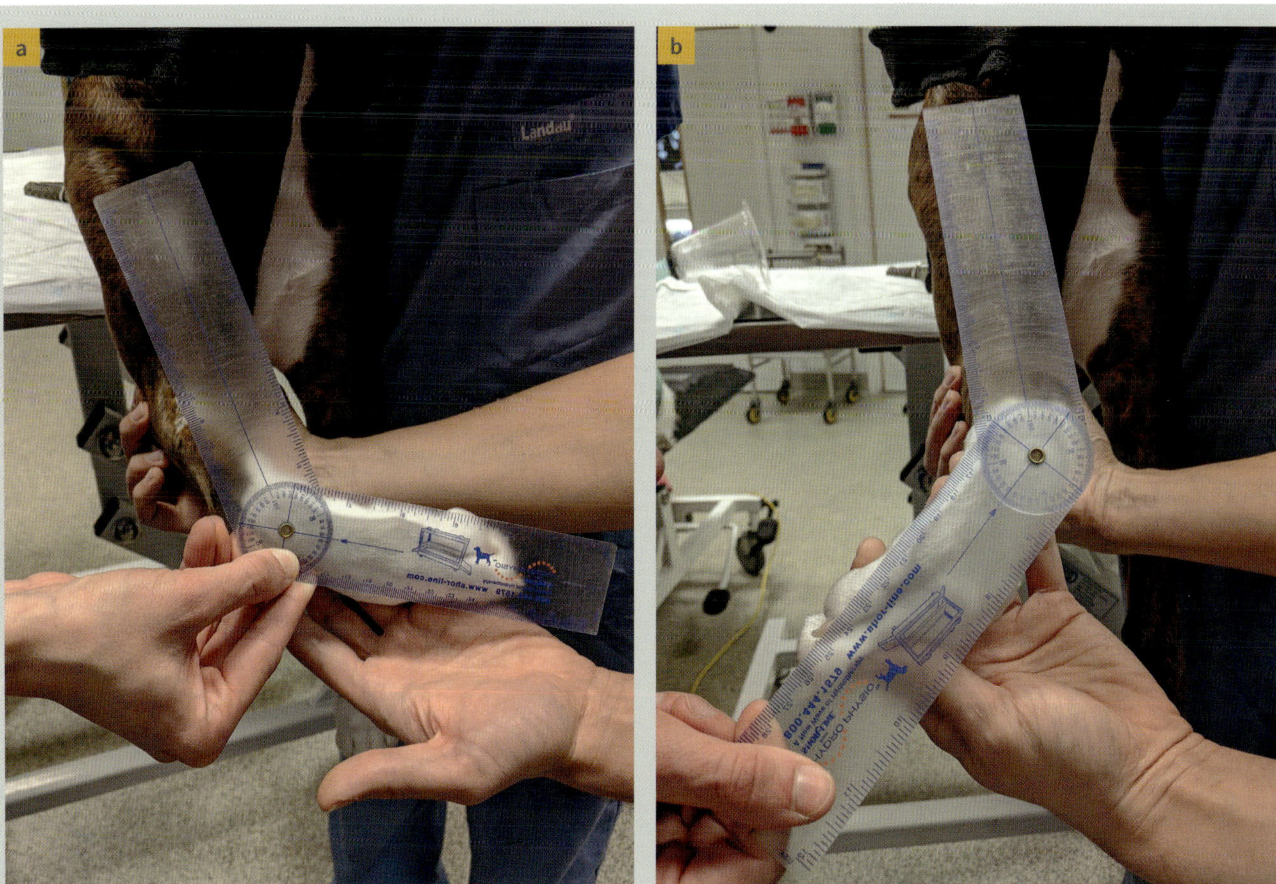

Figure 5. Campbell's test: measurement of elbow supination (a) and pronation (b) using a goniometer.

Postreduction management

If the elbow is palpably stable, a spica splint is applied for 2 weeks (Fig. 6). Crate rest is recommended for 4 weeks, with on-lead walks for toilet purposes only. The patient is then gradually returned to normal activity over the following 4 weeks.

If the elbow remains unstable after closed reduction, the author prefers to apply a transarticular external skeletal fixation (TAESF) for 4 weeks (Fig. 7). This technique relies on periarticular fibrosis to regain stability. As such, the range of motion of the elbow is often very limited after TAESF removal. Following TAESF removal, the patient is restricted to short lead walks for a further 4 weeks. Passive range of motion physiotherapy during this time helps restore the normal range of motion.

Extended periods of joint immobilisation may have a detrimental effect on joint cartilage. Use of a TAESF with a hinge placed at the centre of rotation of the joint may allow for early mobilisation and reduce the requirement for physiotherapy after TAESF removal.

If closed reduction is not possible, open reduction and internal fixation is indicated.

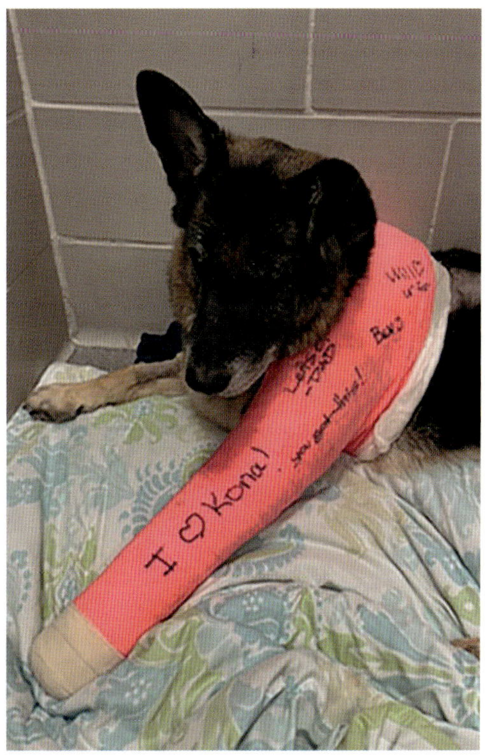

Figure 6. Spica splint. Image courtesy of W. M. Karlin.

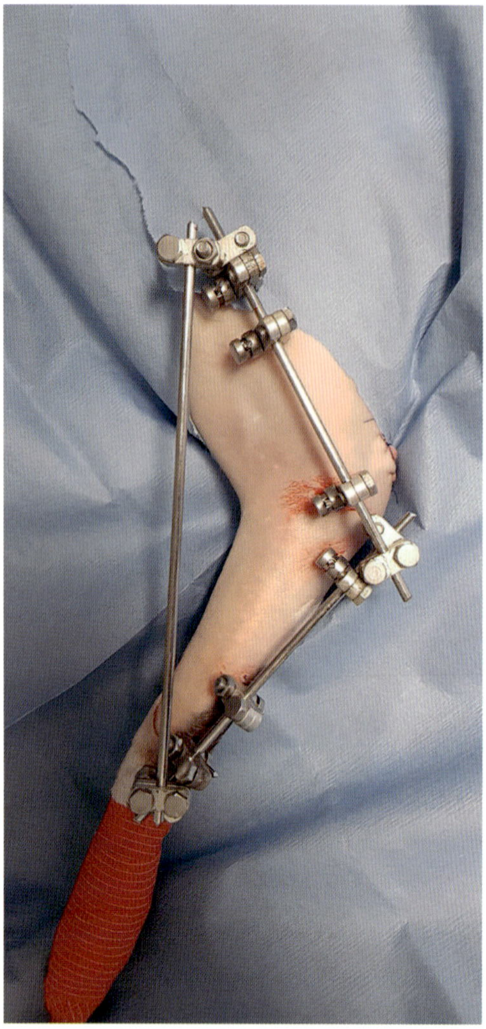

Figure 7. Transarticular external skeletal fixation.

INTERNAL FIXATION

Multiple internal fixation techniques have been described. These include isolated ligament reconstruction using suture prostheses anchored at the ligament origins and insertion points with screws and washers (Fig. 8). Reattachment of avulsed ligament origins/insertions can also be carried out using spiked washers and screws.

The author prefers performing internal fixation with circumferential suture prostheses as described by Farrell et al. (2007), as this can be used with elbow luxations in any direction.

Ligament reconstruction via tunnelled suture prostheses

With the patient positioned in dorsal recumbency, the affected limb is hung and then aseptically prepared. A skin incision is made from the lateral epicondyle of the humerus extending caudodistally to a point midway between the radial head and the caudal aspect of the ulna. The brachial fascia is incised along the same path to expose the lateral epicondyle, the origin of the extensors, and the anconeus muscle.

Elbow reduction is achieved through the same process as described for closed reduction. A small blunt Hohmann retractor or periosteal elevator can be used to help reduce the joint.

A skin incision over the medial aspect of the elbow is then performed extending distally 2–3 cm from the medial epicondyle of the humerus.

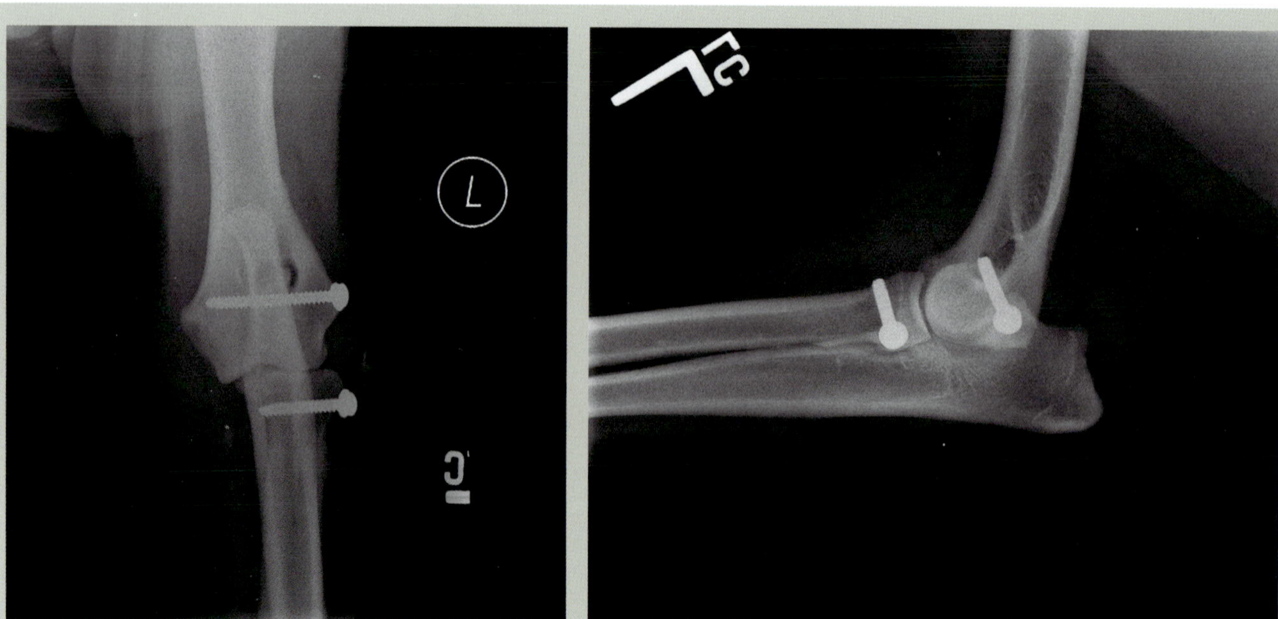

Figure 8. Orthogonal radiographs of an elbow after ligament repair with screws and washers. Images courtesy of W. M. Karlin.

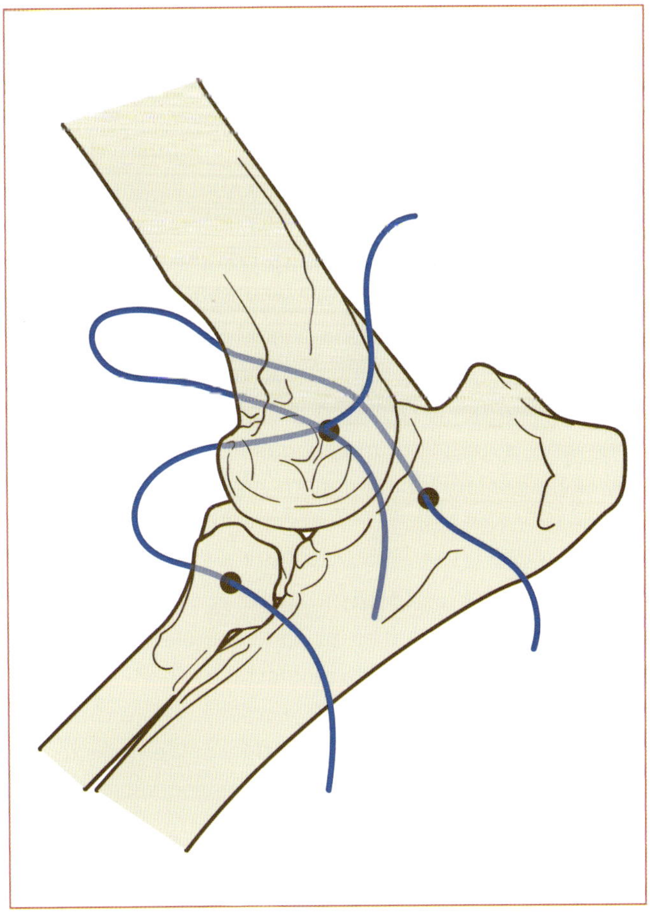

Figure 9. Lateral view of an elbow with placement of ligament prostheses. Adapted from: Farrell M et al., In vitro validation of a technique for assessment of canine and feline elbow joint collateral ligament integrity and description of a new method for collateral ligament prosthetic replacement, *Vet Surg* (2007).

In cats, the approach can be simplified with a single caudal approach which allows for access to both aspects of the elbow (see Fig. 11).

Three lateral to medial bone tunnels are made as follows (Fig. 9):

- A transhumeral bone tunnel is drilled from the origin of the lateral collateral ligament (immediately craniodistal to the lateral epicondyle) to a point immediately craniodistal to the medial epicondyle.
- A transradial bone tunnel is drilled from the insertion of the lateral collateral ligament. The tunnel should be made cranially enough to avoid inadvertently drilling the medial coronoid process (Fig. 10).
- A transulnar bone tunnel is drilled from the midpoint of the ulnar trochlear notch, centred between the articular surface and the caudal cortex.

The diameter of the bone tunnels depends on the material used for ligament reconstruction and on the size of the patient. Whilst other nonabsorbable materials, including monofilament nylon, can be utilised, the author prefers to use 7.0 metric FiberTape (Arthrex) in medium- to large-breed dogs, which requires 2.4 mm diameter bone tunnels. The author uses 4 metric polydioxanone in cats. This

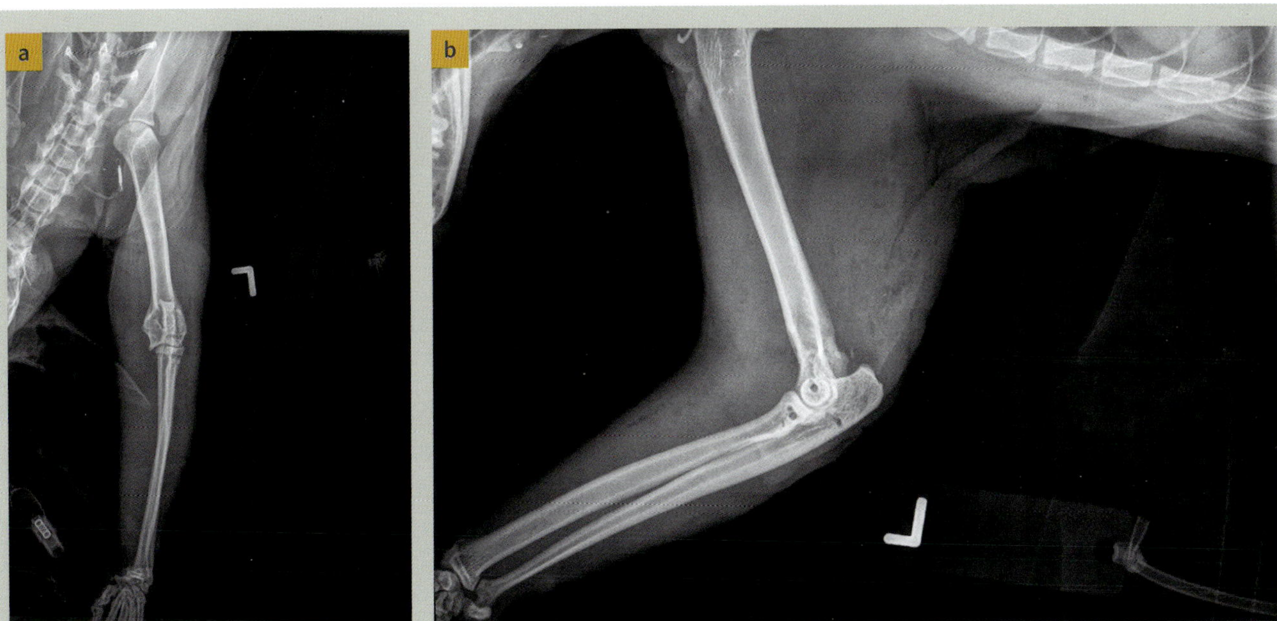

Figure 10. Craniocaudal (a) and mediolateral (b) postoperative radiographs of a cat showing inadvertent drilling through the medial coronoid process.

requires a 2.0 mm transhumeral tunnel and 1.5 mm transradial and transulnar tunnels.

When using FiberTape (Arthrex) or other soft, braided materials, a nitinol suture passing wire is useful to help pull it through the bone tunnels (Fig. 11a). Harder materials like monofilament nylon or polydioxanone can be threaded through by hand or guided with the bevel of an 18- or 20-gauge needle (Fig. 11b).

The suture prosthesis is passed through the loop in the nitinol suture passing wire and then doubled over the loop into equal halves. The wire is then passed in a lateral to medial direction through the transhumeral bone tunnel (see Fig. 11a). The suture is cut at the level of the nitinol loop, and the free ends are passed in a medial to lateral direction: one strand through the transradial bone tunnel and the other through the transulnar bone tunnel.

> Finding the transradial and transulnar bone tunnels from the medial aspect of the joint can be challenging. Passing the nitinol wire from lateral to medial prior to collecting the free end of the FiberTape strand can make this easier. Passing the suture under soft tissues should also be performed, if possible, to minimise impingement during suture tightening. To achieve this, curved mosquito haemostatic forceps or a 20-gauge needle can be useful.

The result is separate humeroradial and humeroulnar circumferential loops. With the elbow held at 135 degrees of extension, each loop is secured with a self-locking knot. If necessary, adjustment in suture positioning can be performed prior to securing the knot to avoid soft tissue impingement. If a monofilament nylon suture is used, the author recommends utilising crimps and a tensioning device. Crimps may impinge the joint in small dogs and most domestic cats and should be avoided in these cases.

The elbow range of motion is then assessed in flexion, extension, supination and pronation. Once satisfactory stability is confirmed, the wounds are lavaged and closed routinely.

Postoperative management

Patients should have their activity restricted for 8 weeks after surgery. This involves restriction to short lead walks for toilet purposes for the first 4 weeks before gradually increasing the duration and frequency of the walks for the following 4 weeks. Passive range of motion exercises can begin at hospital discharge.

In patients with significant concurrent orthopaedic injuries to other limbs, it is the author's preference to immobilise the elbow with a TAESF (Fig. 12) or spica splint for 2–3 weeks postoperatively before starting rehabilitation as outlined above.

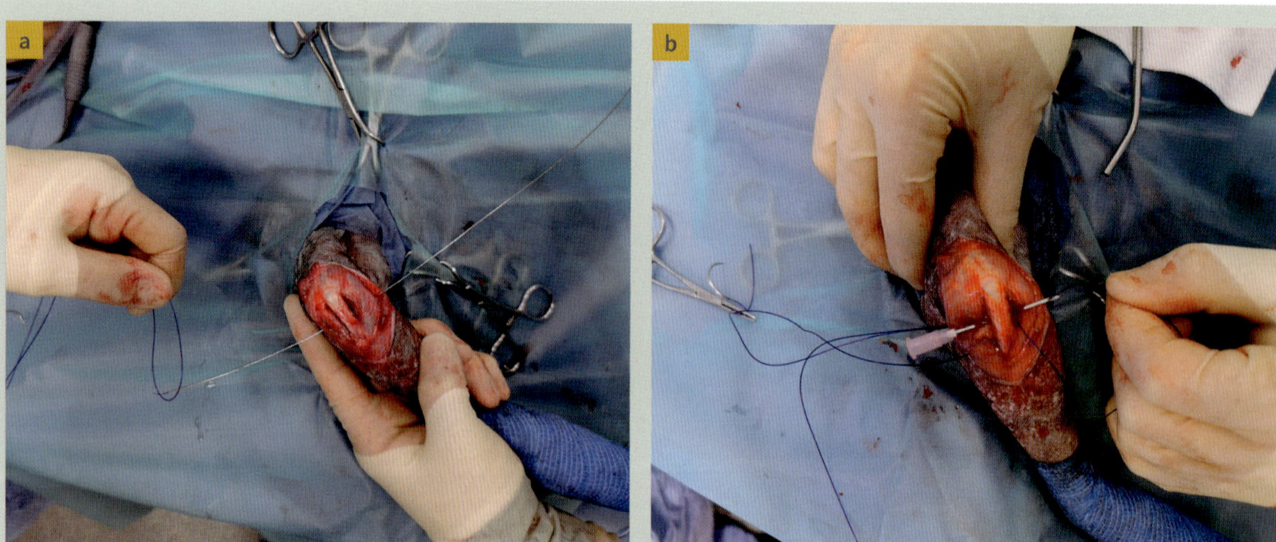

Figure 11. Caudal approach in a cat showing the use of a suture passing wire to help pull through the suture prosthesis (a). For the transradial and transulnar tunnels, 20- or 18-gauge needles can be used (b).

OUTCOME

Closed reduction and management generally carries a good prognosis in dogs, with the larger studies consistently reporting good to excellent outcomes in around 88 % of cases (Schaeffer et al., 1999; Sajik et al., 2016).

Some studies have suggested poorer outcomes in surgically managed cases (O'Brien et al., 1992; Mitchell, 2011). However, case numbers in these studies were limited.

A recent study reported that 15 out of 17 (88 %) closed-managed dogs and 18 out of 20 (92 %) surgically managed dogs had good to excellent owner-assessed function (Sajik et al., 2016).

COMPLICATIONS

Reluxation is the most common complication. Whilst the case numbers in published studies are limited, there may be an increased risk of reluxation in patients with concurrent orthopaedic injuries to other limbs (Sajik et al., 2016; Mitchell, 2011). Therefore, robust fixation should be considered in these cases.

Poorer outcomes have also been reported in closed-managed cases in which instability persisted following initial closed reduction (Schaeffer et al., 1999).

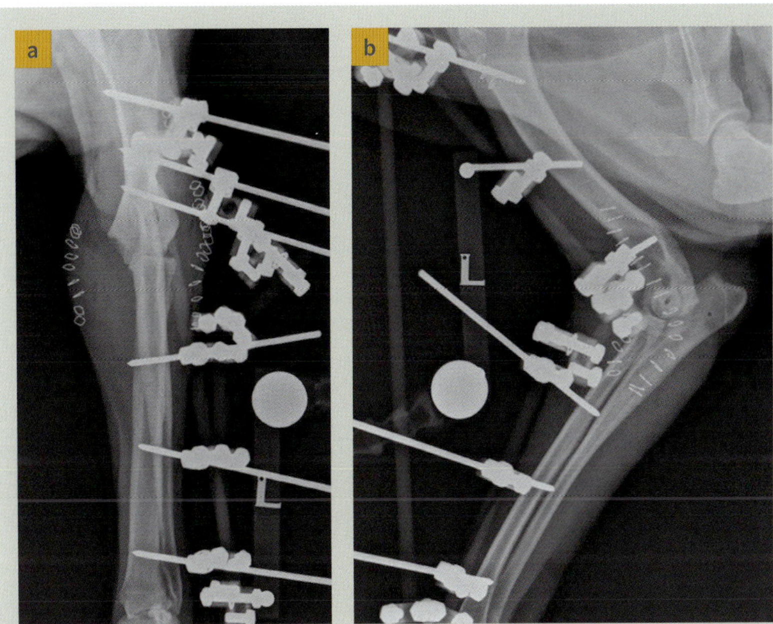

Figure 12. Postoperative craniocaudal (a) and mediolateral (b) radiographs of a dog after elbow luxation reduction using circumferential suture prostheses augmented with transarticular external skeletal fixation.

UNUNITED ANCONEAL PROCESS

Felipe de Vicente

INTRODUCTION

The anconeal process is an extension of the olecranon that inserts into the supracondylar foramen of the humerus when the elbow is in extension. Thus, the anconeal process collaborates in stabilising the elbow while in extension, mainly by providing mediolateral stability. In addition, the anconeal process is the main stabiliser of the elbow in pronation, and the second most important in supination when the limb is bearing weight (Krotscheck and Böttcher, 2018; Talcott et al., 2002).

During the development of the animal, only in large-breed dogs, the anconeal process has its own ossification centre (Cawley and Archibald, 1959). This ossification centre should close before 20 weeks of life under normal conditions. If this does not occur, ununited anconeal process (UAP) is diagnosed. UAP is common in large or giant breeds. Its incidence is high in the German Shepherd breed and it is less frequent in other large or giant breeds, such as Great Danes, St Bernards or Newfoundlands. The presence of UAP has also been described in small breeds, such as the Basset Hound, French Bulldog or Dachshund. The incidence of this disease is twice as high in males as in females, and in 20–35 % of cases the disease is bilateral (Krotscheck and Böttcher, 2018).

The exact cause for why large-breed dogs may develop UAP is unknown. There are several theories in this regard. The most popular is an asynchrony in the growth of the radius and ulna in the early stages of development. According to this theory, this asynchrony causes the ulna to be shorter than the radius in the early stages of development, causing the humeral condyle to exert more pressure on the anconeal process, which gives rise to UAP.

It is possible that some patients may exhibit a compensation for this asynchrony in the later stages of development, which would account for the presence of UAP in animals that do not present joint incongruence at the radioulnar level when the disease is diagnosed (Vezzoni and Benjamino, 2021). The presence of joint incongruence has been described in 50–100 % of UAP patients (Gasch et al., 2012; Meyer-Lindenberg et al., 2006). Thus, while one study reported an incidence of 50 %, with all incongruences being negative (short ulna) (Meyer-Lindenberg et al., 2006), another study showed an incidence of 100 %, with 77 % of radioulnar incongruences being positive (short radius) and 23 % negative (Gasch et al., 2012).

Regardless of the presence or absence of radioulnar incongruence at the time of diagnosis, these patients have persistent joint incongruence due to the UAP itself, resulting in joint instability, cartilage damage and degenerative joint disease (Vezzoni and Benjamino, 2021).

CLINICAL PRESENTATION AND DIAGNOSIS

Patients with UAP present with lameness of variable intensity in the affected limb. This lameness usually appears when patients are between 4 and 10 months of age. Occasionally, abduction of the elbow can be observed when the dog is in a standing position. Upon orthopaedic examination, it is common to find joint effusion and pain throughout the range of motion of the elbow (mainly in extension).

Although this disease is most commonly diagnosed in young animals, it can occasionally be diagnosed in adult animals. In these animals, the clinical signs are due to an exacerbation of a chronic underlying process (osteoarthritis) or to an increase in the mobility of the UAP.

Diagnosing UAP is relatively simple and is based on the verification of the persistence of the anconeal process growth centre in animals older than 5 months. This diagnosis can be established via plain lateral radiographs of the elbow. It is important to perform two lateral radiographs, one in a neutral position and the other in maximum flexion (Fig. 1). In the former, it may be possible to detect an UAP, but sometimes it is difficult to fully assess the anconeal process due to the overlapping of the humeral condyle. However, the lateral radiograph with the elbow in a neutral position is very useful in assessing joint incongruence and deciding whether these should be treated in the same surgery.

> A lateral radiograph of the elbow in maximum flexion allows for appropriate assessment of UAP, as it avoids the overlapping of the humeral condyle and the anconeal process.

It has also been suggested that the degree of mobility of the anconeal process can be compared by assessing the space between the anconeal process and the olecranon when comparing radiographs of the elbow in neutral position and in extension (Vezzoni and Benjamino, 2021). Thus, in some patients with UAP, increased space between the anconeal process and the olecranon is seen on lateral radiographs during elbow extension (compared to neutral radiographs). This increased space seems to be due to the pressure that the humeral condyle exerts on the anconeal process, and indicates a very mobile anconeal process.

Another relatively common way to diagnose UAP is via a CT scan of the elbow (Fig. 2). This technique allows for a more accurate assessment of the structure of the anconeal process and its congruence with the olecranon, which can be very useful when deciding what type of surgical treatment to perform (excision or stabilisation of the anconeal process). A CT scan of the elbow can also be used to assess the presence or absence of joint incongruence in the elbow, and to decide whether surgical treatment is necessary to improve joint congruence. Finally, a CT scan of the elbow also makes it possible to check for other concurrent diseases, such as fragmentation of the medial coronoid process or suspected disease of the medial compartment of the elbow.

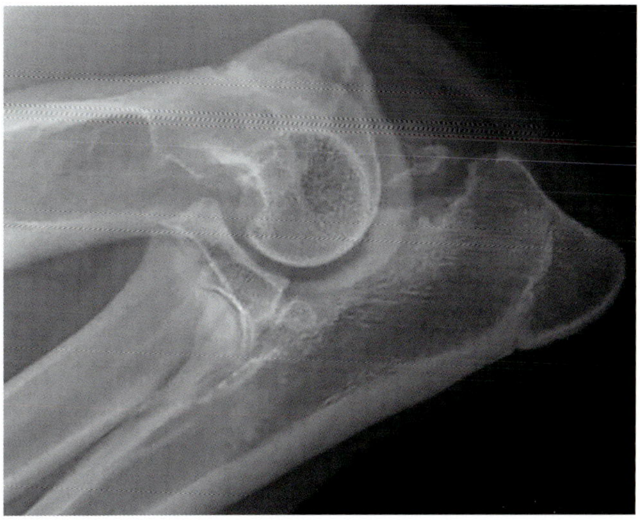

Figure 1. Lateral radiograph of the elbow showing an ununited anconeal process (UAP). The radiograph was taken in flexion to avoid the overlapping of the humeral condyle.

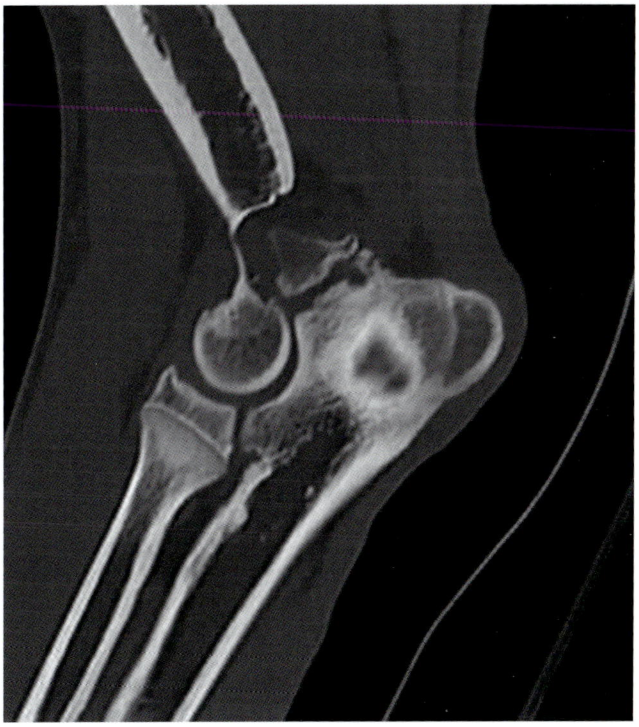

Figure 2. CT scan image of the elbow of a patient with UAP.

TREATMENT

TREATMENT IN YOUNG ANIMALS

In young animals with UAP, surgical treatment is usually recommended. The choice of treatment in these patients will depend on the patient's age, the degree of joint congruence and the mobility between the anconeal process and the olecranon. It is possible to subjectively assess the mobility of the anconeal process via arthroscopy during surgery (Video 1), and sometimes the anconeal process can even be palpated during surgery to assess its degree of stability. Surgical treatment will be aimed at the union of the anconeal process and the olecranon or its excision.

Video 1. Elbow arthroscopy in a dog with UAP. Note the ununited part of the ulna on the upper left side of the image and pathological changes in the cartilage in the intercondylar region of the humerus.

The ultimate goal of treatment in young animals without significant osteoarthritis should be to achieve union between the anconeal process and the olecranon. Performing a proximal ulnar osteotomy has been proposed (Sjöström et al., 1995; Turner et al., 1998) to correct articular incongruence and reduce the pressure exerted on the anconeal process, thus facilitating its union to the olecranon. Treating patients with UAP by stabilising the anconeal process with compression screws has also been proposed (Pritchard, 1976; Fox et al., 1996), in addition to combining both techniques with an ulnar osteotomy and stabilisation of the anconeal process (Meyer-Lindenberg et al., 2001; Krotscheck et al., 2000). Studies evaluating the union rate for the anconeal process in patients treated solely by ulnar osteotomy have shown highly variable results, with union rates ranging from 17–22 % (Turner et al., 1998; Meyer-Lindenberg et al., 1999) to 95 % (Sjöström et al., 1995). Another study reported a union rate for the anconeal process of 50 % when ulnar osteotomy was performed as treatment for UAP, with the union rate increasing to 84 % when stabilisation of the anconeal process with a compression screw was added to the ulnar osteotomy (Pettitt et al., 2009). This high union rate when combining a proximal ulnar osteotomy with stabilisation of the anconeal process has also been reported in other studies, with union rates between 89 % (Ferrigno et al., 2007) and 100 % (Krotscheck et al., 2000). Finally, studies evaluating the union rate for the anconeal process in patients treated solely via stabilisation with compression screws have reported a union rate of between 11 % (Meyer–Lindenberg et al., 1999) and 60 % (Fox et al., 1996) (in the latter study, 40 % of dogs did not have the recommended radiographic follow-up, so this 60 % union rate represents the totality of dogs that underwent medium-term radiographic follow-up). In patients with bilateral UAP, it is recommended to perform both surgeries 2–3 weeks apart.

If the anconeal process shows advanced degenerative signs and, thus, does not have congruence with the olecranon, or presents very high mobility, anconeal process excision should be considered. It is important to remember that when the anconeal process is removed, there is an increase in joint instability and, therefore, it is to be expected that the patient will continue to develop osteoarthritis and may have long-term impaired functionality of the joint. It has been reported that, although 70 % of patients improve clinically after excision of the anconeal process due to UAP, 50 % continue to present limb lameness (Guthrie, 1989).

TREATMENT IN ADULT ANIMALS

In adult animals diagnosed with UAP, the most common cause of clinical signs is a worsening of osteoarthritis secondary to UAP. In these cases, conservative treatment should be attempted first, with the typical recommendations for dogs with osteoarthritis, and surgical treatment should be considered if they do not respond. However, in adult animals in which a significant separation of the anconeal process is evident, the clinical signs may arise due to an acute separation of the anconeal process, in which case surgical treatment is recommended, usually via excision of the anconeal process.

SURGICAL TECHNIQUE

Excision of the anconeal process

With the patient positioned in lateral recumbency, a lateral approach to the elbow is performed by making a curved incision immediately caudal to the humeral epicondyle, following the lateral epicondylar crest (Fig. 3). After dissecting the subcutaneous tissue, the brachial fascia is incised at the level of the cranial border of the lateral head of the triceps brachii muscle (Fig. 4). The anconeus muscle, located

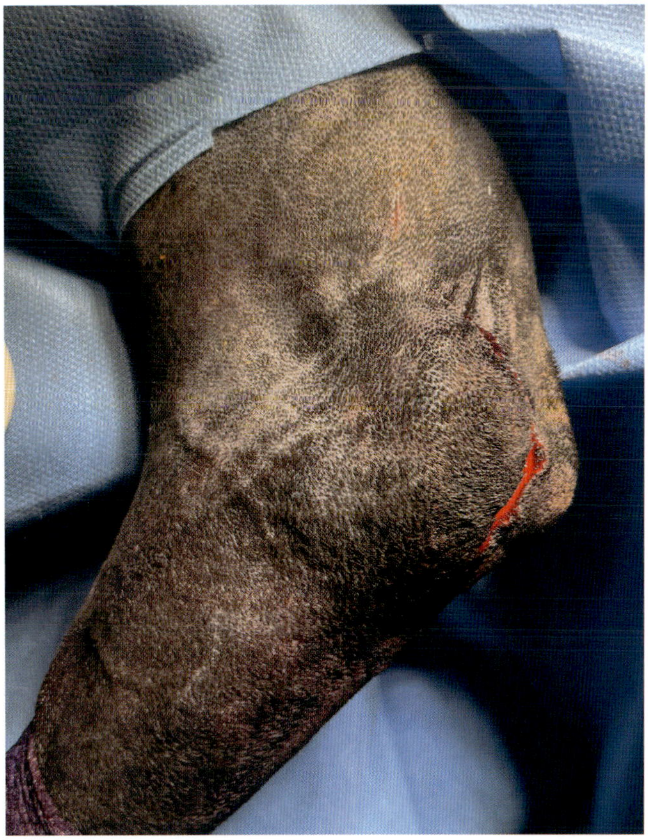

Figure 3. Lateral approach to the elbow. A curved incision is made, caudal to the humeral epicondyle, following the lateral epicondylar crest.

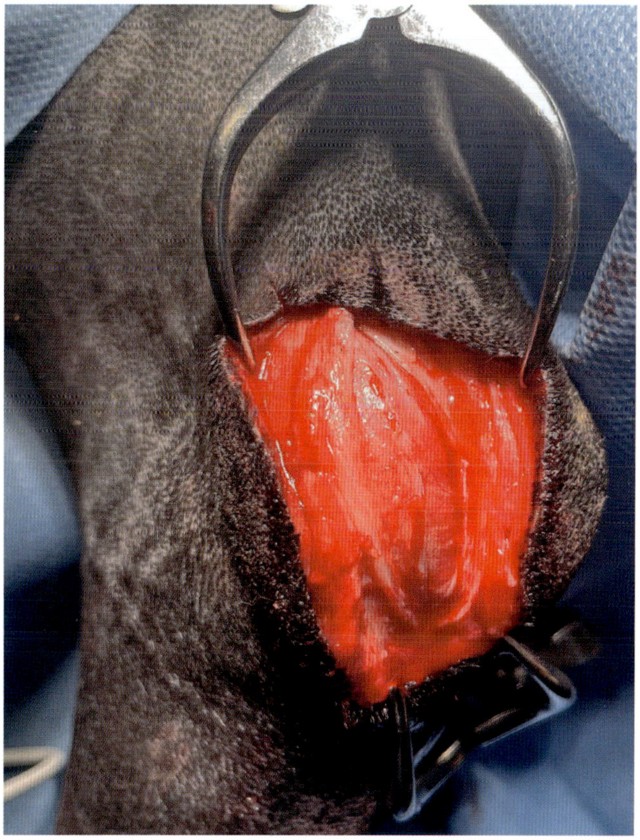

Figure 4. After dissecting the subcutaneous tissue, the brachial fascia is incised at the level of the cranial border of the lateral head of the triceps brachii muscle, visualising the anconeus muscle immediately underneath.

immediately below the brachial fascia, is incised at its origin (on the lateral epicondylar crest). The anconeus muscle is retracted and the joint capsule is incised, exposing the humeroulnar joint and achieving direct visualisation of the anconeal process (Fig. 5).

The fissure between the anconeal process and the olecranon is usually evident. Possible adhesions and fibrosis between the anconeal process and the olecranon are released by means of a periosteotome or osteotome, using a scalpel for minor adhesions. Once freed from the olecranon, the anconeal process is removed with the aid of bone reduction forceps (Fig. 6). Sometimes the ununited area of the anconeal process is not clearly visible, but when pressure is exerted with a probe a depression is seen in the ununited area, and an osteotome can be gently used to release the anconeal process from the olecranon without difficulty.

Once the anconeal process has been removed, the joint is lavaged copiously with sterile saline, the joint capsule is sutured and the anconeus muscle is reinserted into the remnants of the epicondylar crest or, failing that, into the

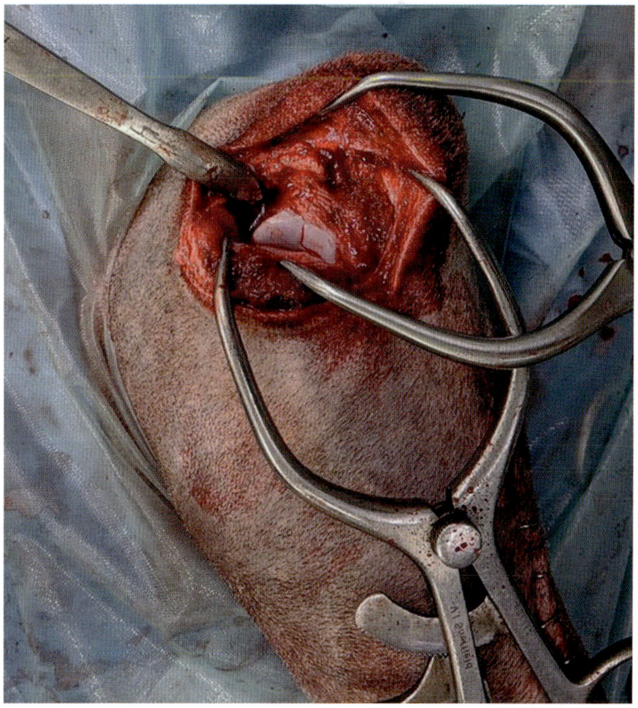

Figure 5. Visualisation of the anconeal process in a patient with UAP. The anconeus muscle is retracted, exposing the humeroulnar joint and achieving direct visualisation of the anconeal process.

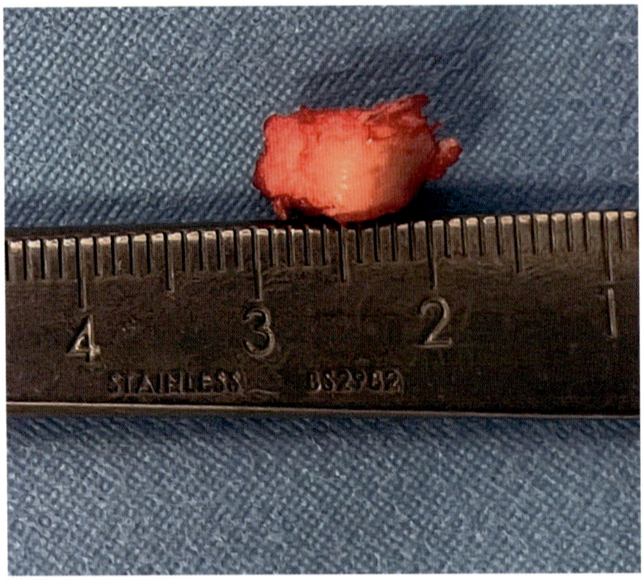

Figure 6. Anconeal process removed from a patient with UAP.

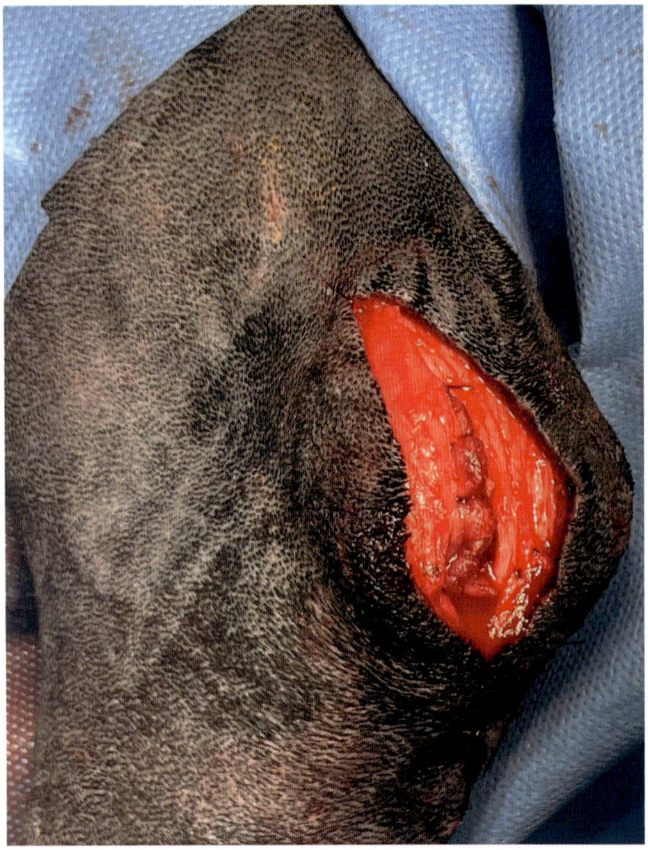

Figure 7. Closure of the lateral approach to the elbow. Suture reconstruction of the anconeus muscle.

extensor muscles of the antebrachium, at their origin on the lateral epicondyle, using an absorbable monofilament suture (the author usually uses polydioxanone) (Fig. 7). The brachial fascia is then sutured (the author uses polydioxanone in a simple continuous pattern), followed by the subcutaneous tissue (the author's preference is polyglecaprone 25 in a simple continuous pattern) and the skin (with surgical staples or nonabsorbable monofilament suture; the author uses nylon in a interrupted cruciate pattern).

Stabilisation of the anconeal process

The approach used to stabilise the anconeal process is identical to that described above.

Once the anconeal process is visualised, a compression screw is placed following the axis of the anconeal process. The original technique was described as placing the screw in a craniocaudal direction from the anconeal process to the caudal area of the olecranon (Herron, 1970; Fox et al., 1996). This technique involved the screw head being placed intra-articularly. Therefore, the caudocranial placement of the screw has also been described, a manoeuvre that avoids the presence of intra-articular implants.

Once the surgical approach has been performed, the anconeal process is visualised and carefully palpated with a periosteotome to assess its degree of mobility. The skin and subcutaneous tissue should be rotated medially to obtain direct access to the caudal part of the olecranon. The position of the anconeal process can be maintained and, at the same time, compression can be exerted by placing reduction forceps between the cranial edge of the anconeal process and the caudal aspect of the ulna. C-shaped guides can also be used for this purpose, while simultaneously ensuring the correct orientation of the screw. If the screw is to be placed in a craniocaudal direction, the tip of the anconeal process is drilled in the direction of the caudal aspect of the olecranon using the appropriate drill bit (Fig. 8). If the screw is to be placed in a caudocranial direction, a drill guide is placed on the caudal aspect of the ulna, determining the exact point by applying the measurements taken on the preoperative radiographs (or CT scans) and using the most proximal part of the olecranon as a reference. The size of the drill bit to be used depends on the type and size of the screw and on its mode of application.

The size of the screw depends on the size of the patient. Usually, a 3.5 mm screw is used in the breeds and ages typically associated with this disease. There are several possibilities regarding the type of screw that can be used for stabilisation of the anconeal process. Cortical screws can be placed in a positional mode, provided that the necessary compression is applied with reduction forceps (this

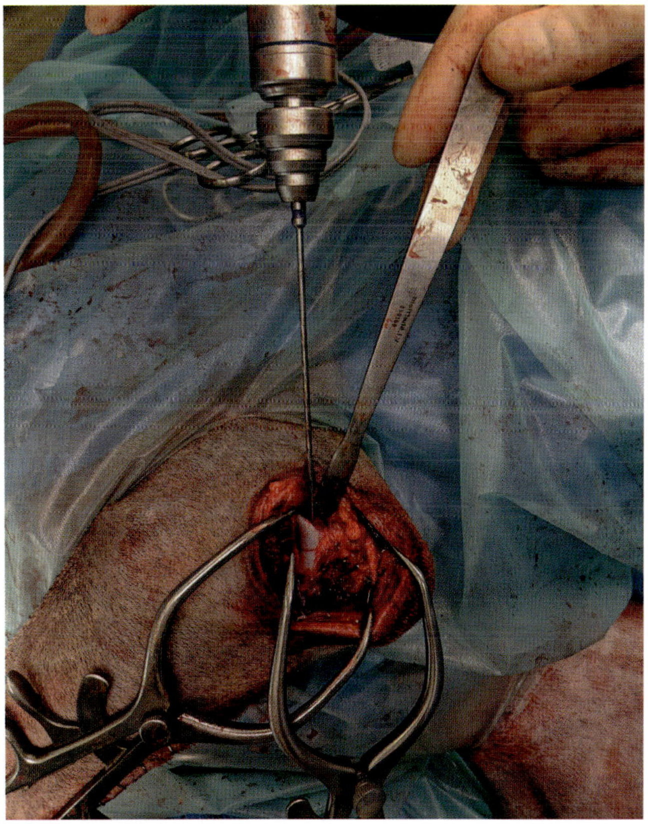

Figure 8. Placement of a compression screw in a craniocaudal direction in a patient with UAP. Initial drilling is done with the appropriate drill bit for the selected screw size and mode of use.

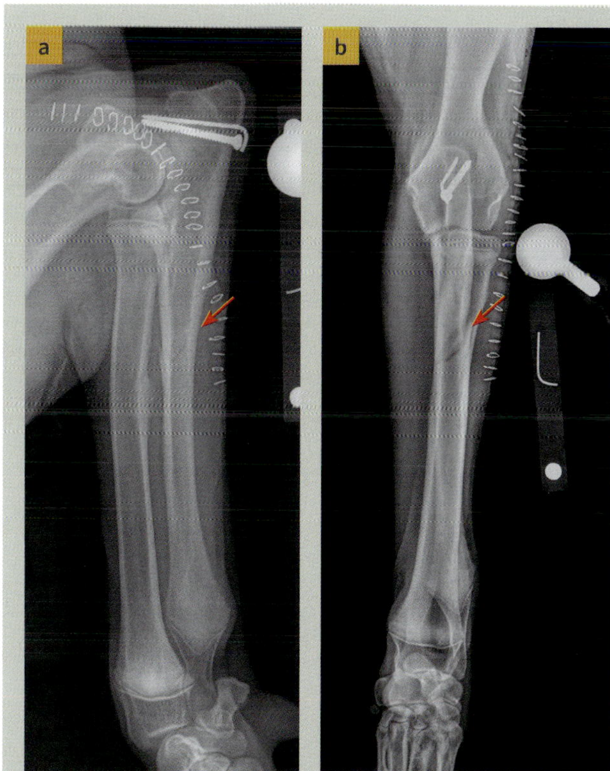

Figure 9. Lateral (a) and craniocaudal (b) radiographs of an UAP treated with a compression screw and a Kirschner wire parallel to the screw to provide an antirotational effect. A bi-oblique ulnar osteotomy was also performed (arrows).

is the author's preference). Another possibility is to use cortical screws in a compression mode, or partially threaded cancellous screws (usually 4.0 mm in size). Finally, it is possible to place an additional implant (usually a Kirschner wire) parallel to the screw to exert an antirotational effect (Fig. 9).

> It is important that the implants maintain the anconeal process in an anatomically accurate position, as inadequate reduction will cause excessive friction between the anconeal process and the humeral condyle, which could lead to implant fatigue and rupture.

Proximal ulnar osteotomy

Ulnar osteotomy can be performed alone or in combination with anconeal process stabilisation. This technique is usually applied when there is articular incongruence, with the aim of reducing the pressure exerted by the humeral trochlea on the anconeal process due to articular incongruence. By relieving the pressure on the anconeal process, direct union of the anconeal process can sometimes be achieved without additional treatment. When this technique is used in conjunction with compression screw stabilisation, on the one hand, it facilitates the union of the anconeal process by relieving the pressure on it secondary to articular incongruence, and on the other hand, it protects the screw from excessive pressure, fatigue and rupture.

Traditionally, performing a transverse proximal ulnar osteotomy was proposed, but this technique fell into disuse due to a relatively high complication rate (mainly nonunion or delayed union of the osteotomy, and excessive inclination of the proximal ulnar segment). Currently, oblique or bi-oblique dynamic ulnar osteotomy is recommended, performed between the middle third and the proximal third of the ulna (see Fig. 9). This osteotomy must have a very marked inclination to increase the contact surface between the two parts of the bone at the level of the osteotomy, thus reducing its instability. Oblique or bi-oblique ulnar osteotomy has a lower complication rate than traditional transverse ulnar osteotomy.

The location of the osteotomy must be planned on preoperative imaging tests (radiographs or CT scans), and the landmarks should be used intraoperatively to determine the appropriate osteotomy site. Usually the lateral humeral epicondyle and the most proximal part of the ulna are taken as anatomical landmarks for measurements.

> To determine the correct location of the osteotomy, it is important to plan the procedure and determine the anatomical landmarks using preoperative imaging.

The approach to perform ulnar osteotomy is through an incision in the skin caudolateral to the antebrachium, long enough to perform the planned osteotomy (previously determined using imaging tests). Periosteal incisions are made in the caudal surface of the ulna, which is easily palpable, and the flexor carpi ulnaris and extensor carpi ulnaris muscles are elevated and retracted medially and laterally, respectively. Retraction of these muscles must be maintained throughout the osteotomy; therefore, manual retractors (usually Hohmann) and Gelpi retractors are utilised. This manoeuvre will expose the proximal ulnar diaphysis during surgery. The author routinely places Hohmann retractors with their tips on the cranial aspect of the ulna, at the level of the end of the osteotomy, thus avoiding damage to the radius.

Oblique dynamic proximal ulnar osteotomy should be performed in a proximocaudal to craniodistal direction, starting at the caudal surface of the ulna, 1–3 cm distal to the radial head, at a 45-degree angle. Bi-oblique dynamic proximal osteotomy should be performed in a proximocaudolateral to distocraniomedial direction, applying as much angulation as possible in the osteotomy.

> To perform oblique ulnar osteotomy, it is safer to use an oscillating saw than a Gigli saw or an osteotome, since with the former it is difficult to obtain the desired osteotomy angle, and with the latter there is an increased risk of creating fissures in the ulna.

POSTOPERATIVE MANAGEMENT

PATIENTS TREATED VIA EXCISION OF THE ANCONEAL PROCESS

Patients who have undergone excision of the anconeal process do not require strict postoperative treatment. The indicated follow-up consists of postoperative radiographs to assess the completeness of the excision.

If there are no contraindications, nonsteroidal anti-inflammatory drugs are prescribed for 1–2 weeks. Exercise should be limited for the first 2 months following surgery, and the owner should be instructed to keep their pet at rest and to take controlled walks on a short leash (10–15 minutes, 3–4 times a day, for 3–4 weeks). For the first 4 weeks, gentle physiotherapy can be performed. It is then recommended to gradually increase the duration of controlled leash walks over the next 3–4 weeks and to progressively introduce periods of off-leash exercise.

PATIENTS TREATED TO ACHIEVE UNION OF THE ANCONEAL PROCESS

In these cases, the follow-up consists of postoperative radiographs to evaluate the position of the implants in the anconeal process and to assess the location and length of the ulnar osteotomy. It is also recommended to apply a protective bandage (modified Robert Jones) for the first 10 days after ulnar osteotomy.

If there are no contraindications, nonsteroidal anti-inflammatory drugs are prescribed for 2–3 weeks. Exercise should be limited for the first 3 months following surgery, instructing the owner to keep their pet on strict cage rest (or in a small room if the patient is large) for the first 3–4 weeks, with very short walks on a short leash (5–10 minutes, 3–4 times a day). For the first 4 weeks, gentle physiotherapy can be performed.

The author performs radiographic evaluation of the anconeal process, osteotomy and implants at 6 weeks postoperatively or earlier if the patient shows clinical deterioration. Once the anconeal process is fused (and the ulnar osteotomy consolidated), very short periods (initially 5 minutes) of off-leash exercise can be introduced at the end of each walk and rehabilitation exercises (physiotherapy or hydrotherapy) can be intensified. The duration of off-leash exercise is progressively increased over a period of 3–4 weeks, after which the patient can resume normal activity.

OUTCOME

The prognosis is excellent for patients in whom union of the anconeal process is achieved and the disease is detected in its very early stages (before the development of osteoarthritis). It is very important to take into account the patient's age and the degree of mobility of the anconeal process when considering the patient's prognosis. Union of the anconeal process is more frequently achieved in young animals, with animals under 6 months of age in large breeds and under 9 months of age in giant breeds being established as a reference (Vezzoni, 2016; Vezzoni and Benjamino, 2021). The mobility of the anconeal process also influences the success rate of the surgery and union is more frequently achieved when instability is mild (because it is attached with firm fibrous tissue). If the anconeal process is unstable and mobile, the rate of success is reduced.

When patients are treated by excision of the anconeal process, the instability of the elbow increases; therefore, a degenerative process of the joint (osteoarthritis) continues to develop in the long term (Roy et al., 1994). Thus, the long-term prognosis after excision of the anconeal process is worse, with decreased range of motion in the elbow and altered limb function.

The prognosis of patients treated via anconeal process excision is worse than that of those in which union of the anconeal process has been achieved via stabilisation.

COMPLICATIONS

The most common complication is nonunion of the anconeal process and loosening or breakage of the implants. In these cases, it is necessary to reoperate on the patient using the approaches described above and assess the need to restabilise the anconeal process, versus excision of the anconeal process and removal of the implants.

Patients that have undergone ulnar osteotomy surgery usually have a continuous lameness until the osteotomy has healed. This process may require up to 12–16 weeks, depending on the age of the patient and the location of the osteotomy. Although rare due to the age of UAP patients, it is possible for ulnar osteotomy to result in nonunion. In these cases, it is necessary to treat the nonunion as appropriately as possible, most commonly by means of a reintervention for bone graft application and osteotomy stabilisation.

MEDIAL COMPARTMENT DISEASE

Alan Danielski

INTRODUCTION

Medial compartment disease is the term used to describe erosion of the articular cartilage of the medial compartment of the elbow joint secondary to incongruence (due to elbow dysplasia or angular limb deformities), traumatic injury (e.g. elbow luxation or fractures) or, in a few cases, iatrogenic damage (due to malpositioning of implants). This erosion usually affects the medial humeral condyle and the medial coronoid process, but it can also extend to the abaxial side of the radial head or to the medial aspect of the ulnar notch.

The severity of cartilage damage has been described and scored using a modified Outerbridge classification system (Farrell et al., 2014):

0. Normal cartilage.
I. Cartilage softening and swelling (chondromalacia).
II. Partial-thickness surface defects with cartilage fibrillation.
III. Deep fibrillation to the level of the subchondral bone.
IV. Full-thickness cartilage erosion.
V. Subchondral bone eburnation.

Due to the loss of cellular components, grades III to V are believed to be irreversible and progressive. The term medial compartment disease can be applied to all those joints with arthroscopically confirmed grade IV or V cartilage damage affecting the medial compartment. Subchondral bone devoid of protective articular cartilage is exposed to inflammation and constant stimulation of the joint nociceptors, resulting in debilitating elbow pain.

TREATMENT

CONSERVATIVE TREATMENT

Conservative treatment can be adopted in all those cases that are considered poor surgical candidates, and it usually involves a multimodal approach. These nonsurgical strategies usually include:

- Weight control.
- Exercise control (low-impact activity, shorter and more frequent walks rather than longer and fewer walks).
- Joint supplements containing omega-3 essential fatty acids (EFAs), glucosamine sulphate and glucosamine hydrochloride, chondroitin sulphate and avocado and soybean unsaponifiables (ASUs).
- Nonsteroidal anti-inflammatory drugs (NSAIDs).
- Nonopioid analgesic drugs such as amantadine, gabapentin, acetaminophen (paracetamol) and tramadol.
- Monoclonal antibody therapy (bedinvetmab).
- Intra-articular injections (hyaluronate acid, polyacrylamide hydrogel).
- Regenerative medicine (platelet-rich plasma, stem cell therapy).

SURGICAL TREATMENT

The principal aims of the currently available techniques to treat medial compartment disease are to shift the weight-bearing axis of the thoracic limb (sliding humeral osteotomy [SHO], New Generation Devices), to shift the load from the medial compartment by causing a slight abduction of the ulna (proximal abducting ulnar osteotomy [PAUL], Kyon) or to partially resurface the damaged articular surfaces and limit bone-on-bone friction by stopping further collapse of the medial compartment (compartmental elbow replacement, Arthrex). A biomechanically anatomical, nonconstrained compartmental (BANC) partial elbow replacement (Kyon) is also currently being clinically tested. In those cases in which both the medial and lateral elbow compartments are affected, a total elbow replacement may be required.

Sliding humeral osteotomy (SHO)

This technique relies on the ability to redistribute the major joint forces from the medial compartment (where profound cartilage and subchondral bone pathology is present) to the lateral compartment (Fig. 1). This shift reduces the mean forces transmitted through the medial compartment of the elbow by 25–28 % (Mason et al., 2008), allowing the reduction of pain in the medial compartment due to an increase in the fibrocartilaginous healing of the articular surfaces (Fitzpatrick et al., 2009).

The ideal candidate for SHO is a skeletally mature dog with damage to the medial compartment only (modified Outerbridge grade III or IV cartilage damage or "kissing lesions"). This procedure is not advised in skeletally immature dogs because the open physeal regions could develop abnormally with the change in force through the elbow joint.

The SHO stepped plates accept 3.5 and 4.0 mm screws (cortical and locking), and there are three variants of the plates, 7 (miniplate), 7.5 and 10 mm, according to the step size desired (Fig. 2). The 7.5 mm plate is usually used in medium-sized dogs, whilst the 10 mm plate is usually employed in large-breed dogs. Although a minimum bone overlap of one-third is needed, ideally the surgeon should aim to achieve 50 % contact between the humeral surfaces at the level of the cut.

Surgical technique

The patient is placed in lateral recumbency with the affected limb near the operating table, and a standard approach to the medial humerus is performed. The plate is positioned on the medial aspect of the humerus and secured using locking screws in the proximal humeral segment and cortical screws in the distal humeral segment. A mid-diaphyseal osteotomy is then performed using the step of the plate as a cutting guide. The cortical screws are tightened sequentially, drawing the bone to the plate and providing the offset sliding motion of the humerus. All the cortical screws are

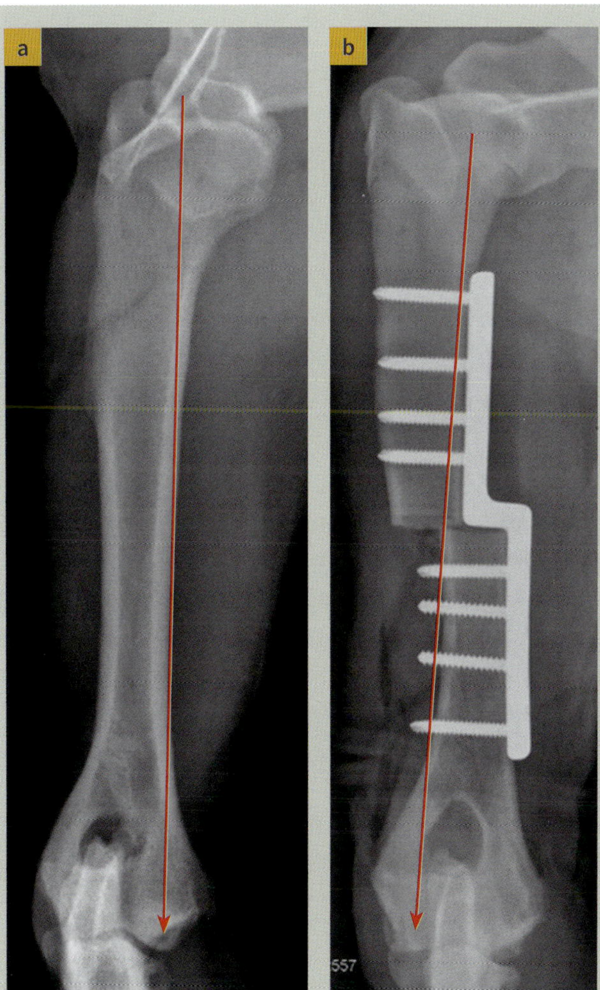

Figure 1. The medial elbow compartment of a dog suffering from medial compartment disease is usually overloaded and collapsed. The aim of the sliding humeral osteotomy procedure is to shift the weight-bearing axis from the medial (diseased; a) to the lateral (healthy; b) compartment.

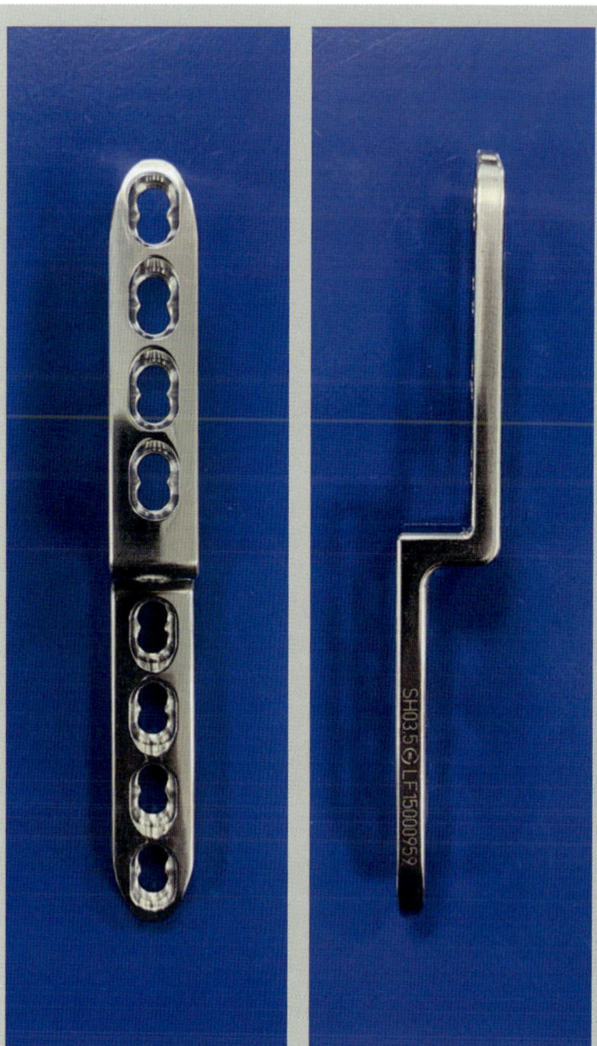

Figure 2. 3.5 mm, 10 mm stepped sliding humeral osteotomy plate (New Generation Devices).

then replaced by locking screws. Soft tissue closure is performed in a routine fashion.

Outcome and complications

Only two peer-reviewed studies have evaluated the clinical outcome of dogs undergoing SHO. Wendelburg and Beale (2014) evaluated the medium- and long-term outcome following SHO. At over 1 year after surgery, 7 out of 35 elbows did not reveal osteophytosis progression, and out of 32 dogs, 3 achieved significant improvement in peak vertical forces and 2 achieved significant improvement in vertical impulse when compared with the ipsilateral limb preoperatively. Major complications were experienced in 17 % of cases (infection, broken/loose screws, humeral fracture), and one case had a catastrophic complication (euthanised following a humeral fracture). In the second study (Fitzpatrick et al., 2015), which involved 46 dogs (60 elbows), lameness improved in all limbs by 12 weeks and resolved in 49 limbs. No major complications were noted, and only minor complications (4.2 %) were reported. In a previous study testing the different previous generations of SHO implants, the same research group reported major complications in 15.2 % of cases (Fitzpatrick et al., 2009).

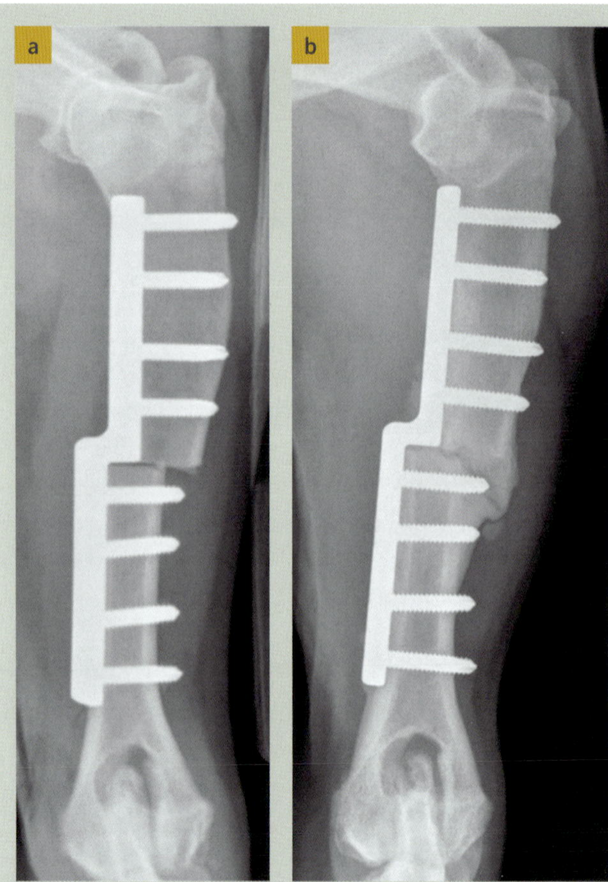

Figure 3. Immediate postoperative (a) and 6-week follow-up (b) radiographs of a dog that had a sliding humeral osteotomy procedure performed. Note the large amount of callus formation at the humeral osteotomy site.

> Although the current SHO technique and the development of new stronger implants have decreased the complication rate and early results suggest it is effective in relieving pain associated with medial compartment disease in dogs, this procedure has a steep learning curve and remains technically very challenging.

Proximal abducting ulnar osteotomy (PAUL)

The proposed biomechanics of PAUL are similar to those of high tibial osteotomy for the treatment of varus deformity of the knee associated with medial compartment syndrome in humans: a medial open wedge osteotomy of the tibial plateau leads to elevation of the medial tibial plateau with subsequent lateralisation of the distal limb, loading of the lateral compartment of the knee and unloading of the medial compartment. In dogs, the application of a stepped plate on the lateral aspect of the ulna should similarly raise the ulna on the medial humeral compartment and result in lateralisation of the paw. This should subsequently increase the load through the lateral compartment and unload the medial compartment, alleviating pain.

This technique is best suited for skeletally mature patients, not older than 8 years, with full-thickness cartilage damage to the medial compartment of the elbow. Surgery is not indicated in dogs older than 8 years because of irreversible joint changes and the difficulty to achieve the desired degree of abduction due to loss of elasticity of the interosseous ligament and chronic periarticular changes. Cartilage damage to the lateral humeral condyle or to the abaxial/oblique aspect of the radial head are a contraindication to perform this surgery. Arthroscopy – to fully assess the status of the elbow joint – is mandatory prior to surgical intervention (Fig. 4), and the presence of osteophytosis on radiographs cannot be considered a justification to perform this surgical procedure without previous arthroscopic inspection.

Four different PAUL plate sizes are available: 8 and 9, which accept 3.5 mm locking screws and are typically used in dogs under 25 kg, and 10 and 11, which accept 4.5 mm locking screws and are used in dogs over 25 kg. Plates are available with a 2 or 3 mm step (Fig. 5). The angle of abduction achieved is approximately 4 degrees with the 2 mm step plate and 6 degrees with the 3 mm step plate. Due to the extra 4–5 degrees attributable to the natural curvature of the ulna, the final lateral shift is approximately 8 degrees with the 2 mm step plate and 11 degrees with the 3 mm step plate.

Surgical planning

Preoperative planning involves measurement of the mechanical medial elbow angle (mMEA) on a craniocaudal radiograph of the entire antebrachium (including the elbow and the carpal joint). A line is drawn from the centre of the humeral condyle to the centre of the antebrachiocarpal joint. A second line is drawn tangential to the articular surface of the medial and lateral humeral condyles. The medial angle resulting from the intersection of these two lines represents the mMEA, which in normal dogs has a range of 81.5 ± 2.5 degrees. A 2 mm step plate should be used in cases with an mMEA of more than 82 degrees, whilst a 3 mm step plate should be used in cases with an mMEA of less than 82 degrees (Fig. 6). Implant size selection can be determined by using specific plug-in software or by superimposing acetate templates over conventional radiographs.

Surgical technique

The ulna is palpated at the caudolateral aspect of the antebrachium, and a skin incision is performed directly over the ulna. The muscles on the lateral aspect are elevated and the osteotomy site is located. This should always be approximately 4 cm distal to the articular surface of the radial head. In those cases in which the medial compartment is severely collapsed and the mMEA is less than 79 degrees, the cut should be made slightly more proximal (≈3.5 cm) to achieve additional ulnar abduction. The plate is centred on the lateral aspect of the bone, making sure that the most distal hole is centred on the ulna and will accommodate the correct size screw.

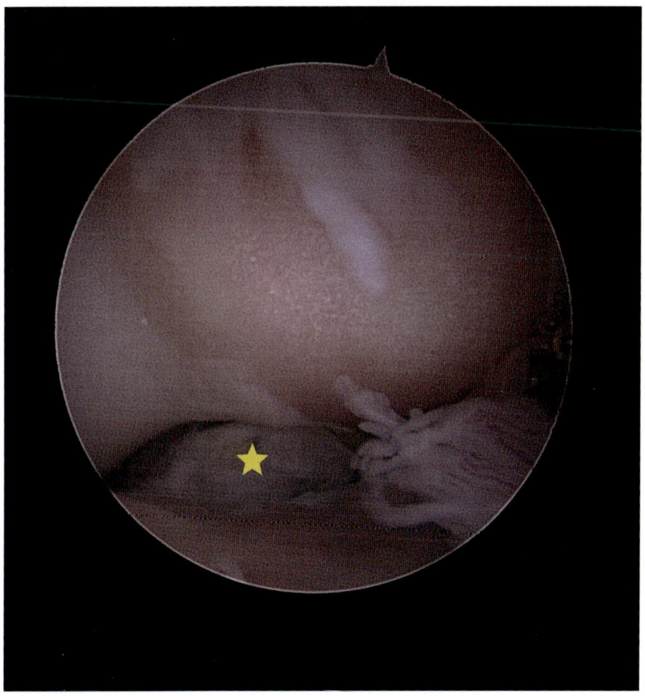

Figure 4. Arthroscopic image of the left elbow of a 16-month-old Labrador Retriever. Note the diffuse full-thickness cartilage damage (modified Outerbridge grade IV) affecting the medial humeral condyle and medial coronoid process. A completely detached tip-radial incisure fragment of the medial coronoid process is also visible (star).

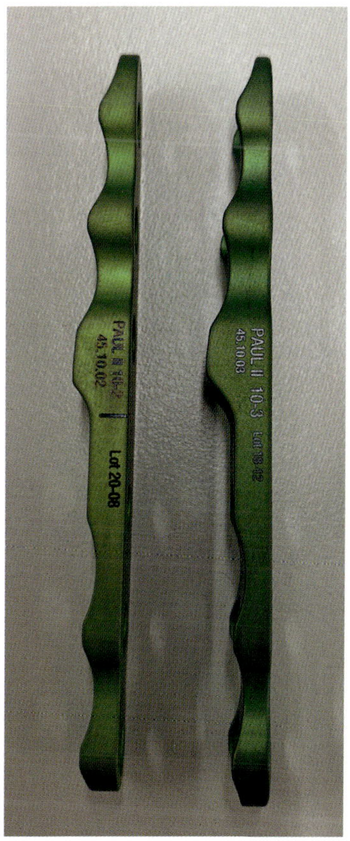

Figure 5. PAUL-II 10 plates with a 2 mm step (left) and 3 mm step (right). The black line immediately distal to the step should be aligned with the osteotomy cut in order to provide the correct and desired angle of abduction of the proximal ulna.

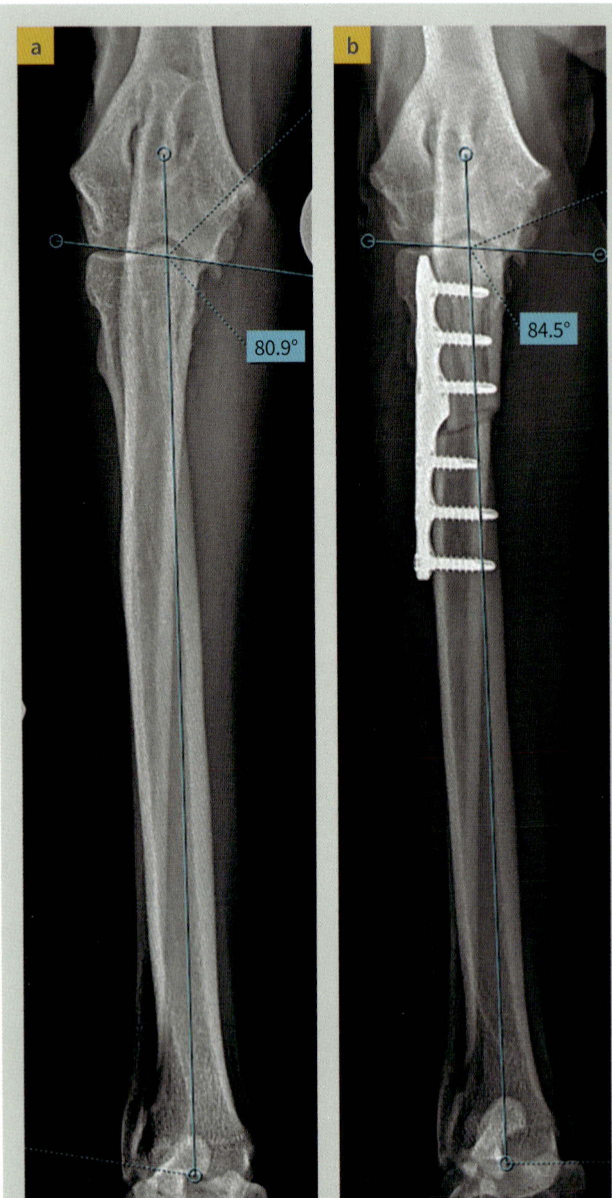

Figure 6. Preoperative (a) and postoperative (b) measurement of the mechanical medial elbow angle. A PAUL 9-3 mm plate (with 3.5 mm locking screws) was used. Note that the osteotomy cut was performed at a slightly oblique angle to help displace the proximal ulnar segment laterally.

The osteotomy is then performed with an oscillating saw, taking care to protect the surrounding soft tissue and interosseous vessels.

The plate is then secured in place with a pointed forceps, and the distal end of the plate is inspected again to ensure that the most distal hole is centred on the bone (which can be particularly thin at that level).

> The plate must be parallel to the sagittal plane (not facing cranially or caudally) so as to achieve proper abduction. The lateral surface of the ulna is very often curved, which can be misleading when the surgeon secures the plate. To avoid this mistake, the sagittal plane of the limb should always be assessed with respect to the plate.

With the plate holes numbered from 1 to 6 from the most proximal to the most distal, the cortical screws are sequentially inserted into holes 6 and 4, making sure that the caudal margin of the distal portion of the plate is parallel to the caudal margin of the distal ulnar segment.

The proximal end of the plate is secured again against the bone using point-to-point forceps, making sure that the most proximal portion of the plate is in strict contact with the bone (if this is not the case, the degree of abduction achieved will not be the desired one). A caudal tilt (1–2 mm) is then applied to the proximal ulnar segment at level of the osteotomy site to help increase the distance between the medial coronoid process and medial humeral condyle. After sequentially drilling holes 1 and 3, the appropriate cortical screws are inserted to secure the plate against the bone (Fig. 7). Holes 2 and 5 are then drilled, and the appropriate-sized locking screws are inserted after measuring the depth of the hole. It is important to ensure that the tip of the locking screws fully exits the transcortex in order to achieve the desired holding power. The cortical screws are then removed, the bone tunnels are overdrilled using the appropriate-sized drill bit, and the drill guide and locking screws are inserted (Fig. 8).

> If the proximal end of the plate is impinging on the side of the radial head and it becomes difficult to place the drill guide into the most proximal hole, it means that the proximal end of the plate is tilted too cranially or that the osteotomy site is too proximal, so plate inclination and osteotomy location should be rechecked.

> If the ulnar bone at the level of the most distal plate hole is too thin or if the hole is not perfectly centred, the cortical screw should be left in place and not replaced by a larger-size locking screw that could put the integrity of the cortex at risk of fracturing.

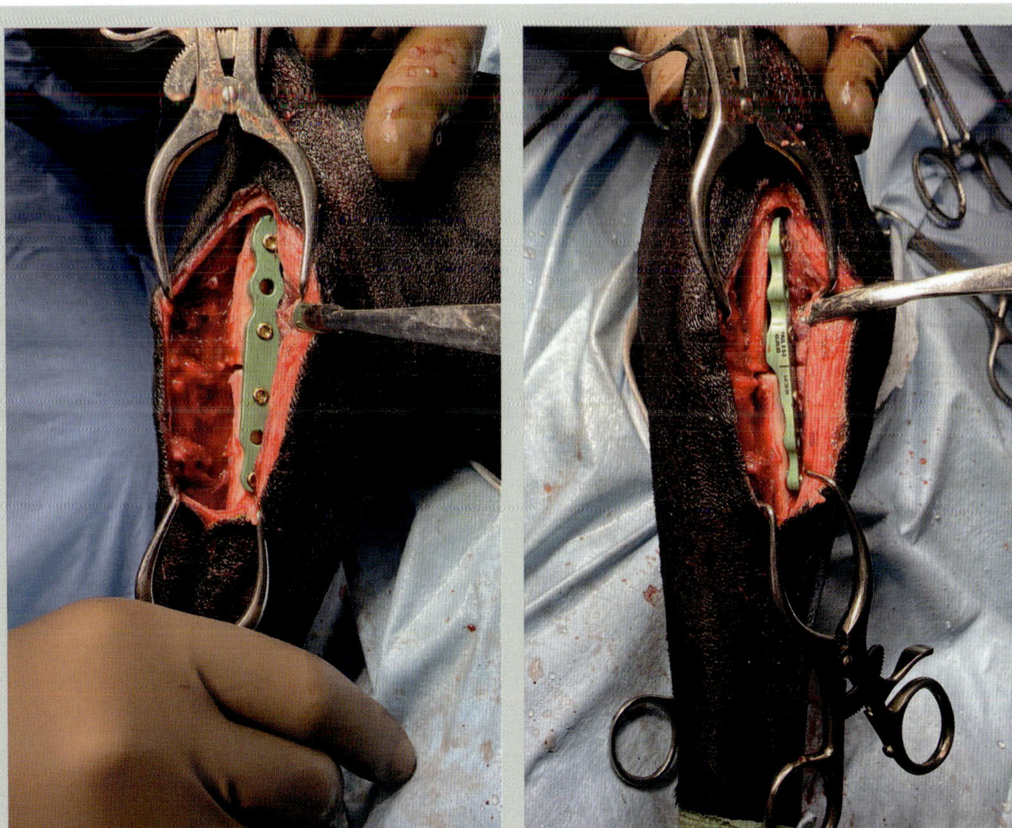

Figure 7. Intraoperative images of a 19-month-old Labrador Retriever undergoing proximal abducting ulnar osteotomy (PAUL) surgery. After performing the osteotomy, the PAUL 9-3 mm plate is being kept in position by four 2.4 mm cortical screws. A small step has been created at the caudal aspect of the ulna to move the medial coronoid process away from the humerus. Care must be taken not to exceed 4 mm of tilt.

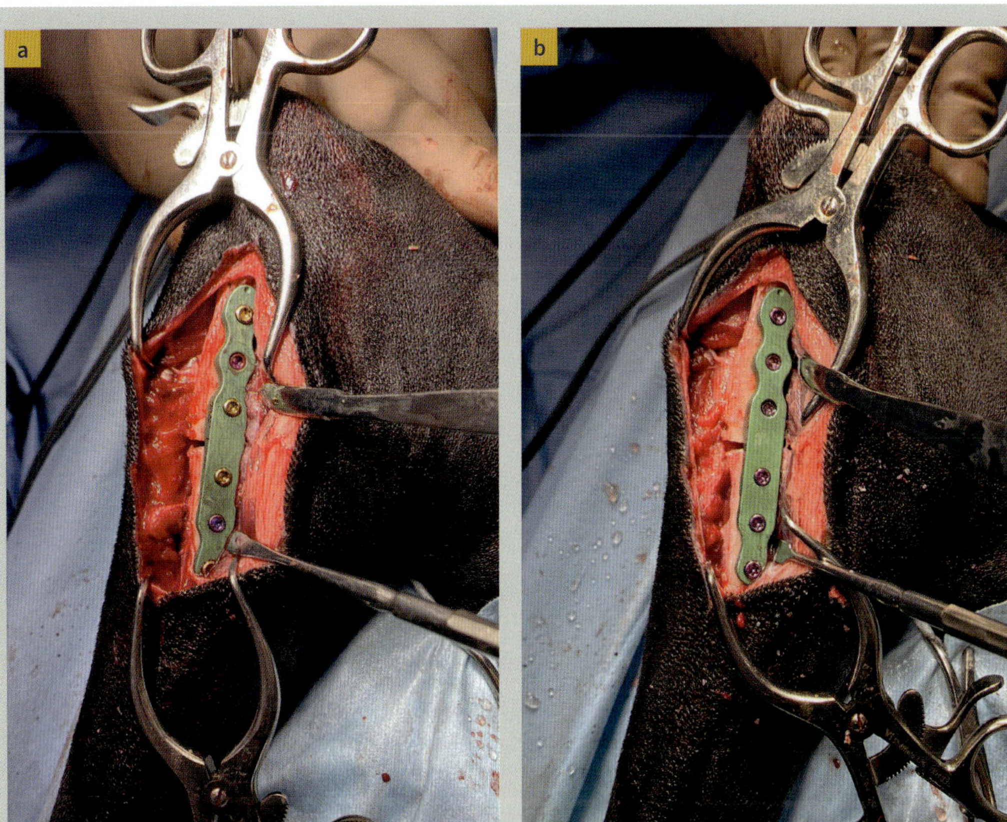

Figure 8. The two remaining empty holes are filled with 3.5 mm locking screws (a). Once the two locking screws are in place, the 2.4 mm cortical screws are sequentially removed and replaced with 3.5 mm locking screws (b). The most distal 2.4 mm cortical screw can be left in place if the drill hole is not perfectly centred in the middle of the ulna but in a position that risks fracturing the cortex.

The antebrachial fascia is then closed using long-lasting absorbable suture material in a continuous pattern, followed by closure of the subcutaneous tissue and skin as per routine.

Outcome

Although this technique has been available for several years, there are very few peer-reviewed scientific clinical studies, and the reported outcomes are mostly based on anecdotal experience of single surgeons. This undoubtedly reflects the difficulty in isolating and objectively assessing a complex disease such as medial compartment disease. One recent study concluded that PAUL had no significant benefits over arthroscopy alone in a cohort of dogs with medial compartment disease when the outcome was assessed by canine brief pain inventory (CBPI) grading, NSAID use and owner-assessed questionnaires (Coghill et al., 2021). Increased age (>3 years) at the time of surgery was associated with an increase in the CBPI score and incidence of NSAID use at follow-up in all dogs. Another recent study assessed the type of complications arising from performing PAUL in 74 limbs (Danielski et al., 2022). Major complications were reported in 13 out of 74 limbs (17.5 %), with 10 limbs needing revision surgery. Increased body weight was the only variable significantly associated with an increased risk of postoperative complications. This study did not attempt to evaluate clinical outcome following PAUL surgery.

In the author's opinion, this is undoubtedly an efficacious technique that is available for the treatment of medial compartment disease, but case selection and precise surgical technique are paramount. Whilst in some cases the author documented formation of de novo fibrocartilage covering the previously completely damaged medial compartment following PAUL, in other cases only small islands of presumed fibrocartilage covering the damaged medial compartment were reported. The former cases had an excellent outcome, whereas the latter cases showed only mild clinical improvement, which is most likely related to the fact that the subchondral bone is still exposed to the inflammatory agents present in the joint fluid.

Compartmental elbow replacement

The canine unicompartmental elbow (CUE) is a joint replacement system which uses humeral and ulnar implants to partially resurface the eburnated joint surfaces of the medial compartment of the elbow with the aim to eliminate bone-on-bone contact throughout the normal stance phase. The two implants are purposefully slightly proud in order to address the collapse of the medial compartment that is so often seen in advanced stages of the disease. When compared to load-shifting osteotomies and total elbow replacement, the CUE has the theoretical advantages of maintaining physiological load transmission and distribution through the joint (while preserving anatomical joint stabilisers), preserving physiological kinematics among humeroulnar, humeroradial and radioulnar joints and avoiding the catastrophic complications related to total joint replacement. A successful CUE surgery leads to the promotion of fibrocartilage ingrowth around the implants by stopping bone-on-bone contact, which also reduces the stimulation of subchondral bone nociceptors and, therefore, pain.

The CUE was developed with the intention of having a straightforward and repeatable procedure, with simple instrumentation and limited implant inventory needs. The humeral component, which has a curvilinear snowman shape, is made of a cobalt-chrome alloy surface mounted on a Biosync porous titanium base that provides good corrosion resistance and enables rapid osseous ingrowth to stabilise the implant (Fig. 9). The ulnar component, in turn, is made of ultrahigh-molecular-weight polyethylene mounted on the same base of Biosync to provide an osseous ingrowth surface (Fig. 10). Both implants are press-fit. The humeral and ulnar components are available in two sizes: medium and large (Franklin et al., 2014; Cook et al., 2015).

The ideal candidates for this procedure are adult dogs (typically between 4 and 12 years of age) with moderate to severe osteoarthritic changes affecting the elbow, lameness and pain poorly responsive to medical treatment, and full-thickness cartilage damage (modified Outerbridge grade IV or V) affecting the medial humeral condyle confirmed by arthroscopy (Fig. 11). Damage to the abaxial side of the radial head is not considered a contraindication for this surgery.

> CUE surgery is not recommended in dogs younger than 4 years, as it is unknown what the effect of wear is on the ulnar implant in the long term.

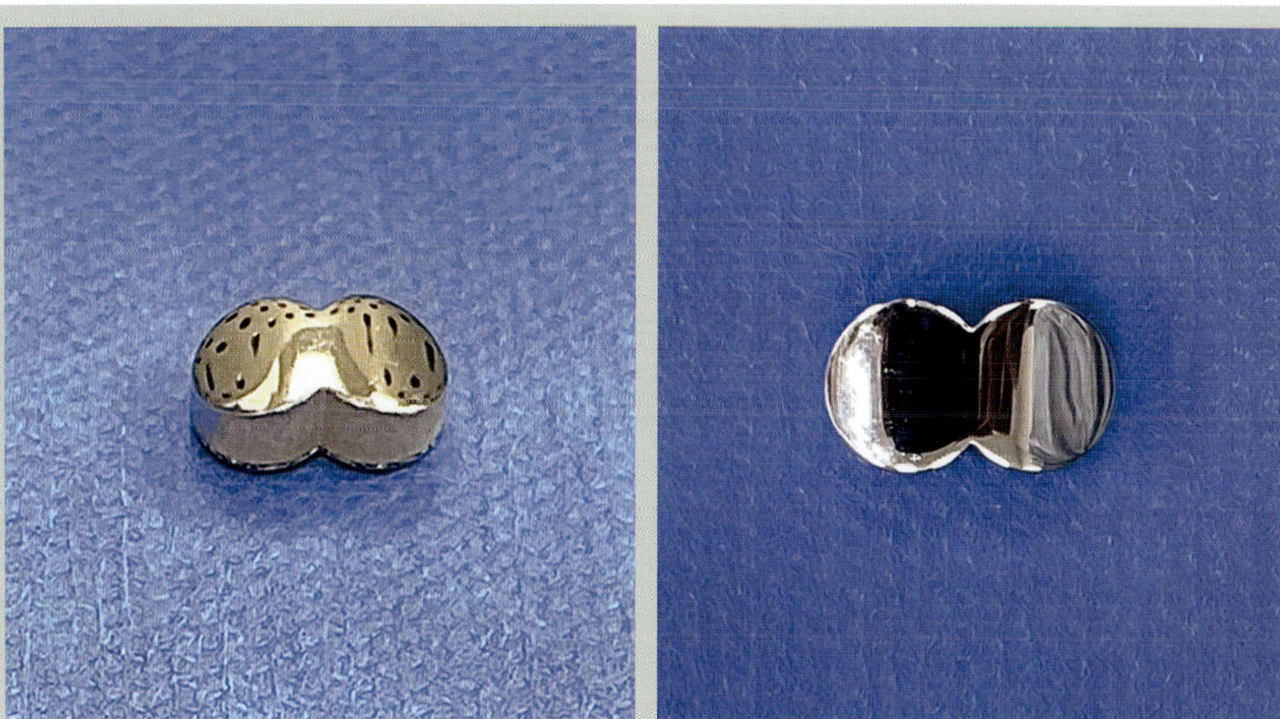

Figure 9. Canine unicompartmental elbow, humeral component. This implant, shaped like a snowman, has a biradial arc of curvature to replicate the normal curvature of the humeral articular surface and allows contact with the ulnar component throughout the stance-phase range of motion of the elbow joint. Note the slightly raised central region of the implant (to stop the collapse of the medial compartment) and the Biosync porous titanium base (to facilitate bone ingrowth).

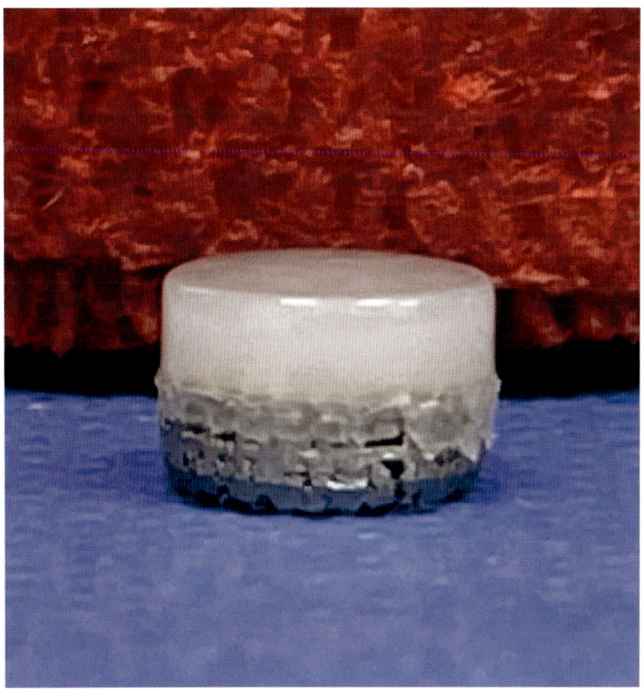

Figure 10. Canine unicompartmental elbow, ulnar component. Single cylindrical implant made of ultrahigh-molecular-weight polyethylene. It is also slightly raised in the middle to help avoid the collapse of the medial compartment. This implant also has a Biosync porous titanium base to provide an osseous ingrowth surface for subchondral bone.

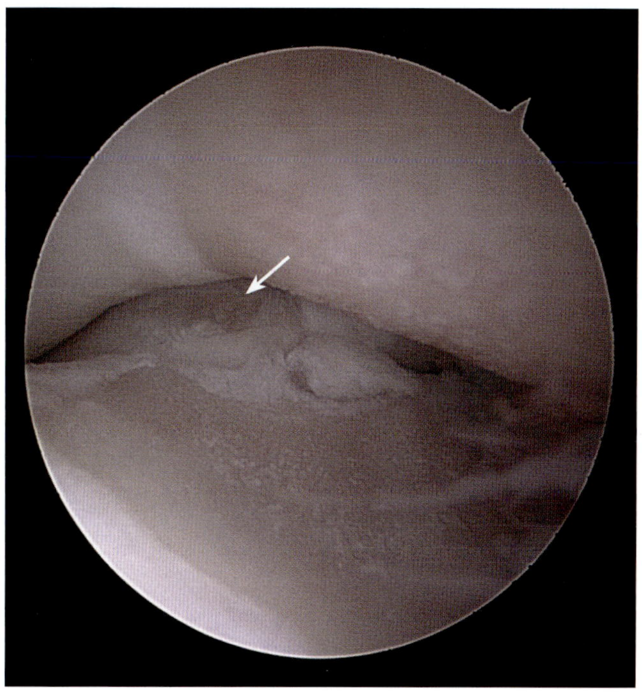

Figure 11. Arthroscopic image of the left elbow of a dog with modified Outerbridge grade IV cartilage damage affecting the medial humeral condyle, the medial coronoid process and the abaxial side of the radial head (arrow).

Surgical technique

Although the original technique describes the use of only one ulnar implant, it is the author's preference to place two implants on the ulna (the second being immediately caudal to the main ulnar implant) to distribute the focal pressure over a larger area and to avoid the superficial wear and plastic deformation of a single implant. The second ulnar implant can be of the same or different size.

The most challenging part of the surgery is usually to achieve adequate exposure of the articular surfaces to allow perpendicular placement of the guide pins and therefore optimal implant placement. A modified Wendelburg caudomedial approach is performed (see chapter "Osteochondrosis of the elbow joint"), allowing subluxation of the ulna and complete access to the coronoid process and humeral surfaces. A 2.4 mm guide pin is inserted perpendicular to the articular surface of the medial coronoid process using an ulnar drill guide to confirm that the ulnar implant will not be too close to the medial or lateral edge of the coronoid process.

If the ulnar drill guide is not sitting in a central position, there is a high risk of breaking the medial or lateral wall of the socket at the time of drilling.

An ulnar socket is then prepared by using a cannulated ulnar reamer inserted over the guide pin (Fig. 12).

When drilling with the reamer, make sure that the hands are kept still and not oscillating; otherwise, the socket will be misshapen and the press-fit effect will be lost (with subsequent movement of the implant).

The guide pin is removed, and the ulnar socket is assessed using a trial ulnar implant. After this, the guide pin is reinserted (blunt side in first) and retrieved on the caudolateral aspect of the ulna (keeping the sharp tip flush with the articular surface), the elbow joint is reduced and put at a weight-bearing angle (135–140 degrees), and the guide pin is driven in to mark on the humeral surface where the centre of the ulnar socket best matches up. The elbow joint is then flexed to approximately 100 degrees and the same operation is repeated. This will ensure correct alignment of the humeral implant reaming and ultimate implant orientation and placement.

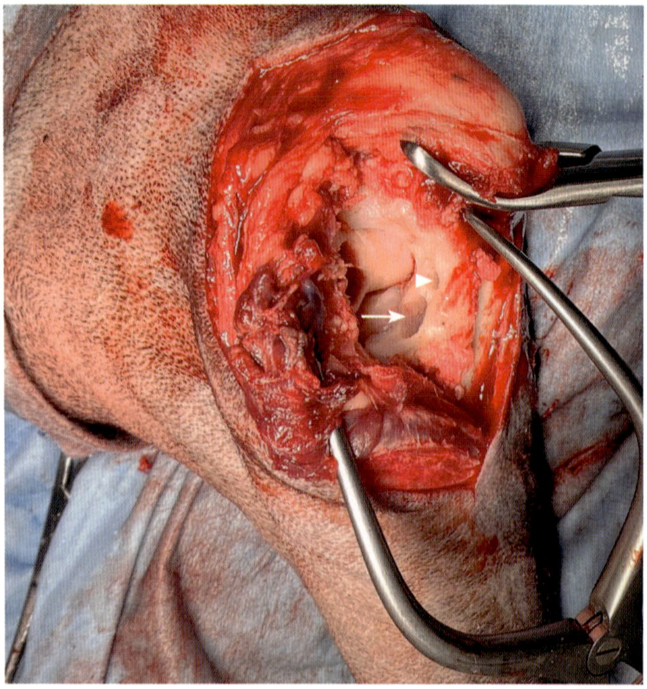

Figure 12. Intraoperative image of a right elbow. A reamer has been used to drill two cylindrical sockets (large, arrow; medium, arrowhead) into the medial ulnar compartment. The exact depth of reaming is guaranteed by the depth stop shoulder of the reamer, ensuring it matches the height of the ulnar implants.

A humeral guide is then placed along the sagittal line created by the previous pin marks, and two guide pins are placed parallel to each other into the guide. A cannulated humeral reamer is inserted over the guide pins and used to drill the humeral sockets (Fig. 13). After flushing the sockets with saline, a humeral template is used to confirm correct reaming depth. The final ulnar and humeral implants are then tapped into the sockets, taking care not to scratch or damage the exposed surface (Fig. 14). The elbow joint is reduced, and the antebrachial fascia is closed with long-lasting absorbable suture material. The rest of the soft tissue is closed as per routine.

Two postoperative mediolateral radiographs, one with the elbow in extension and one with the elbow at approximately 100 degrees, should be taken to confirm appropriate contact between the humeral and ulnar implants throughout the stance phase of the patient (Fig. 15).

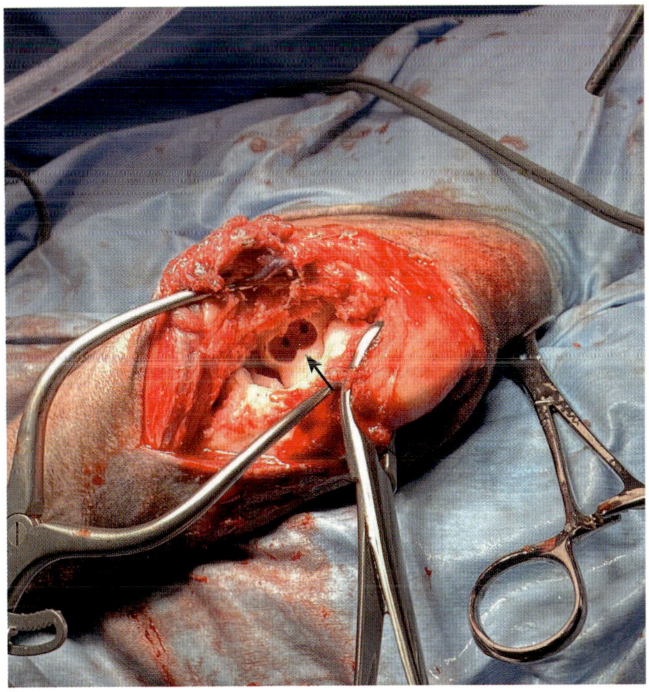

Figure 13. Each humeral socket is reamed sequentially to create the snowman-shaped socket (arrow) that matches the prosthesis. If reaming is adequate, the humeral implant will seat within the sockets such that its cranial and caudal ends are flush with the articular surface and its centre is 0–2 mm proud.

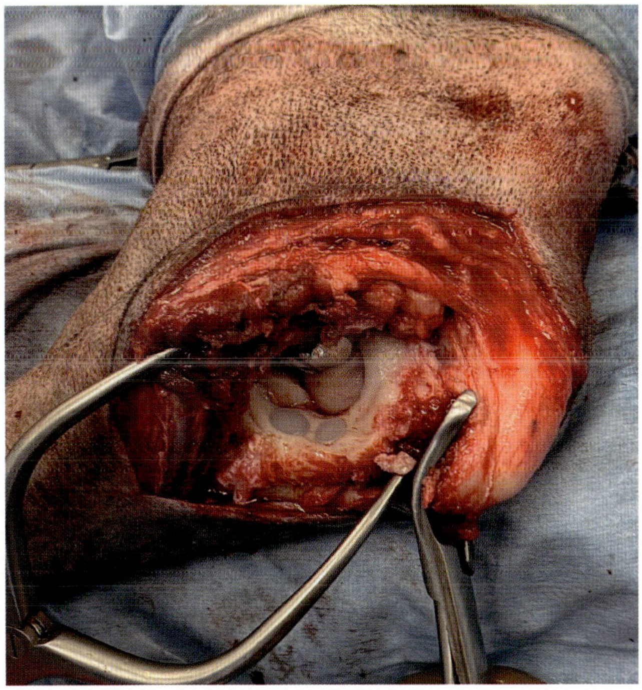

Figure 14. Intraoperative image after placement of the final prostheses (a large humeral implant and two ulnar implants, large and medium).

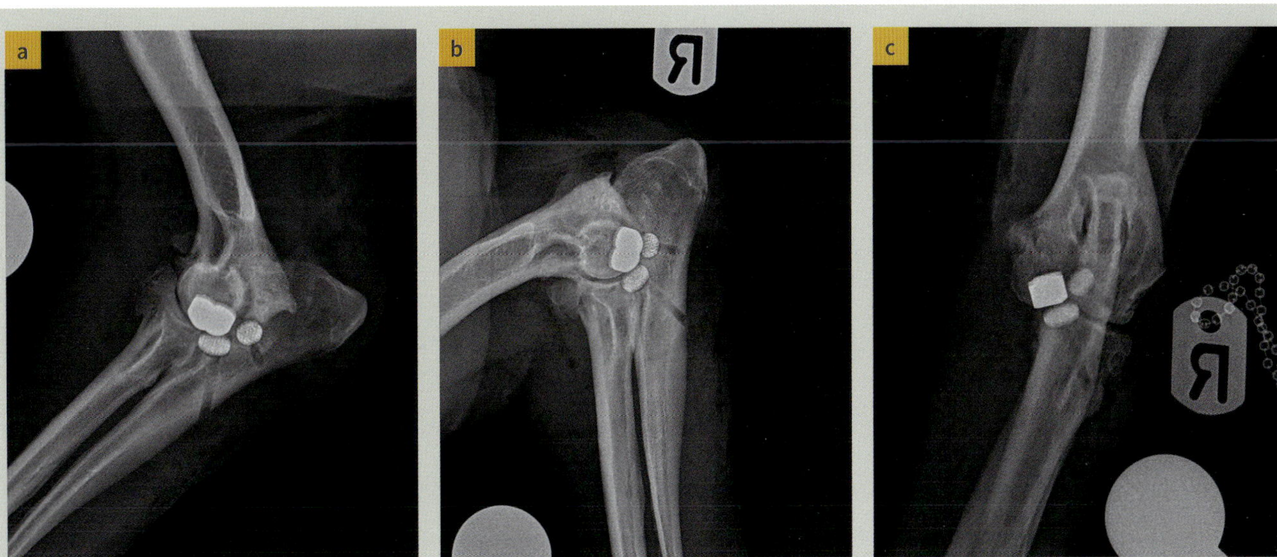

Figure 15. Postoperative mediolateral radiographs are performed to ascertain contact between the humeral and ulnar implants throughout the stance-phase range of motion of the elbow joint (a, b). Implant parallelism can be assessed on a craniocaudal radiograph (c).

Outcome and complications

There are only two scientific articles published analysing the outcome of CUE surgery in dogs. Cook et al. (2015) reported mid- to long-term results of CUE surgeries performed in multiple institutions by several surgeons. The procedure, performed in 103 dogs, was associated with 1 catastrophic (1 %), 11 major (10.7 %) and 28 minor (27.2 %) complications. Outcomes following CUE surgery were reported as full function in 49 cases (47.6 %), acceptable in 45 cases (43.7 %) and unacceptable in 9 cases (8.7 %) at a 6-month or later follow-up. This study involved the use of tenotomy of the flexor tendons at their origin on the medial epicondyle or osteotomy of the medial epicondyle while maintaining the attachment of origin of the flexor muscles. A second more recent study evaluated the clinical outcome in 44 dogs (52 CUE procedures) in which a caudomedial approach (Wendelburg approach) to the elbow joint was instead performed (Bayer et al., 2019). Complications occurred in 11 cases (21 %), being major in 8 (15 %) and minor in 3 (6 %). Major complications included refractory pain and lameness 6–12 months postoperatively (5 cases), intraoperative fracture of the radius or ulna (1 case each) and septic arthritis together with ulnar implant loosening (1 case). At the last follow-up, 12 cases (25 %) were considered to have full function, 35 cases (73 %) had acceptable function and in 1 case the function was considered unacceptable. The results suggested that older dogs might be at risk of having an inferior clinical outcome when compared to young patients. Second-look arthroscopy in 5 cases with delayed or disappointing functional improvement showed evidence of implant-related contact lesions and progressive erosion of the medial coronoid area in three elbows.

The latter finding is probably the most important limitation to this technique and the reason why patient selection is so critical. The author recommends not to perform this technique in dogs younger than 4 years, as it is unknown what the life span of the implants or the percentage of cases suffering from progressive cartilage/implant erosion are. In the author's experience, in such cases, although persistent mild lameness is present at a walk, orthopaedic examination usually reveals significant improvement of the degree of discomfort associated with elbow manipulation.

OSTEOCHONDROSIS OF THE ELBOW JOINT

Alan Danielski

INTRODUCTION

As previously discussed in chapter "Generalities of osteochondritis dissecans", osteochondrosis (OC) is an abnormality of the endochondral ossification process that can affect, among other areas, the medial humeral condyle. It is frequently recognised in young, large-breed dogs and is more common in male dogs. The pathogenesis and aetiology of OC is not fully understood, but it is believed to be a multifactorial condition. Genetics, diet (excessive intake of calcium and/or vitamin D_3), excessive exercise in skeletally immature dogs, rapid growth rate and trauma have been implicated. The shoulder is the most commonly affected joint followed by the elbow, stifle and tarsus.

TREATMENT

CONSERVATIVE TREATMENT

Conservative management of elbow OC includes body weight control, exercise modification, nutraceutical supplementation and administration of nonsteroidal anti-inflammatory drugs.

SURGICAL TREATMENT

Traditional surgical treatment involves removal of the cartilage flap and debridement of the subchondral bone arthroscopically or via medial arthrotomy. The aim of this procedure is to allow fibrocartilaginous infilling of the osteochondral defect. Although there is no clinical evidence supporting the superiority of hyaline cartilage over fibrocartilage, this technique has been questioned because of the inferior biomechanical properties of fibrocartilage in experimental models (Minas and Nehrer, 1997). In fact, it has been reported that although dogs may improve clinically after surgical treatment, many have ongoing lameness and degenerative joint disease is progressive despite surgical treatment (Minas and Nehrer, 1997).

Restorative techniques have been developed to address this problem. Osteochondral autograft transfer involves transplantation of one or more cylindrical cores of articular cartilage harvested from the stifle joint. However, several important limitations to this technique need to be acknowledged. These include the morbidity associated with osteochondral graft collection and the nonhomogeneous distribution of cartilage thickness harvested from donor sites in the distal aspect of the canine femur. Consequently, research has focused on synthetic osteochondral implants in humans, horses and dogs. The use of a synthetic implant consisting of a surface layer of polycarbonate urethane and a bone ingrowth material (SynACART, Arthrex Vet Systems) for the treatment of OC lesions in the shoulder and stifle in dogs has been reported with favourable results (Danielski and Farrell, 2018; Egan et al., 2018). This is the author's preferred treatment technique and is described below.

A modified Wendelburg approach to the caudomedial aspect of the elbow is used. With the dog in dorsal recumbency, standard arthroscopy is performed to confirm presence of the OC lesion. A sandbag placed next to the patient's body under the distal humerus is used as a fulcrum during arthroscopy and during the procedure to help gain access to the joint. Perfect patient positioning is mandatory to maximise visualisation of the joint structures once the approach has been performed. The caudal ulnar spine, medial humeral epicondyle and medial olecranon ridge are palpated (the ulnar spine goes from the tip of the olecranon to the proximal third of the caudal ulna and is easily palpable below the skin, especially at its proximal aspect). The skin incision starts slightly medial to the ulnar spine at the level of the proximal third of the ulna. The incision continues proximally between the olecranon and the medial humeral epicondyle to the point over the olecranon ridge along the medial border of the triceps muscle (Fig. 1). The antebrachial fascia is exposed and incised directly over the ulnar spine. The incision is then extended proximally towards the olecranon. This will expose the flexor carpi ulnaris muscle just cranial to the incision. This muscle is elevated all the way up to the tubercle where it is attached (ulnar head). The muscle is then elevated from the bone in a caudocranial direction with a freer or an AO periosteal elevator

(Fig. 2). Gelpi retractors are helpful to retract the belly of the flexor carpi ulnaris muscle cranially and expose the caudal aspect of the elbow joint. The joint capsule attachment to the ulna should then become visible. Elevation is continued more cranially in the direction of the medial coronoid process until the fan-shaped attachment of the biceps ulnaris tendon on the medial coronoid process becomes visible (Fig. 3).

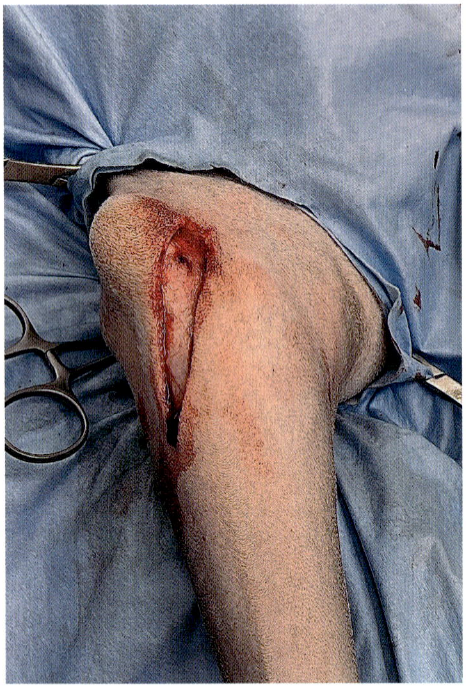

Figure 1. The skin is incised on the caudal aspect of the antebrachium along the spine of the ulna.

The joint capsule is then incised near the attachment on the ulnar side, taking care not to damage the surrounding tissue or the articular surface. The incision is continued proximally to the anconeal process, and the articular surface of the medial humeral condyle should become apparent (Fig. 4). The medial collateral ligament is identified just cranial to the tip of the medial coronoid process, and a blunt Hohmann retractor is inserted lateral to the medial collateral ligament in the front of the radial head to retract all soft tissues cranially, including the ulnar nerve, and protect them (Fig. 5). Release of the biceps brachii muscle insertion along the medial aspect of the medial collateral ligament is performed to improve the opening of the joint space when exerting supination of the ulna. A medium-sized bone clamp placed at the level of the olecranon is used to act as a lever arm for further pronation of the ulna, improving access to the medial joint compartment. In dogs with arthritic elbows, marked osteophytosis can be found where the joint capsule inserts onto the ulna. In these cases, the excess osteophytes need to be removed with rongeurs or

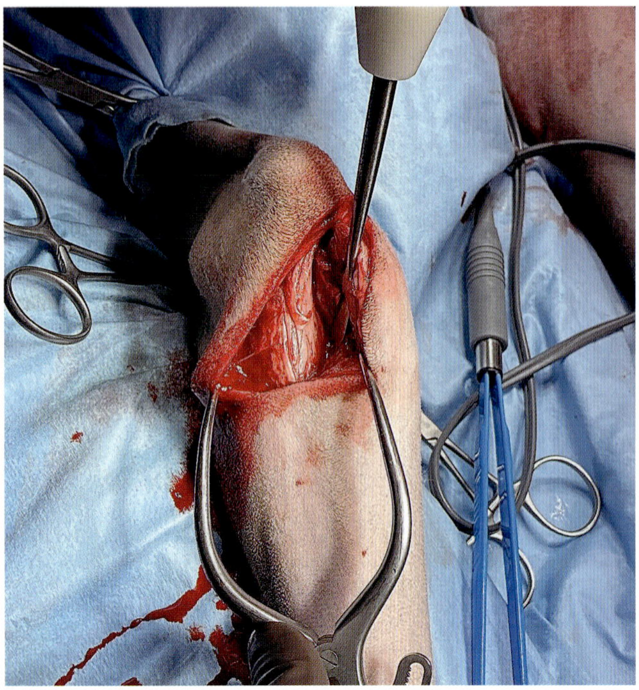

Figure 2. The soft tissues are elevated from the medial aspect of the ulna.

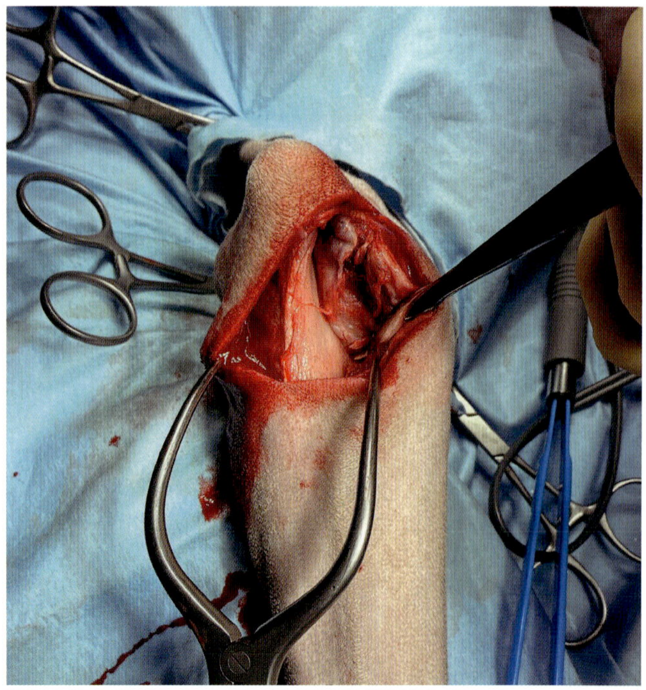

Figure 3. The joint capsule, the medial coronoid process, the medial collateral ligament and the fan-shaped insertion of biceps brachii muscle on the coronoid process are exposed.

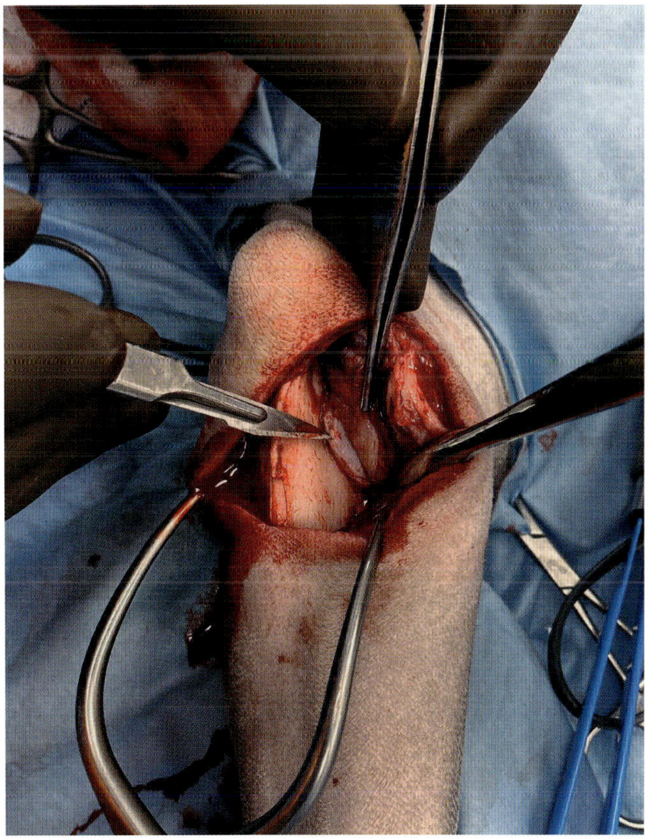

Figure 4. The joint capsule is sharply incised to gain access to the elbow joint.

a high speed burr to allow sufficient access to the joint for implant placement (Fig. 6).

SynACART implants are available in diameters of 8, 10, 15, 20 and 22 mm (Fig. 7). A guide is first placed against the humeral trochlea. It is very important to ensure that the guide is perfectly perpendicular and as flush as possible to the articular surface and not tilted in any direction.

A 2.4 mm drill guide pin is driven through the guide to secure the site. For this, the guide is held perpendicular against the joint surface and held securely into position at the correct location. The pin is then driven into the humeral condyle whilst the pin and the area are irrigated with sterile saline.

> It is mandatory to have the guide and the pin perfectly perpendicular to the articular surface in order to allow the implant to sit flush to the articular surface.

An appropriately sized reamer is then advanced over the guide pin until it reaches the joint. Once the reamer is in place, drilling commences and the recipient socket for the implant is created (Fig. 8). Once the reaming process

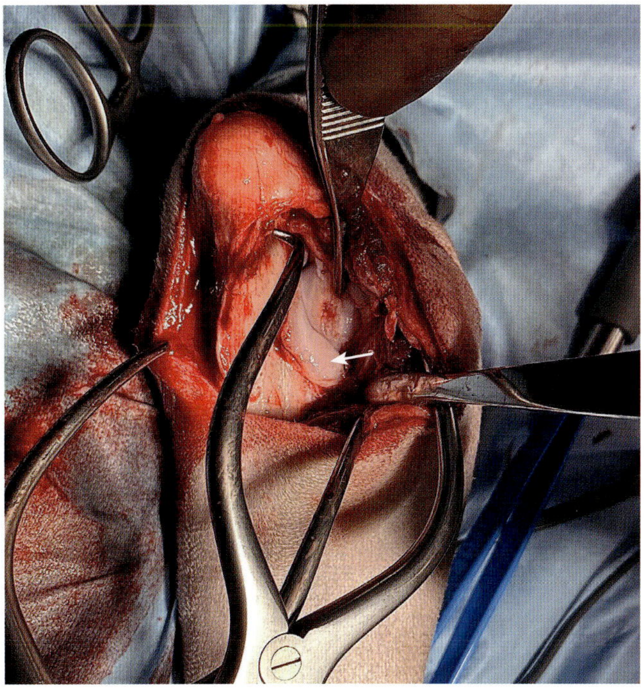

Figure 5. The OC lesion on the humeral condyle becomes visible when the elbow is flexed to about 90–110 degrees. Note the large number of osteophytes present on the ulna at the level of the insertion of the joint capsule (arrow).

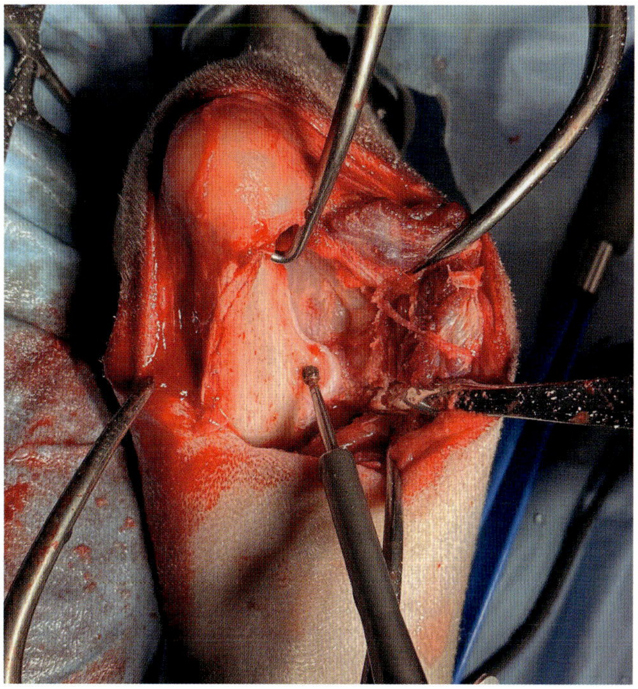

Figure 6. Osteophytes are removed with a high-speed burr to allow better access to the elbow joint and to the medial humeral condyle.

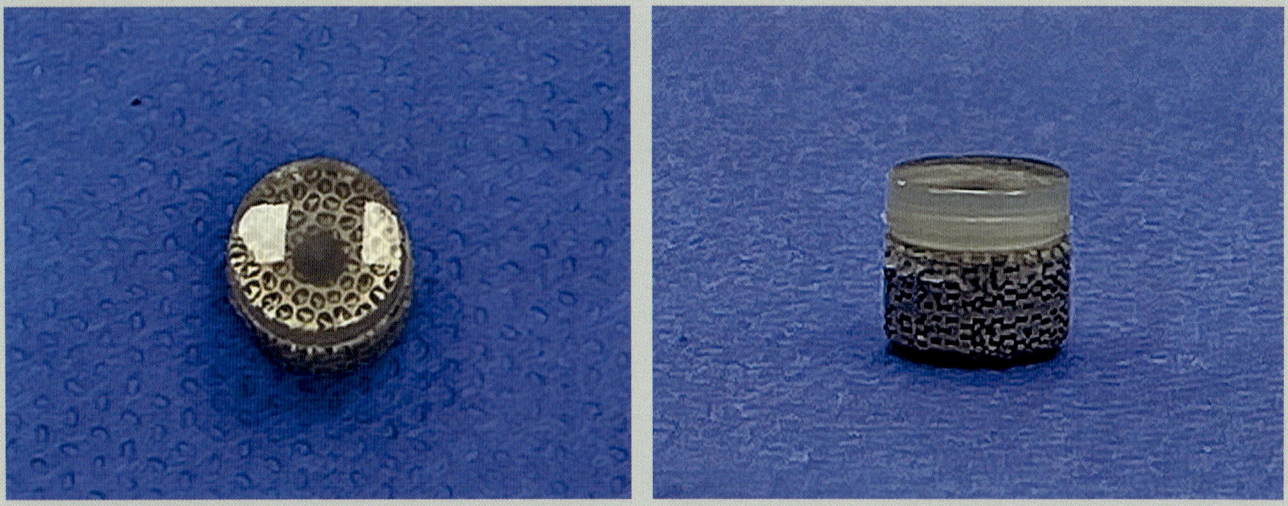

Figure 7. 8 × 8 mm osteochondral implant utilised in this case (SynACART, Arthrex Vet Systems). The deep layer is composed of lattice-type titanium to facilitate bone ingrowth. The surface layer is composed of polycarbonate urethane.

is completed, the reamer is removed along with the guide pin. The socket is inspected, gently cleaned and flushed to remove debris (Fig. 9). The SynACART implant is then placed into the osteochondral defect using a tamped, press-fit technique (Fig. 10). The edges of the implant should be flush with the articular surface and no steps should be present.

Closure is performed as per routine. The antebrachial fascia is identified and closed primarily using long-lasting monofilament suture material such as polydioxanone. It is not necessary to close the joint capsule, nor to suture the flexor carpi ulnaris muscle.

> A strict aseptic technique needs to be used throughout the surgery to avoid the risk of infection. Deep infection leads to bone reabsorption around the titanium mesh and implant loosening, which requires implant removal.

POSTOPERATIVE MANAGEMENT

A compression bandage is applied postoperatively to the limb (making sure that the bandage extends proximally to the elbow joint) and is kept in place for 5 days. Postoperative analgesia is provided by administration of methadone (0.2 mg/kg) followed by buprenorphine (0.02 mg/kg, after

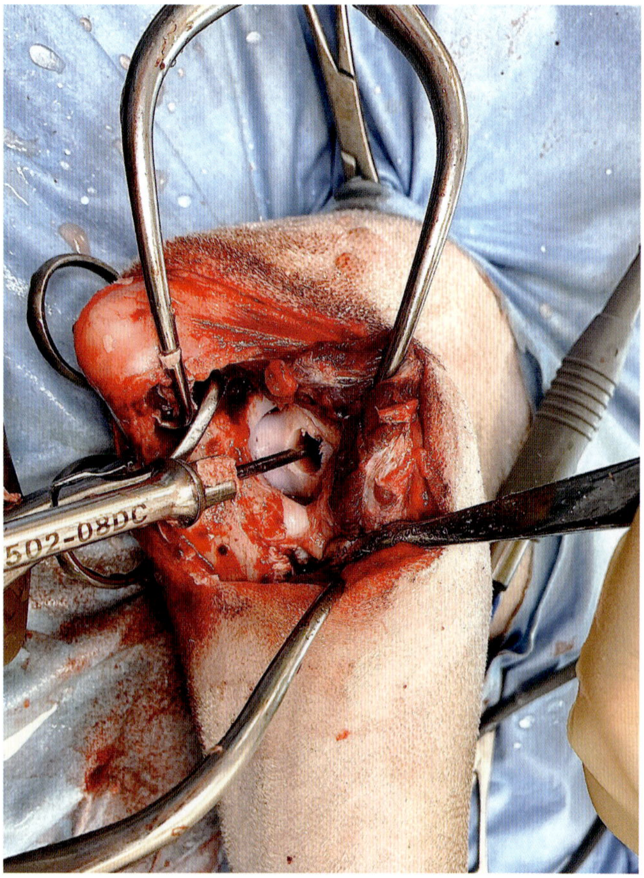

Figure 8. An osteochondral defect is created using an 8 mm alignment guide centred on the exposed OC lesion. A 2.4 mm diameter guide pin is placed through the centre of the alignment guide, perpendicular to the surface of the lesion, and drilled to a depth of approximately 2 cm into the medial humeral condyle. An 8 mm diameter depth-controlled reamer is placed over the guide pin and used to create an osteochondral defect of 8 mm in diameter and 8 mm in depth.

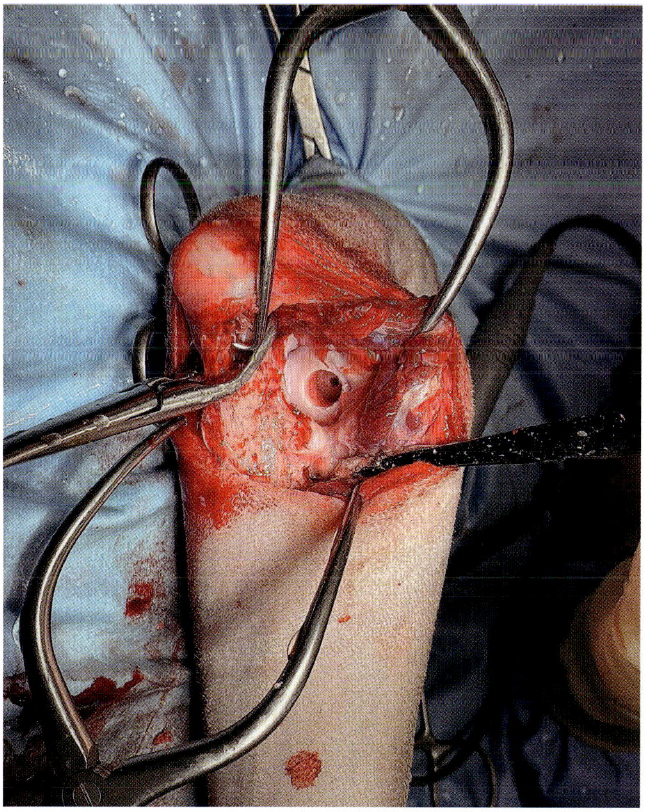

Figure 9. Appearance of the osteochondral defect after being flushed with saline to remove debris.

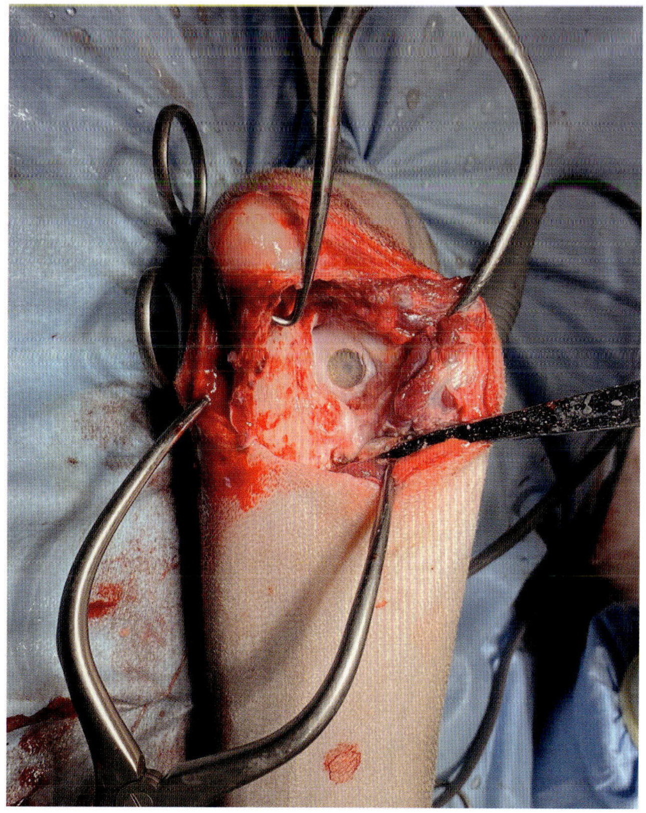

Figure 10. The implant is placed into the osteochondral defect using a tamped, press-fit technique.

6–12 hours). Antibiotic therapy is administered peri- and postoperatively for a total of 7–10 days. Oral nonsteroidal anti-inflammatory drugs are provided for 3 weeks.

The patient is discharged with instructions of cage confinement for 6 weeks and room confinement for 6 more weeks. Slow-paced lead walks are allowed from day one up to three times a day. Lead exercise can be increased by 5–10 minutes per walk on a weekly basis. Hydrotherapy is usually recommended after 6 weeks to increase the muscle tone of the thoracic limbs and eliminate any residual joint stiffness.

OUTCOME AND COMPLICATIONS

Whilst in the veterinary literature there are several reports describing the use of SynACART implants in shoulder and stifle joints as a treatment for OC, there is a lack of scientific studies reporting clinical outcomes and complications following their use in the elbow joint. Infection (with the risk of subsequent implant loosening) is the major postoperative risk, and a strict aseptic protocol is therefore recommended at the time of surgery.

SHORT ULNA SYNDROME

Miguel Solano

INTRODUCTION

Radioulnar incongruence is the most common form of elbow incongruence. This can be caused by physeal trauma or congenital factors (DeCamp et al., 2015). Chondrodystrophoid breeds are predisposed to asynchronous growth of the radius and ulna, generally resulting in a shorter ulna relative to the radius. Premature closure of the distal physis of the ulna has been reported as the most common growth plate injury in dogs (Johnston and Tobias, 2018). The V shape of the distal ulnar physis is likely to play a role in the high incidence of its premature closure versus the relatively flat shape of the proximal and distal radial physes (Fig. 1). In addition to this morphological difference, the distal physis of the ulna is responsible for 100 % of the growth in length below the elbow joint. Therefore, disturbances in the distal ulnar physis result in greater alteration than the ones involving the radial physis.

After premature closure of the distal ulna, the radius typically continues to grow, often leading to radial procurvatum, radial torsion, carpal valgus and elbow incongruence.

> Short ulna syndrome may lead to elbow incongruence and abnormal carpal loading, subsequently leading to the development of elbow and carpal osteoarthritis (OA).

CLINICAL PRESENTATION AND DIAGNOSIS

> Early diagnosis of short ulna syndrome simplifies its management.

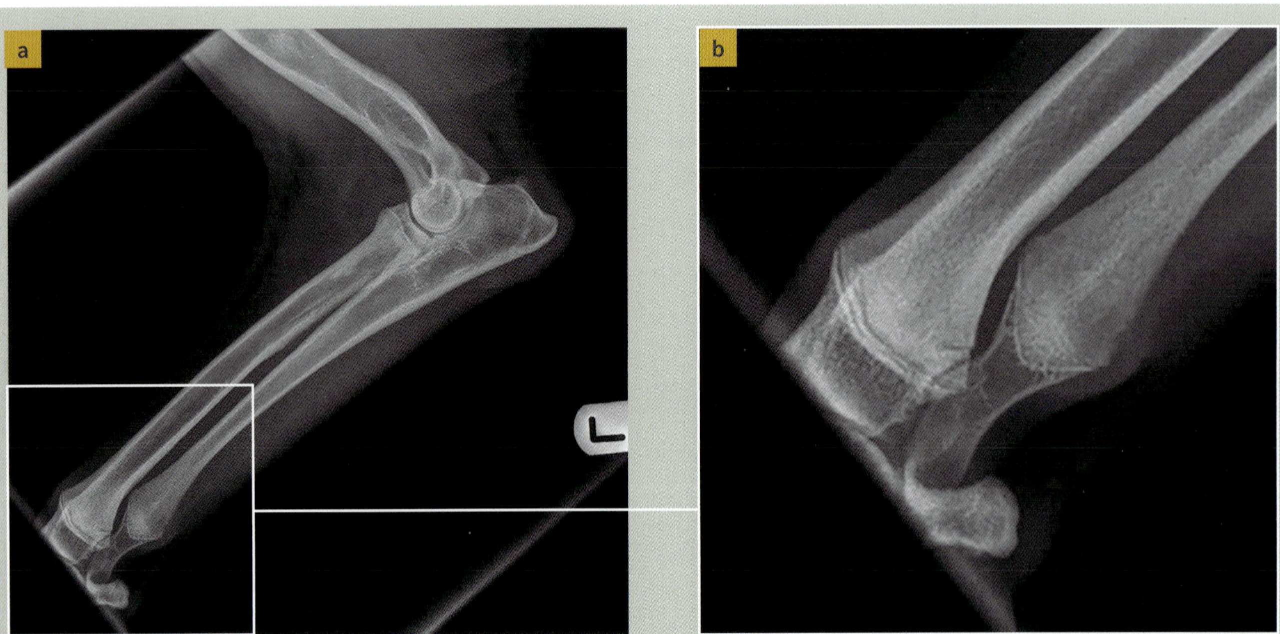

Figure 1. Mediolateral radiograph of the antebrachium of a skeletally immature dog showing a V-shaped distal ulnar physis versus a relatively flat distal radial physis (a). Detail of the distal ulnar and radial physes (b).

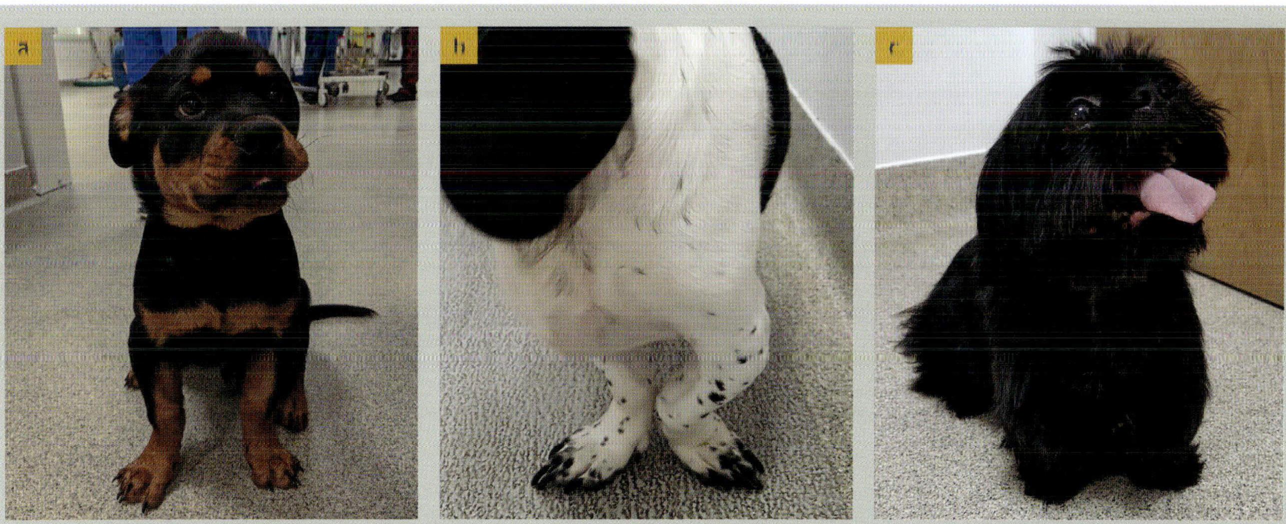

Figure 2. Rottweiler puppy with signs of carpal valgus in the right thoracic limb (a). Basset Hound with severe signs of carpal valgus, radial procurvatum and torsion in the left thoracic limb (b). Shih Tzu with bilateral signs of antebrachial limb deformity (c).

Lameness associated with elbow incongruence is the most common reason for clinical presentation of skeletally immature dogs. On some occasions, the owners may have noticed a disparity/deformity involving the two thoracic limbs, with or without witnessing lameness (Figs. 2 and 3), although noticing some degree of deformity beyond the "standard" of a particular chondrodystrophoid breed can be particularly challenging for owners. In older patients, lameness may be associated with elbow and/or carpal OA.

On physical examination, patients generally have pain associated with elbow manipulation (Video 1). Some dogs may show signs of partial lateral subluxation of the radial head.

Video 1. Same dog as in Figure 3 showing significant pain on carpal manipulation.

Orthogonal radiographs of the full antebrachium (from elbow to carpus) of both the affected and contralateral limbs should be taken to assess elbow incongruence. In patients with short ulna syndrome, the medial coronoid process tends to be located lower than the radial head. In addition, the space surrounding the humeral condyle may be reduced close to the anconeal region and widened distally (Fig. 4).

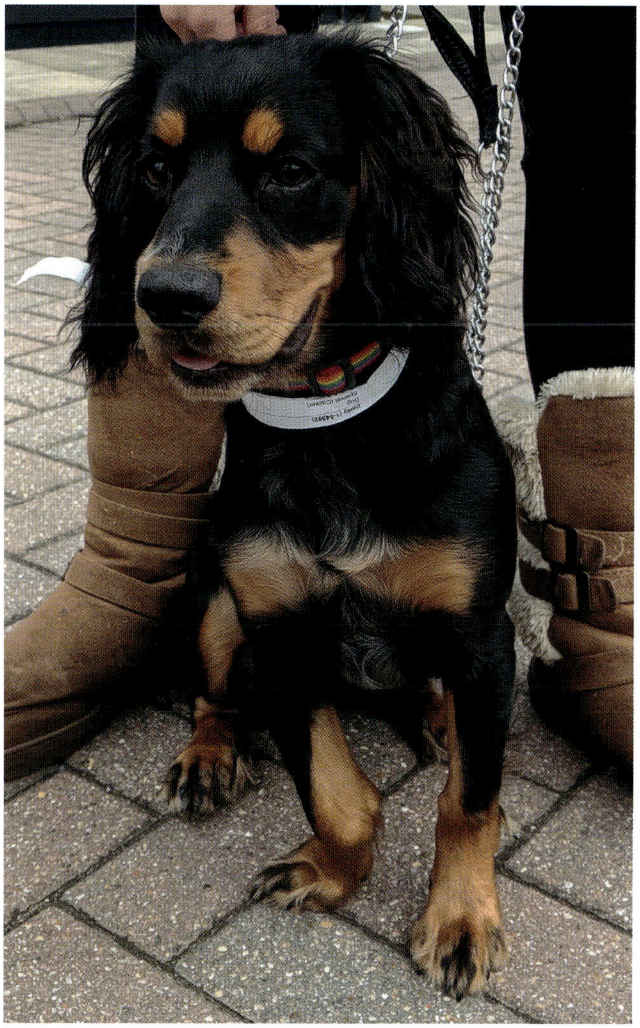

Figure 3. Young dog with a severe antebrachial limb deformity. Note the marked carpal valgus and radial procurvatum.

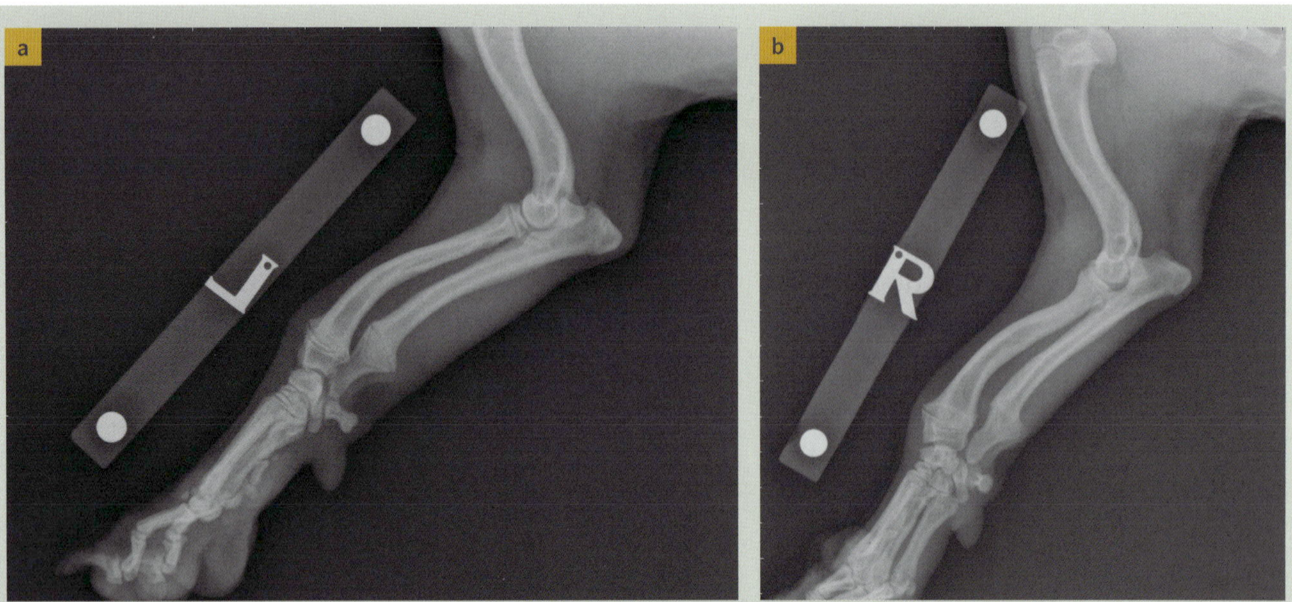

Figure 4. Mediolateral radiograph of the left antebrachium of a skeletally immature chondrodystrophoid dog (a). Mediolateral radiograph of the right antebrachium of the same dog showing short ulna syndrome (b). Note the degree of humeroulnar and radioulnar incongruence and the reduced joint space between the humeral condyle and anconeal process. The position of the medial coronoid process is lower than that of the radial head.

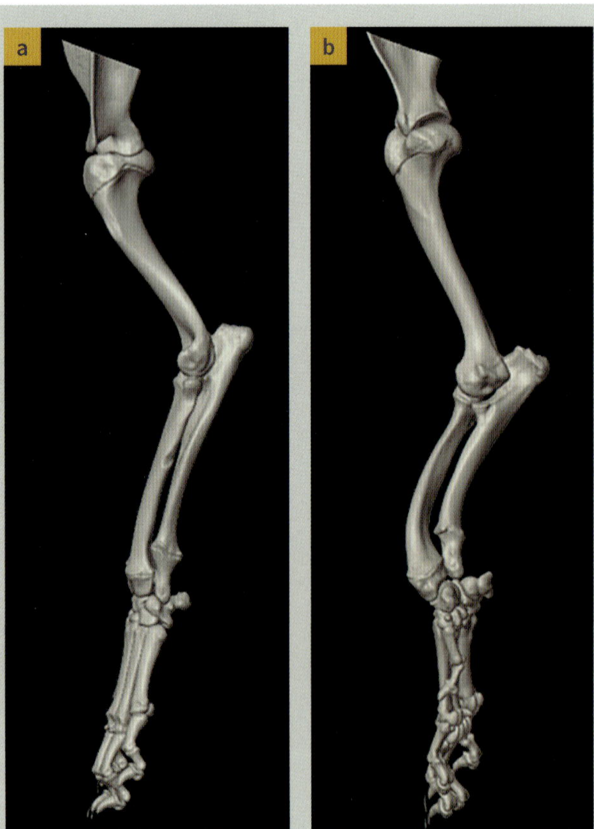

Figure 5. Three-dimensional volume-rendered CT images of a dog with a normal left antebrachium (a) and a contralateral thoracic limb showing a shorter ulna, elbow incongruence, radial procurvatum and radial torsion (b).

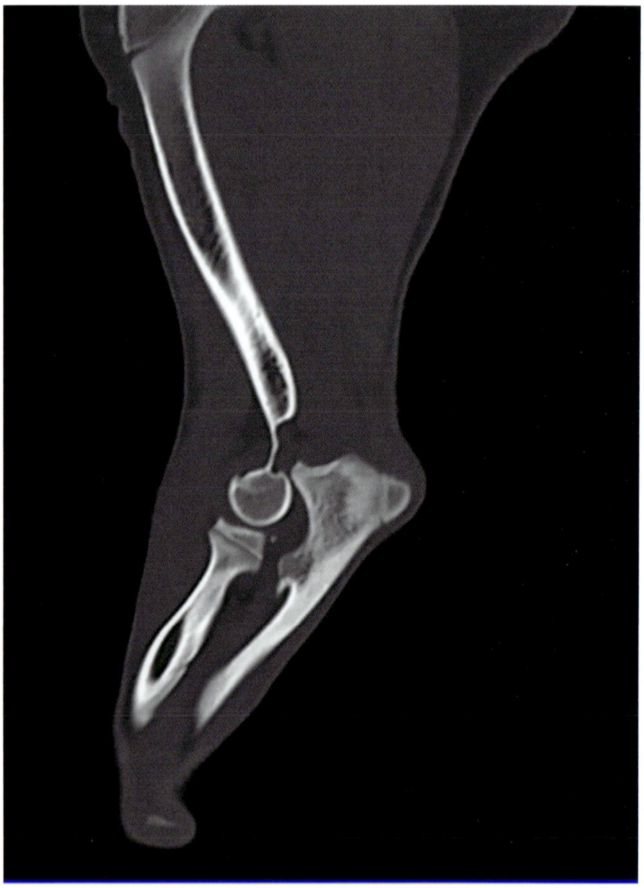

Figure 6. Sagittal plane CT image of the same dog as in Figure 2b showing humeroulnar and radioulnar incongruence.

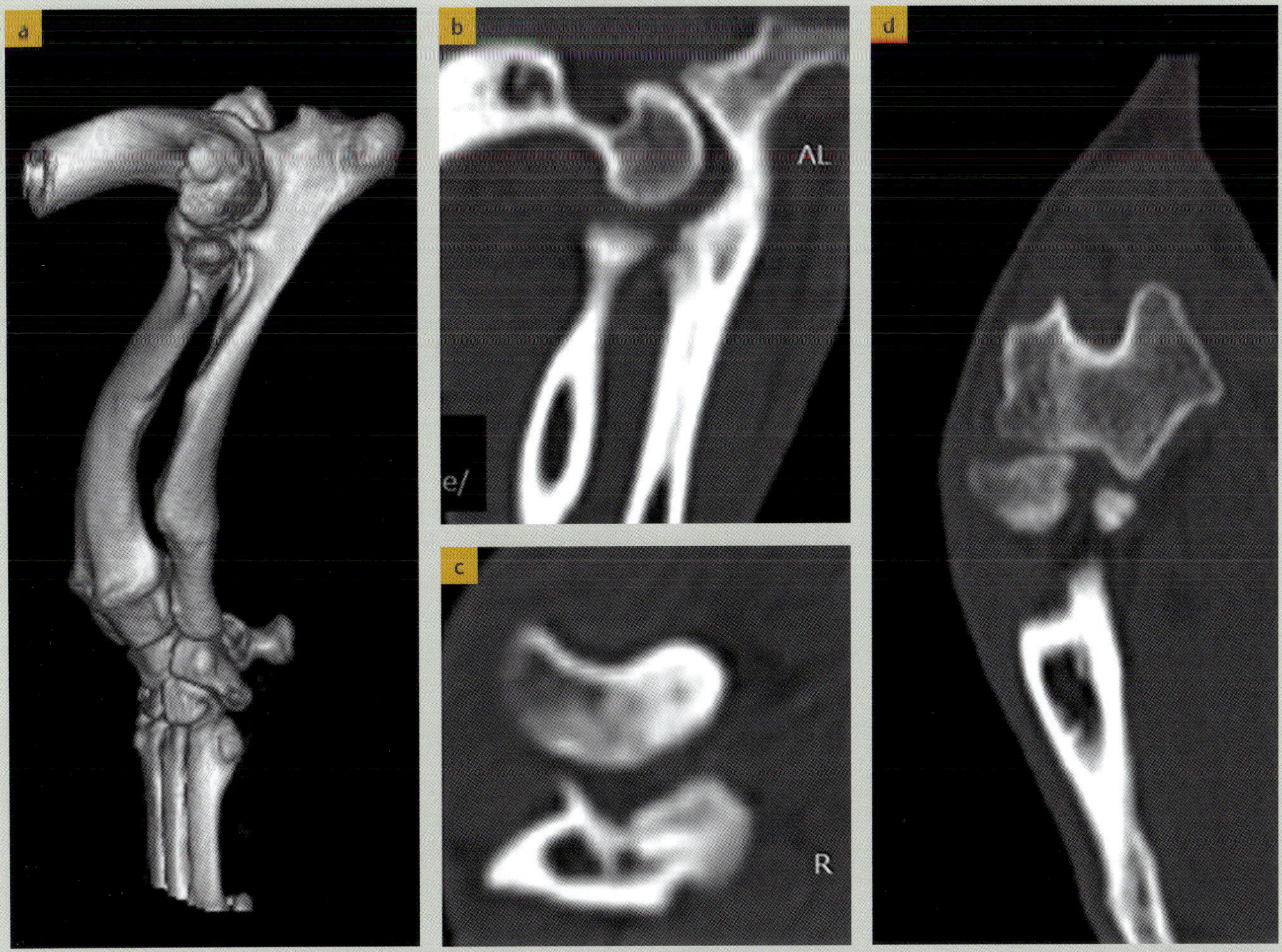

Figure 7. Three-dimensional volume-rendered CT image (a) and sagittal (b), transverse (c) and frontal (d) plane CT images of a skeletally mature dog with short ulna syndrome. Radial deformity leading to elbow incongruence can be seen.

Dogs predisposed to ununited anconeal process (UAP) can present with concurrent classic signs of short ulna syndrome (see chapter "Ununited anconeal process").

CT is an ideal tool to precisely quantify multiplanar deformities associated with short ulna syndrome (Figs. 5–7). It can also be used for accurate planning of the surgical correction, for creating three-dimensional printed guides and custom implants and for practising the execution of the correction in stereolithographic models (Worth et al., 2019) (Fig. 8).

> The use of CT for multiplanar deformity quantification and three-dimensional printing-assisted surgical corrections leads to excellent outcomes in dogs with angular and rotational limb deformity (ARLD).

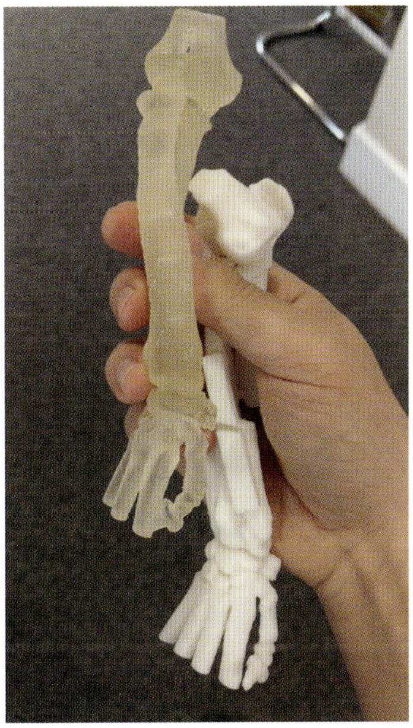

Figure 8. Three-dimensional printed stereolithographic models of the antebrachium of a dog with an antebrachial limb deformity before (left) and after (right) correction.

TREATMENT

SURGICAL TREATMENT

Corrective surgery is advised when there is altered mobility and exercise intolerance or to reduce the progression of secondary OA of the carpus and elbow (Fox, 1984; Ramadan and Vaughan, 1978; O'brien et al., 1971).

Key factors in decision-making in the management of short ulna syndrome are patient skeletal maturity (open versus closed radial physis), the presence of a significant radial deformity leading to carpal valgus and, in older patients, the presence of severe carpal OA/pain. The current evidence on decision-making is sparse and rather poor. The expected displacement on a proximodistal and mediolateral plane after ulnar osteotomy/ostectomy is likely influenced by several factors (e.g. age of the patient, angle of proximal ulnar osteotomy [PUO], height of PUO, postoperative activity, interosseous ligament disruption) and is not well defined in the literature. Figure 9 presents the author's proposed guidelines for the management of short ulna syndrome based on the current literature and personal experience. These guidelines are likely to change over time as our understanding of the condition improves.

Skeletally immature dogs with an open distal radial physis and no obvious signs of bone deformity nor elbow incongruence

In these patients, a distal ulnar ostectomy (DUO) can be considered to allow the radius to continue growing without restrictions. The optimal length of the ostectomy has not been established. Factors to take into consideration are the patient's age and breed (small- versus giant-breed dogs). In very young giant-breed dogs (e.g. a 4-month-old Great Dane), multiple ostectomies may be necessary to allow the radius to fully grow without disturbances. Additional ostectomies should be considered in dogs whose ulna heals before the radius completes longitudinal growth. Periodic (every 3–4 weeks) radiographs should be taken to monitor the need for additional ostectomies (Figs. 10 and 11). Disruption of the periosteum at the level of the ostectomy site (Johnston and Tobias, 2017), placement of a graft at the DUO site and performing a DUO of 1.5 times the diameter

Figure 9. Proposed decision-making algorithm for management of short ulna syndrome.

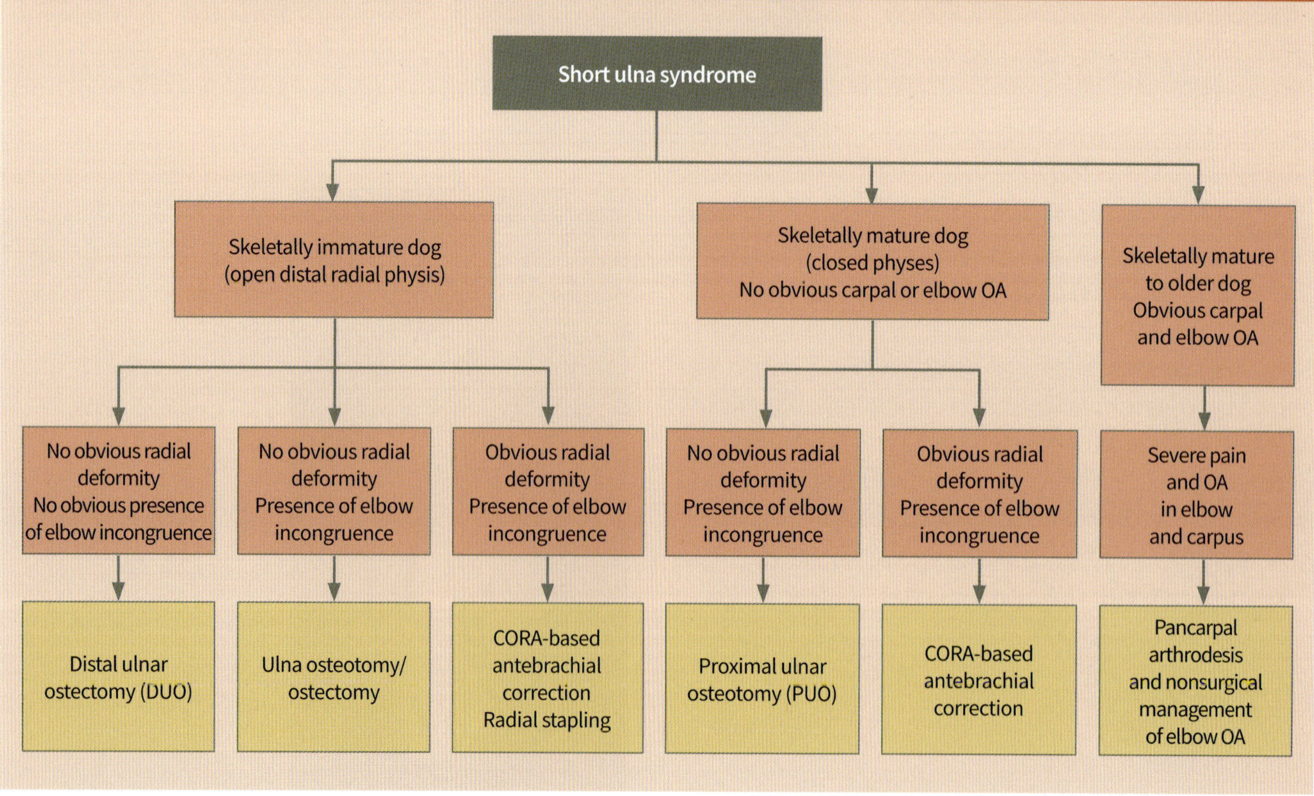

CORA, centre of rotation of angulation; OA, osteoarthritis.

of the ulna have been recommended to delay ulna healing. See chapter "Medial compartment disease" for a detailed description of the DUO procedure.

Skeletally immature dogs with an open distal radial physis, elbow incongruence and minimum to no radial deformity

In these cases, a dynamic ulnar ostectomy has been advocated as the treatment of choice (Johnston and Tobias, 2018). This procedure frees the proximal aspect of the ulna, allowing it to move and improving elbow congruence with the humerus (see chapter "Medial compartment disease"). Simultaneously, the radius can continue to grow without restriction. The execution of the procedure has been reported with the aid of an intramedullary pin to minimise caudoproximal displacement of the proximal segment of the ulna by the action of the triceps muscle (Johnston and Tobias, 2018). Alternatively, a proximal ulnar ostectomy can be considered in dogs with a milder degree of ulnar shortening (see chapter "Medial compartment disease" for a detailed description of the PUO procedure).

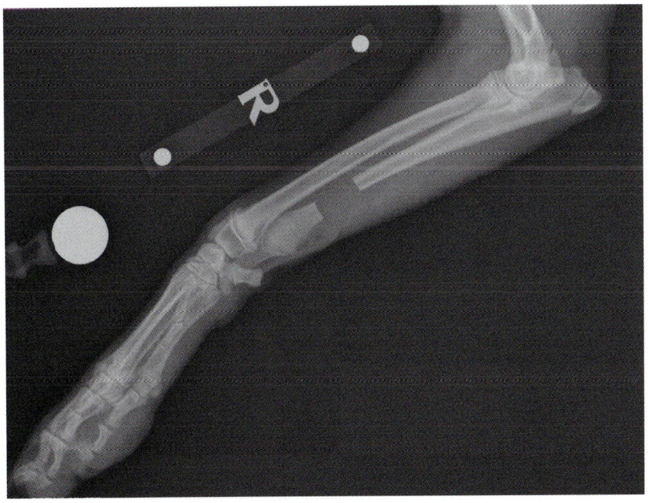

Figure 10. Mediolateral radiograph of the antebrachium of a skeletally immature dog with signs of medial coronoid disease (subtrochlear sclerosis) after distal ulnar ostectomy.

Skeletally immature or young mature dogs with elbow incongruence and noticeable radial deformity but no elbow/carpal OA

A centre of rotation of angulation (CORA)-based corrective surgery has been suggested for patients with a multiplanar deformity (Fox, 1984; Ramadan and Vaughan, 1978; O'brien et al., 1971) (Figs. 12 and 13). Accurate measurements with the help of CT are recommended. CORA-based assessment of antebrachial deformities, surgical planning and execution are beyond the scope of this chapter. CORA-based corrections have been reported with the use of internal fixation, external fixation and three-dimensional printed guides (Carwardine et al., 2021; Crosse and Worth, 2010;

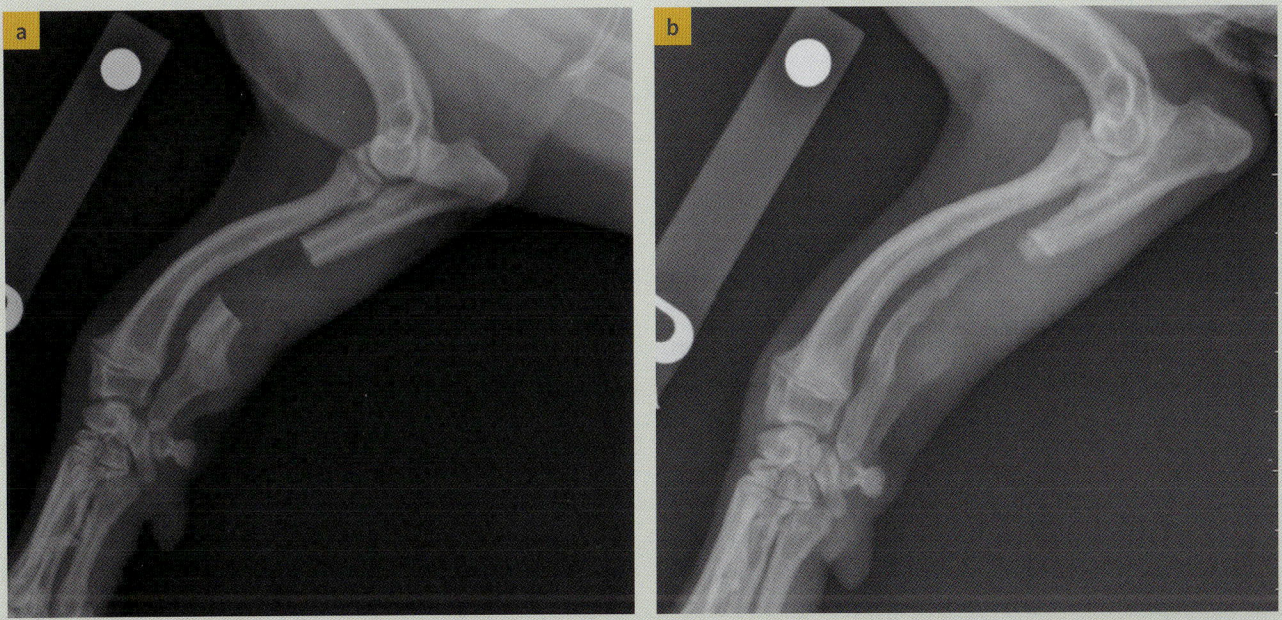

Figure 11. Same patient as in Figure 4. Postoperative radiograph after distal ulnar ostectomy (a). Note the partial improvement in elbow congruence. Radiograph 6 weeks after surgery showing significantly improved elbow congruence (b).

Deruddere and Snelling, 2014; Longo et al., 2019; Fitzpatrick et al., 2011; Marcellin-Little et al., 1998; Quinn et al., 2000).

The development of three-dimensional printing-assisted corrections has simplified surgical execution (Figs. 14 and 15). Potential drawbacks are the cost and the time required for planning and printing the guides.

Coggeshall et al. (2014) reported arthroscopic-guided ulnar distraction for the correction of elbow incongruence in four dogs, with good long-term results based on owner questionnaire. The surgical procedure involved a transverse ulnar osteotomy and a controlled, arthroscopic-guided ulnar distraction with intra-articular assessment of radioulnar congruence, followed by internal fixation (plate and screws).

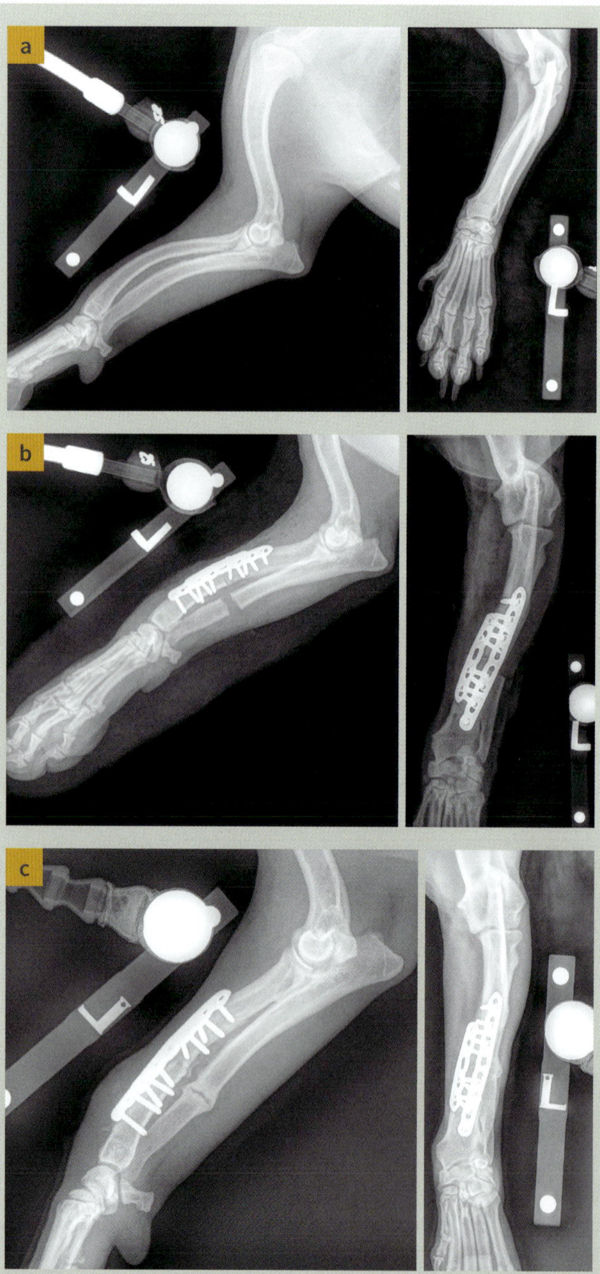

Figure 12. Mediolateral and craniocaudal radiographs of the antebrachium of a dog with an antebrachial limb deformity (a). Postoperative radiographs after CORA-based three-dimensional printing-assisted corrective surgery (b). Radiographs 4 months after surgery showing complete healing of the radius and advanced stage of healing of the ulnar ostectomy (c).

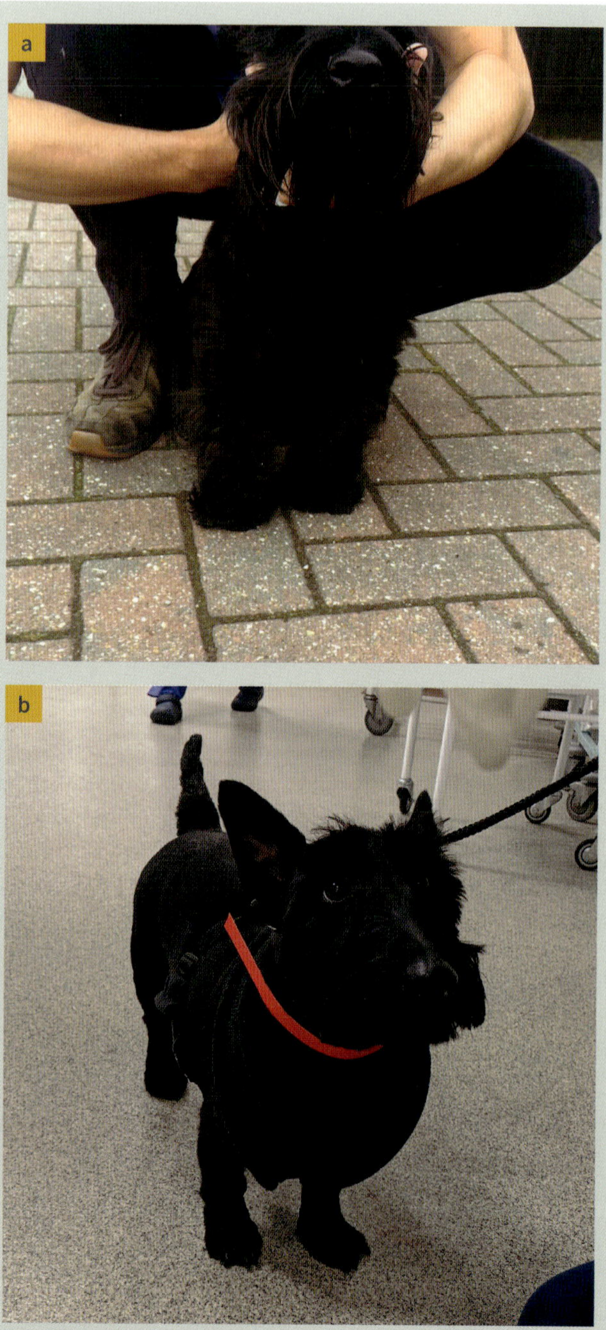

Figure 13. Dog with a deformity of the right thoracic limb (a). Note the degree of torsion and valgus. Same patient 12 weeks after surgical correction (b).

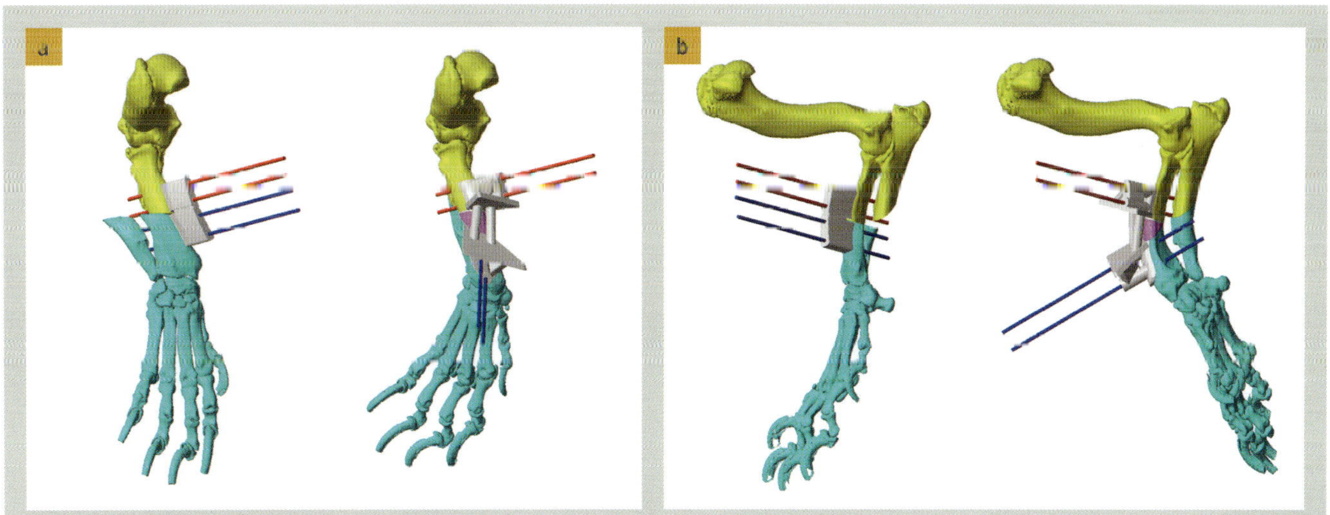

Figure 14. Three-dimensional planning for the design of cutting and reduction guides for correction of an antebrachial limb deformity. Images courtesy of Bill Oxley, Vet3D.

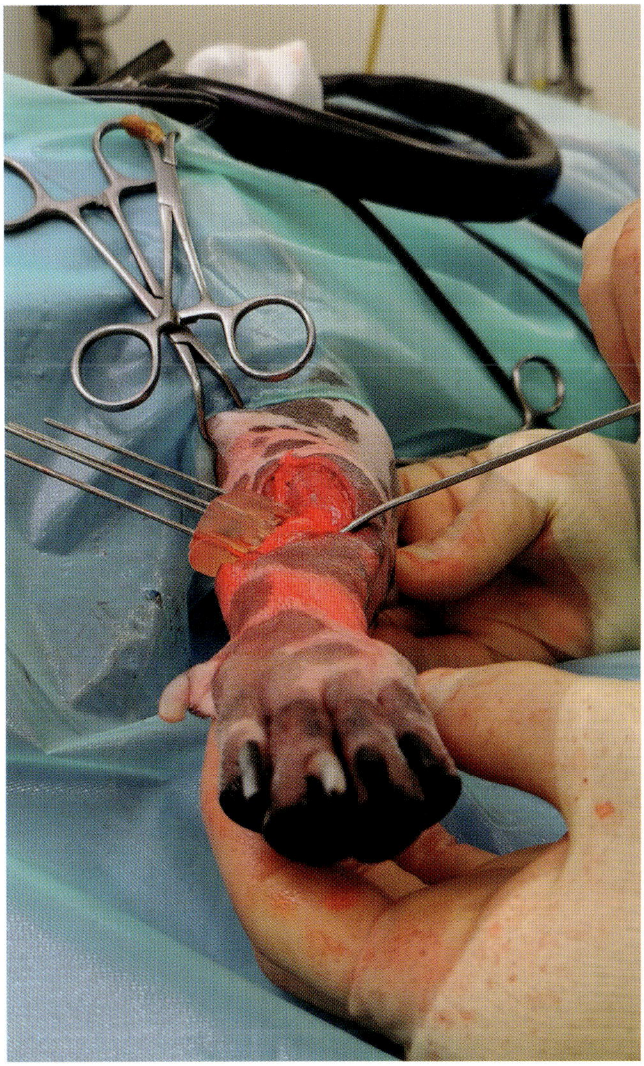

Figure 15. Intraoperative image after resolution of an antebrachial torsional deformity in a dog using three-dimensional printed guides (Vet3D).

Skeletally mature dogs with elbow incongruence and none to minimal radial deformity

For skeletally mature dogs with elbow pain but with minimum to no deformity of the radius, a PUO can provide some degree of clinical improvement (Fitzpatrick and Yeadon, 2009) (Fig. 16). See chapter "Medial compartment disease" for a detailed description of the PUO procedure.

Skeletally mature to older dogs with elbow incongruence and antebrachial deformity that has led to elbow and severe carpal OA

A pancarpal arthrodesis can be considered for these patients. Dogs with pronounced torsional deformity and carpal valgus can, over time, develop carpal OA and failure of the medial collateral ligament complex. These dogs can have pain associated with carpal OA and have poor walking function (they are typically described as buckling over when walking) (Fig. 17). Pancarpal arthrodesis can improve their quality of life (improved function and reduced pain) (Fig. 18). See chapter "Pancarpal arthrodesis" for further details.

During the surgical procedure, an ostectomy of the distal radius can be performed to correct carpal valgus. Torsion is resolved during arthrodesis by derotation of the radiocarpal joint with respect to the radius. Radial procurvatum is generally not corrected during a standard arthrodesis and persists after surgery. The presence of pronounced radial procurvatum in these dogs makes accurate plate contouring paramount to match the local anatomy (see Fig. 18b).

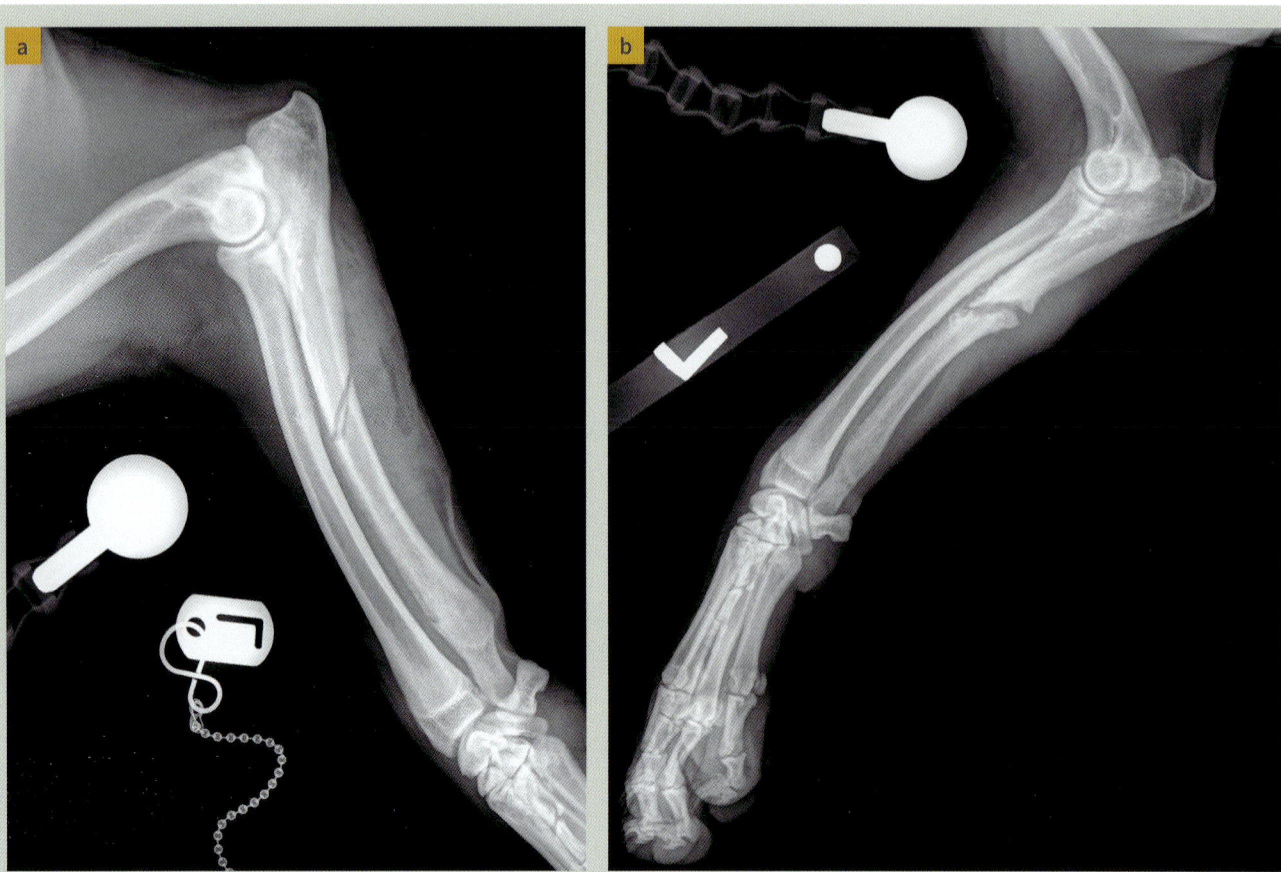

Figure 16. Mediolateral radiograph of a dog with mild premature closure of the distal ulna, minor changes in the radius and elbow pain (subtrochlear sclerosis, medial coronoid disease) after proximal ulnar osteotomy (PUO) (a). Mediolateral radiograph of the same dog 6 weeks after surgery showing an active hypertrophic callus at the PUO site (b).

Pancarpal arthrodesis can be considered as a salvage procedure for older dogs with severe carpal OA and poor function.

Very commonly, elbow OA is present. A nonsurgical management consisting of body weight loss/management, hydrotherapy, daily supplements, therapeutic exercises, judicious use of nonsteroidal anti-inflammatory drugs and/or intra-articular therapy with biological products is recommended.

OUTCOME

Management of dogs with an antebrachial angular and rotational limb deformity (ARLD) with a CORA methodology is well documented (Carwardine et al., 2021; Crosse and Worth, 2010; Deruddere and Snelling, 2014; Longo

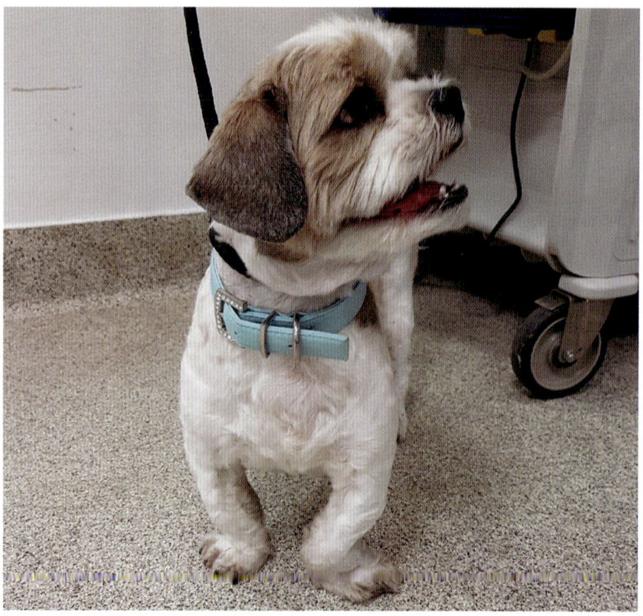

Figure 17. Middle-aged dog with bilateral carpal valgus (more pronounced in the left forelimb). This patient had very poor function and pain on carpal manipulation but tolerated elbow manipulation reasonably well despite the presence of osteoarthritis.

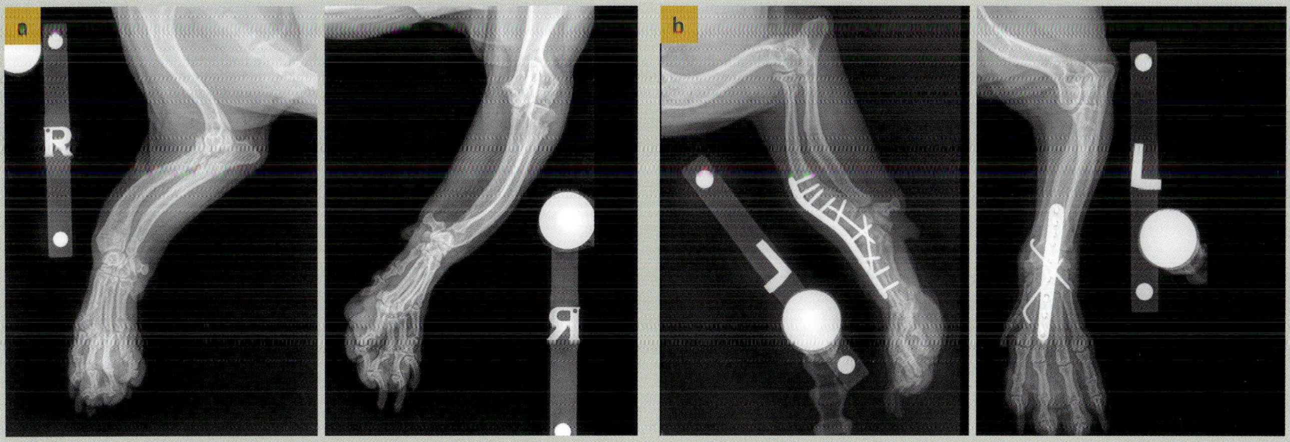

Figure 18. Radiographs of the same dog as in Figure 17 showing pronounced radial torsion, radial procurvatum and elbow OA (a). Postoperative radiographs after pancarpal arthrodesis (b).

et al., 2019; Fitzpatrick et al., 2011; Marcellin-Little et al., 1998; Quinn et al., 2000). This is the subtype of patients with antebrachial limb deformities with the largest number of studies. Short-term outcomes after CORA-based correction with internal and external fixation are good to excellent. Long-term owner questionnaires reported improvement in quality of life and lameness and, interestingly, resolution of buckling over in all cases (Carwardine et al., 2021). The literature for management of patients in other categories is sparser.

It is the author's experience that skeletally immature dogs with an open distal radial physis without obvious signs of bone deformity nor elbow incongruence respond well to DUO, while skeletally mature dogs that have pain associated with elbow incongruence as a consequence of short ulna syndrome are more challenging to treat.

04
CARPUS

ABDUCTOR POLLICIS LONGUS TENOSYNOVITIS

Stephen Kalff

INTRODUCTION

The abductor pollicis longus (APL) muscle originates on the lateral aspect of the radius and ulna, crosses over the distal radius, where its insertional tendon passes through a sulcus and under the medial collateral ligament, and inserts onto the proximal aspect of digit 1 (Fig. 1). In humans, it is one of the extrinsic muscles of the hand and its major role is to abduct the thumb at the wrist. In dogs, digit 1 is primarily vestigial, so this function may be relatively redundant. However, given the relatively large size of this muscle, it may play a role in carpal adduction and/or be an active stabiliser of the carpus.

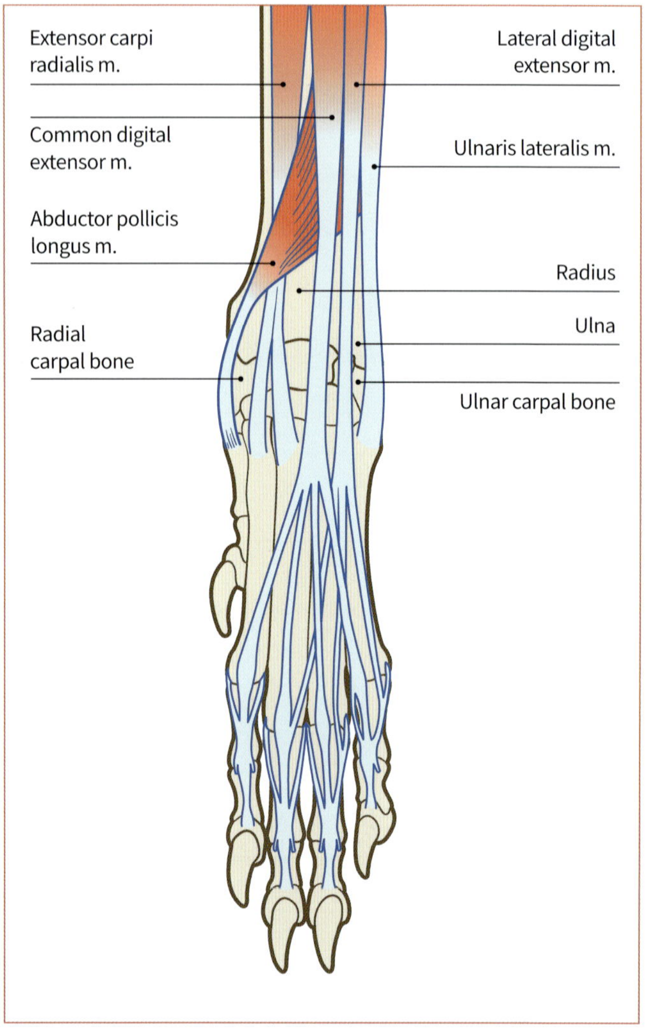

Figure 1. Anatomy of the abductor pollicis longus muscle and tendon.

CLINICAL PRESENTATION AND DIAGNOSIS

APL tenosynovitis (also known as stenosing tenosynovitis of the APL muscle) is thought to be due to a chronic repetitive strain injury of the tendon of insertion and is predominantly seen in active medium- to large-breed dogs (Moores and Comerford, 2005). A similar condition in humans known as De Quervain's syndrome is commonly seen in video gamers. Whilst stereotypically not as active as their canine counterparts, the injury in people is the result of vigorous, repetitive thumb movements.

The resultant proliferation of bone and soft tissue adhesions along the medial sulcus through which the tendon and its sheath run through can cause impingement of the tendon.

Dogs presenting with APL tenosynovitis have soft tissue thickening on the medial aspect of the distal radius and carpus and usually exhibit pain on carpal flexion and often also on firm digital pressure over this swelling (Fig. 2).

Radiographs demonstrate soft tissue swelling over the affected region. More chronic cases also have bone remodelling along the medial aspect of the distal radius (Fig. 3).

Whilst radiographs and physical examination are generally sufficient for a working diagnosis, more advanced imaging techniques such as CT provide detailed information, particularly of the bone changes in the sulcus through which the tendon sheath runs. An experienced ultrasonographer can detect soft tissue changes, such as tendon sheath thickening and fluid in the sheath, and exclude differential diagnoses including chronic collateral ligament sprain (Hittmair et al., 2012).

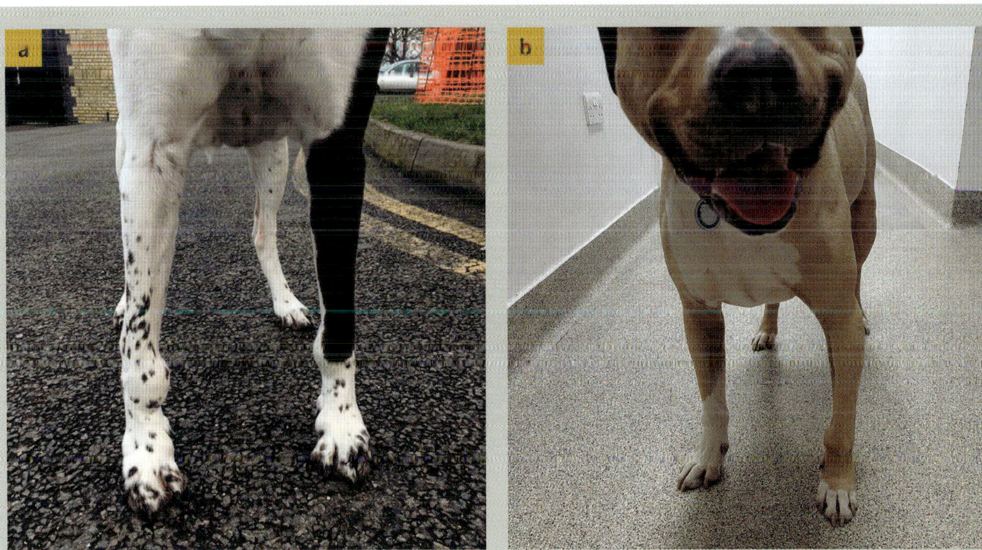

Figure 2. Dog with visible thickening on the medial aspect of the distal radius and carpus (a). Similar clinical presentation in the left thoracic limb of another dog (b).

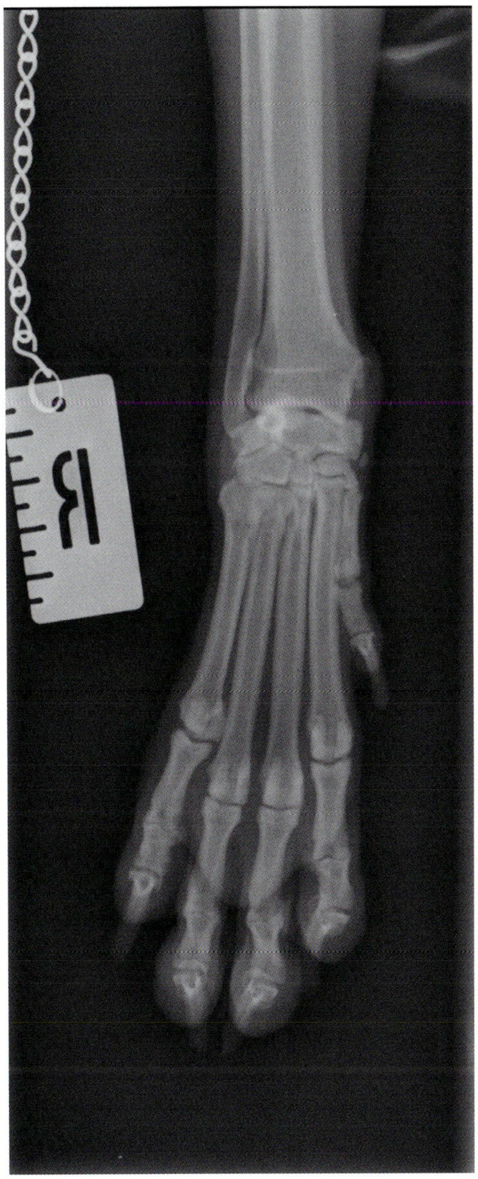

Figure 3. Dorsopalmar radiograph of a dog showing a soft tissue opacity on the medial aspect of the distal radius, with bone proliferation.

TREATMENT

Medical management should be tried initially. This consists of restriction of activity for 4–6 weeks and local injection of up to 0.5 mg/kg of methylprednisolone acetate.

In more chronic cases, surgical intervention can be considered. The author recommends debridement of the sulcus and tendon sheath to free up the tendon.

A longitudinal incision is made on the medial aspect of the distal radius. The sulcus and tendon sheath are identified. An incision is made in the tendon sheath, and the adhesions and impinging bone along the sulcus are debrided (Fig. 4). Flexing and extending the carpus should demonstrate a freely movable tendon once debridement is complete.

After surgery, dogs should have their activity restricted for 4 weeks, with lead walks only. Gentle physiotherapy with frequent flexion and extension exercises can also be helpful.

Tenotomy has also been described with good outcomes. However, this technique can result in significant carpal osteoarthritis. As such, the author reserves its use as a last-resort salvage option.

OUTCOME

There is very limited data published on dogs with APL tenosynovitis. However, in the author's experience the prognosis tends to be good. The author starts with medical management and will move to surgical debridement in refractory cases. Rarely is tenotomy required, although patients undergoing tenotomy tend to do well despite the progression of carpal osteoarthritis.

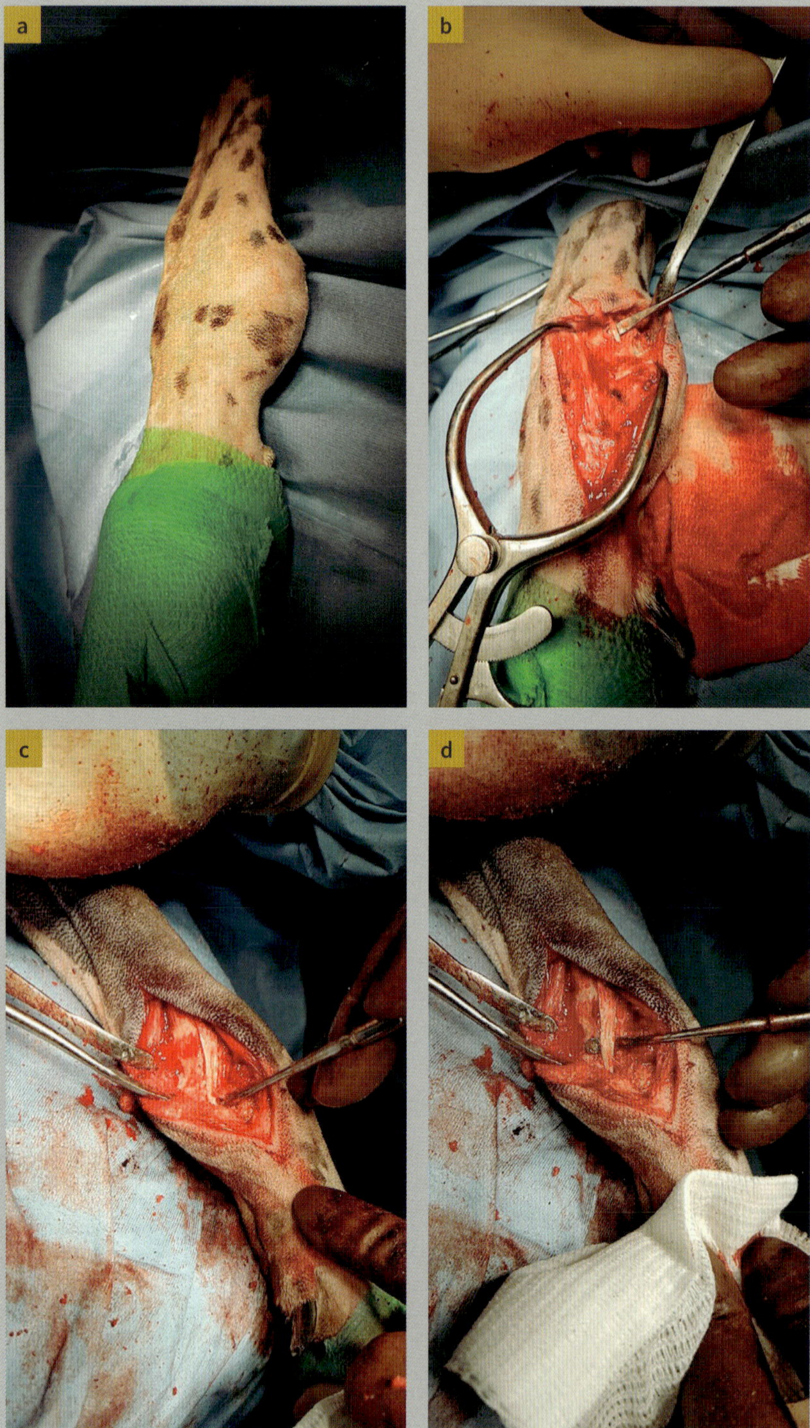

Figure 4. Surgical management of an abductor pollicis longus tenosynovitis by release of the tendon through debridement, in sequence from approach (a) to release (d).

PANCARPAL ARTHRODESIS

Felipe de Vicente

INTRODUCTION

Pancarpal arthrodesis is the surgical fusion of the carpal joint, which is considered a salvage procedure. The ultimate goal of this intervention is to permanently immobilise the carpus, thus relieving the pain associated with various carpal diseases. Fusion should be performed at a physiological weight-bearing angle to achieve the best possible function of the limb.

The carpus consists of several joint lines – antebrachiocarpal, intercarpal and carpometacarpal joints – and has a range of motion in the dog of 164 degrees (Petazzoni and Jaeger, 2008). When establishing the arthrodesis angle, the angle that the joint moves through during the stance phase of the limb should be considered. This angle can be determined from the contralateral limb, or reported angles can be used as a reference.

> The standing weight-bearing angle of the carpus is 10–12 degrees of extension in the dog and 15–20 degrees of extension in the cat (Basa and Johnson, 2019).

Numerous stabilisation methods for pancarpal arthrodesis have been proposed in recent years. Although the use of linear or circular transarticular external fixators has been described (Lotsikas and Radasch, 2006), especially in small animals (cats and small-breed dogs), most of these stabilisation techniques are based on the application of plates and screws. The use of dynamic compression plates (DCP), cuttable plates, hybrid plates and locking plates has been described. The use of orthogonal plates (dorsal and medial) in comminuted articular fractures has also been described (Brown et al., 2016), along with the combination of Kirschner wires or crossed cortical screws with a dorsally applied plate (Arnott et al., 2008; Tuan et al., 2019).

On the other hand, numerous biomechanical studies have been performed comparing the different methods of internal fixation when performing pancarpal arthrodesis. Specifically, it has been shown that hybrid pancarpal plates (HDCP, hybrid dynamic compression plate) are biomechanically superior to classic DCPs (Wininger et al., 2007; Guillou et al., 2012). In addition, HDCPs have been compared to castless (double locking) plates, without demonstrating a significant advantage of this plate type over HDCPs (Meeson et al., 2012). Finally, the effect of adding crossed Kirschner wires to a dorsally placed HDCP was compared and, although the crossed wires increased implant strength by 27.6 %, in both cases the implants resisted more load than a patient could apply (Arnott et al., 2008). In summary, at the time of writing this chapter, it is very difficult to make recommendations on the most appropriate plate of choice for pancarpal arthrodesis. The key is to choose the most appropriate one for the patient and their disease.

> All plates may be suitable depending on the patient and the disease.

INDICATIONS

Pancarpal arthrodesis is recommended in diseases where other medical or surgical treatments have been unsuccessful or as a primary treatment in diseases where the likelihood of achieving optimal results with other medical or surgical treatments is very low. Accordingly, indications for pancarpal arthrodesis include:

- Carpal hyperextension injuries (Fig. 1).
- Nonreconstructable articular fractures or complex fractures of the distal radius (Figs. 2 and 3).
- Severe osteoarthritis not sufficiently responding to medical treatment.
- Joint collapse or pain secondary to immune-mediated arthritis.
- Chronic carpal luxations.
- Angular deformities.

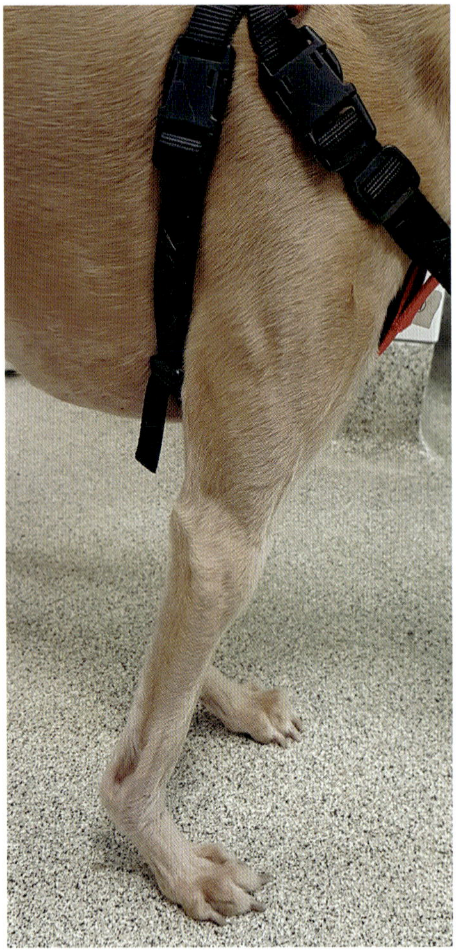

Figure 1. Patient with a carpal hyperextension injury.

- Neurological injuries affecting only the distal part of the forelimb (Kapatkin et al., 2018; Petazzoni and Nicetto, 2014).
- Pancarpal arthrodesis can also be performed in severe carpal collateral ligament injuries, either as a primary treatment or as a secondary treatment if other surgical techniques have been unsuccessful.

CLINICAL PRESENTATION AND DIAGNOSIS

The clinical signs of patients with carpal diseases vary from mild to non-weight-bearing lameness. Upon orthopaedic examination, one or more of the following signs may be detected: periarticular swelling, pain upon flexion or extension of the joint, intra-articular effusion, joint instability, crepitus and inadequate alignment of the limb with deformity at this level.

Diseases for which pancarpal arthrodesis is indicated are diagnosed in the vast majority of cases via conventional orthogonal radiographs. In these cases, it is useful to perform stress radiographs of the carpal joint to determine the location of the instability. In more complex cases, it may be necessary to use advanced imaging techniques, such

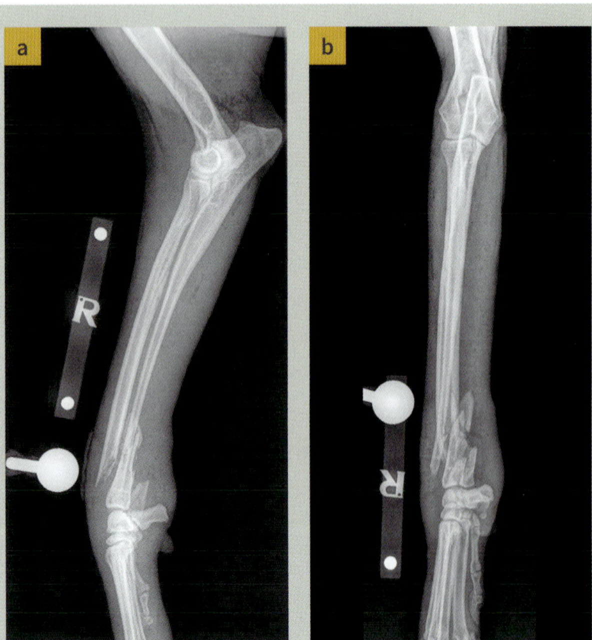

Figure 2. Preoperative mediolateral (a) and dorsopalmar (b) radiographs of a comminuted fracture of the distal radius with intra-articular involvement.

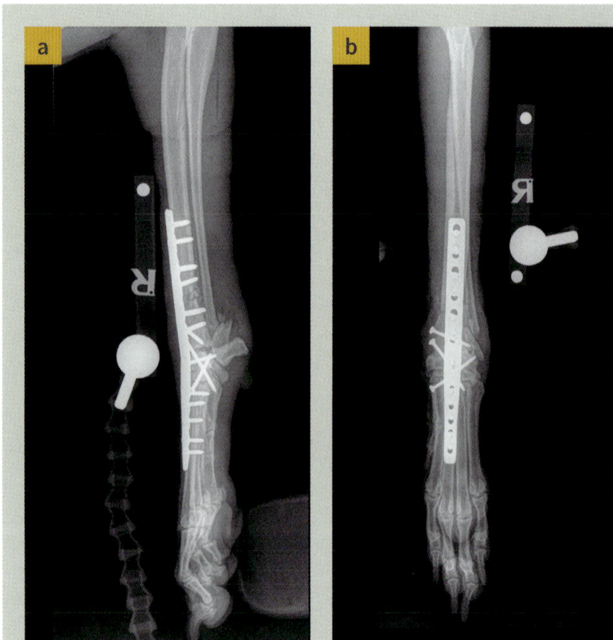

Figure 3. Postoperative mediolateral (a) and dorsopalmar (b) radiographs of the patient from the previous figure. The fracture was stabilised via pancarpal arthrodesis.

as CT (in the diagnosis of some intra-articular fractures or angular deformities) or MRI (in neuropathies).

SURGICAL PLANNING

Orthogonal radiographs of the carpus should be taken, including all of the metacarpal bones and at least half the length of the radius, to determine the size of the implants to be used. In cases of severe osteoarthritis, marked instability or fractures that make it difficult to assess implant placement, radiographs of the contralateral limb are required to establish the surgical plan.

There are currently no clear recommendations regarding which type of plate to use for pancarpal arthrodesis. The author usually uses specific arthrodesis plates, since they are designed as hybrid plates in which the diameter of the screws is smaller in the metacarpals than in the radius.

The plate of choice for each patient must meet certain requirements to minimise the risk of postoperative complications. It is important to select a plate that exceeds 50 % of the length of the third metacarpal bone (Whitelock et al., 1999), and in which the metacarpal screws do not occupy more than 40 % of the diameter of the bone (Koch, 2005), if they are centred on it.

> To reduce postoperative complications, it is recommended to apply plates 50 % longer than the third metacarpal with screws that do not exceed 40 % of the bone diameter.

Irrespective of the type of stabilisation used, it is essential to follow general arthrodesis principles (see chapter "General concepts about arthrodesis"). According to these principles, it is necessary to:

- Meticulously debride the articular cartilage.
- Use bone grafts.
- Stabilise the joint rigidly with interfragmentary compression.
- Stabilise the joint at a functional weight-bearing angle.

SURGICAL TECHNIQUE

Pancarpal arthrodesis is usually performed using internal fixation systems. Dorsal (Johnson, 1980), medial (Guerrero and Montavon, 2005) and palmar (Chambers and Bjorling, 1982) pancarpal arthrodesis techniques have been described. Palmar pancarpal arthrodesis is the most suitable from a biomechanical point of view, since the implants are located on the tension side of the joint. However, this approach is rarely applied due to the anatomical complexity of the palmar aspect of the carpus. For the purpose of this chapter, the pancarpal arthrodesis technique using a dorsal approach is described, as this is the most common technique when performing this procedure.

The limb is surgically prepared, including the shoulder in the surgical field if an autogenous bone graft is to be obtained from the proximal humerus. The patient may be placed in lateral, dorsal or sternal recumbency (Fig. 4) based on the surgeon's preference. It is possible to place an Esmarch bandage up to the elbow (or a tourniquet at that level) to minimise bleeding during the procedure.

A dorsal approach to the carpus is made from the distal third of the radius (avoiding the accessory cephalic vein) to the distal third of the metacarpal bones (Fig. 5). A curve can be made medially or laterally in the distal part of the incision to prevent the suture line from overlapping the plate. The subcutaneous tissue is dissected and the antebrachial fascia is incised between the extensor carpi radialis tendon and the common digital extensor tendon (Fig. 6). To obtain adequate exposure of the distal radius, it is usually necessary to section the tendon of the abductor muscle of first digit. Next, the extensor carpi radialis muscle tendon is identified and its insertion on the second and third metacarpal bones is sectioned (Figs. 7 and 8). The common digital extensor tendon is then identified and retracted laterally, allowing the visualisation of the antebrachiocarpal, intercarpal and carpometacarpal joints. The joint capsule is incised and these joints are exposed. Extensive resection of the joint capsule should be performed to obtain good visualisation of the articular surfaces (Fig. 7).

To perform an arthrodesis, the articular cartilage of all the joint lines must be removed until the subchondral bone is exposed (flexing the carpal joint improves visualisation of the cartilage for this purpose). This process is usually performed using a pneumatic burr (Fig. 9), although the use of gouges or the performance of a small ostectomy on the articular surface with an osteotome or oscillating saw has also been described. At this point in the procedure, some surgeons perform osteostixis on the radius (Fig. 10) and the head of the metacarpal bones to provide a connection to the medullary canals of these bones and create channels for neovascularisation. After copiously lavaging the surgical

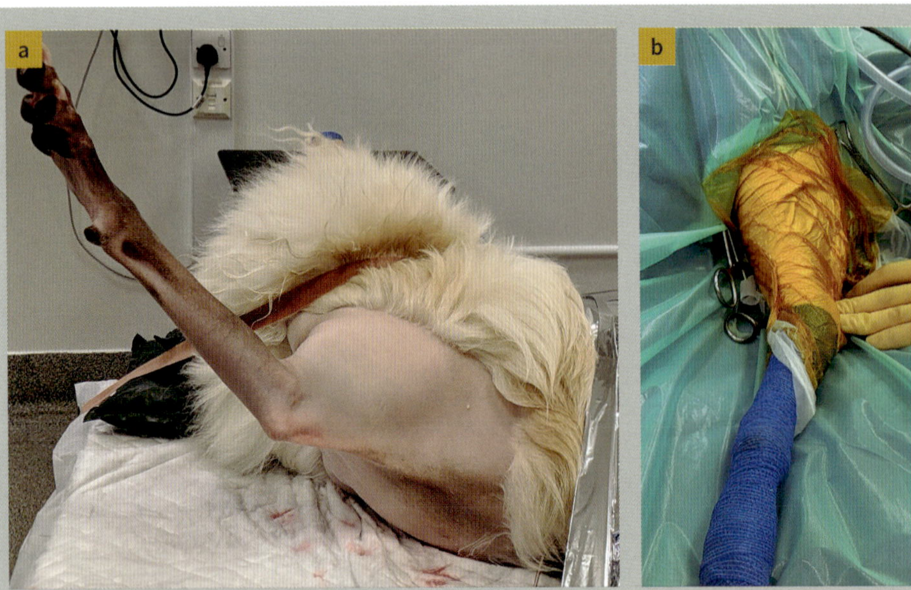

Figure 4. Patient positioning in sternal recumbency to perform pancarpal arthrodesis (a). Preparation of the surgical field (b).

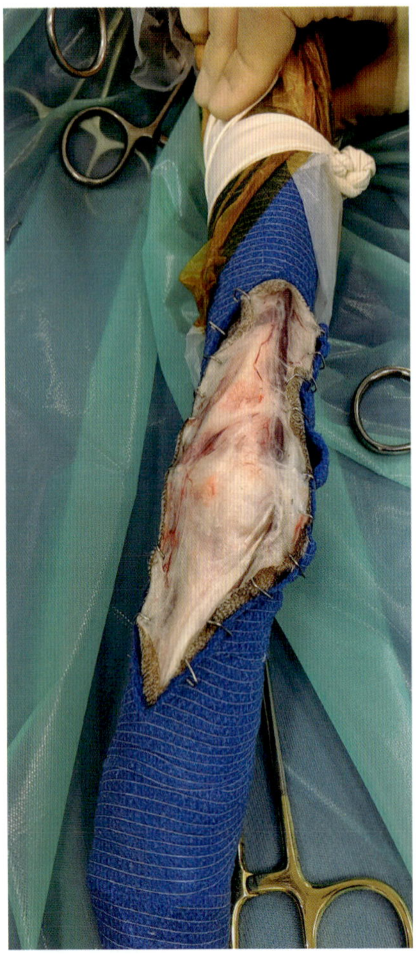

Figure 5. Dorsal approach to the left carpus, from the distal third of the radius to the distal third of the metacarpal bones. An Esmarch-type bandage was applied to the forelimb to minimise bleeding during surgery.

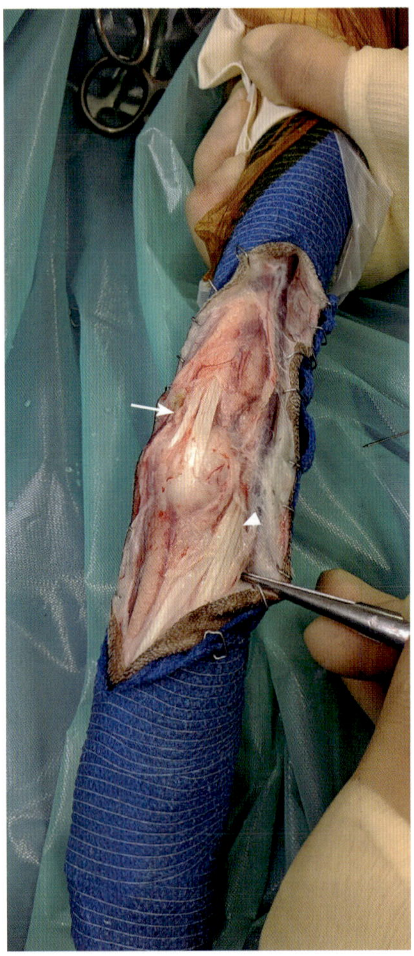

Figure 6. The subcutaneous tissue is dissected and the antebrachial fascia is incised between the extensor carpi radialis muscle tendon (arrow) and the common digital extensor muscle tendon (arrowhead).

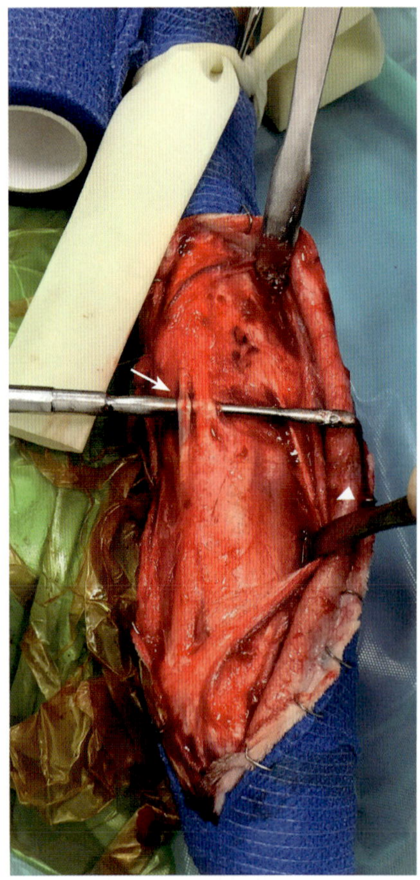

Figure 7. The extensor carpi radialis muscle tendon is identified at its insertion on the second and third metacarpal bones, in the image shown with the help of a periosteal elevator (arrow). The common digital extensor muscle tendon is identified and retracted laterally (arrowhead), allowing the identification of the antebrachiocarpal, intercarpal and carpometacarpal joints.

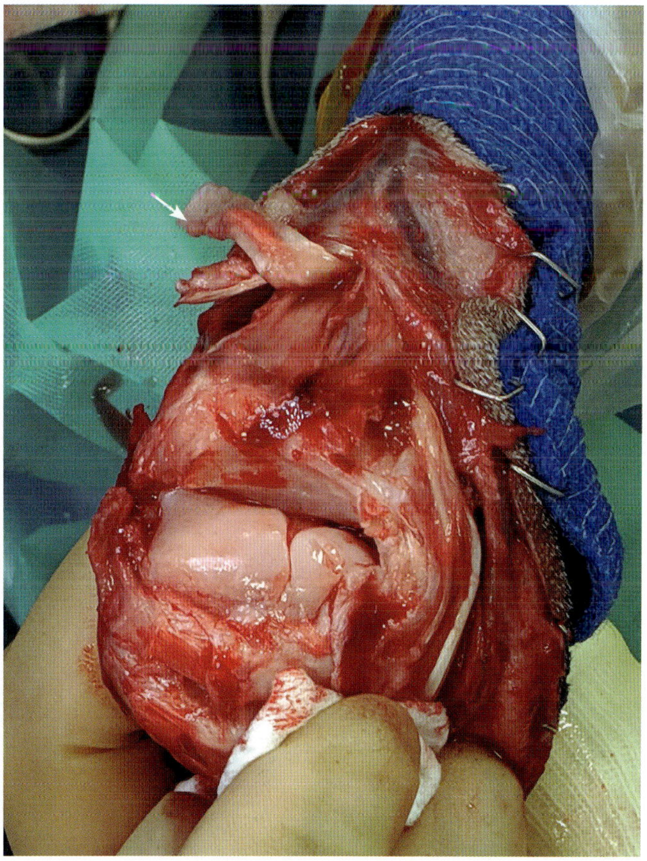

Figure 8. Section of the extensor carpi radialis tendon at its insertion on the second and third metacarpal bones (arrow). The joint capsule is incised and the joints are exposed by flexing the carpus.

site with sterile saline, the bone graft (preferably autogenous) is placed between the different joints (Fig. 11).

> To improve visualisation of the articular cartilage resection and removal process, as well as the exposure of the subchondral bone, it is recommended to flex the joint.

The author routinely harvests an autogenous bone graft from the proximal humerus. For this purpose, an incision is made craniolateral to the greater tubercle of the humerus, separating the brachiocephalic muscle and the acromial part of the deltoideus muscle with surgical retractors (the author usually uses Gelpi retractors). A monocortical hole is drilled in the craniolateral surface of the proximal humerus, using a drill or pneumatic burr. The hole should be of sufficient size to harvest cancellous bone without difficulty using a Volkmann curette. Once a sufficient amount has been removed to fill the carpal joints, the surgical site is lavaged and the wound is sutured using absorbable monofilament material for the muscle layers (the author uses polydioxanone) and subcutaneous tissue (the author uses poliglecaprone 25) and nonabsorbable monofilament material or staples for the skin (the author uses nylon).

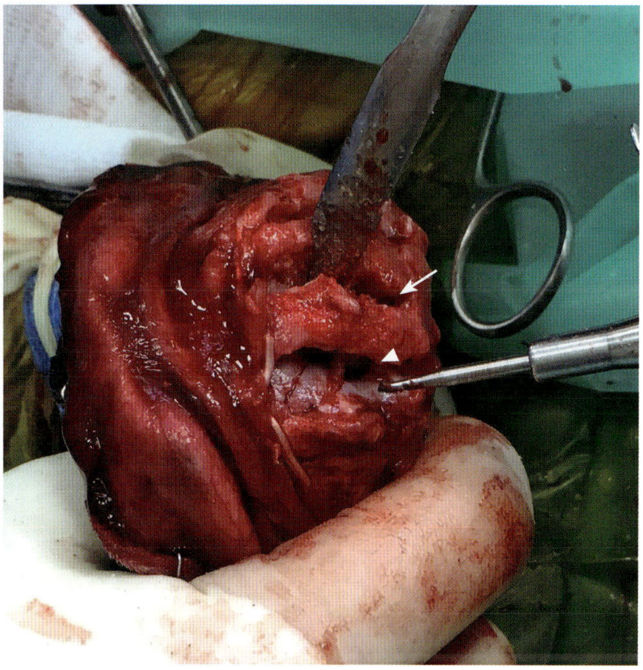

Figure 9. The articular cartilage of the carporadial (arrow) and carpometacarpal (arrowhead) joints is removed until the subchondral bone is exposed. This process is usually performed with the aid of a pneumatic burr.

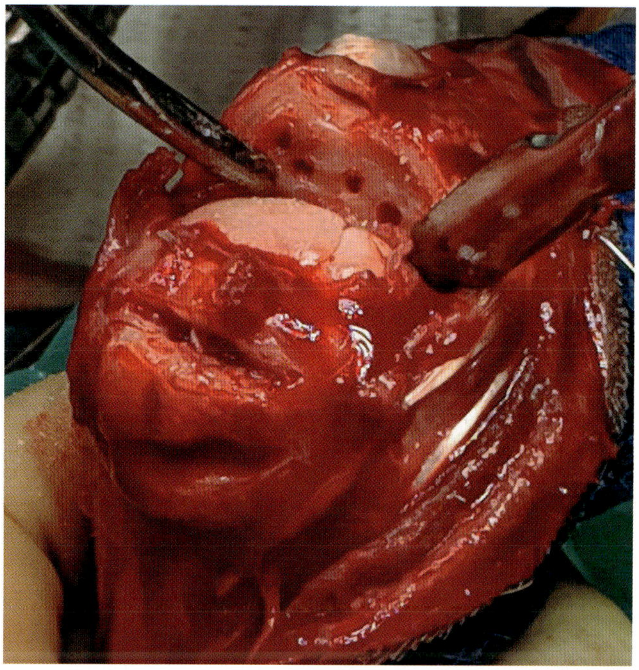

Figure 10. Osteostixis in the radius.

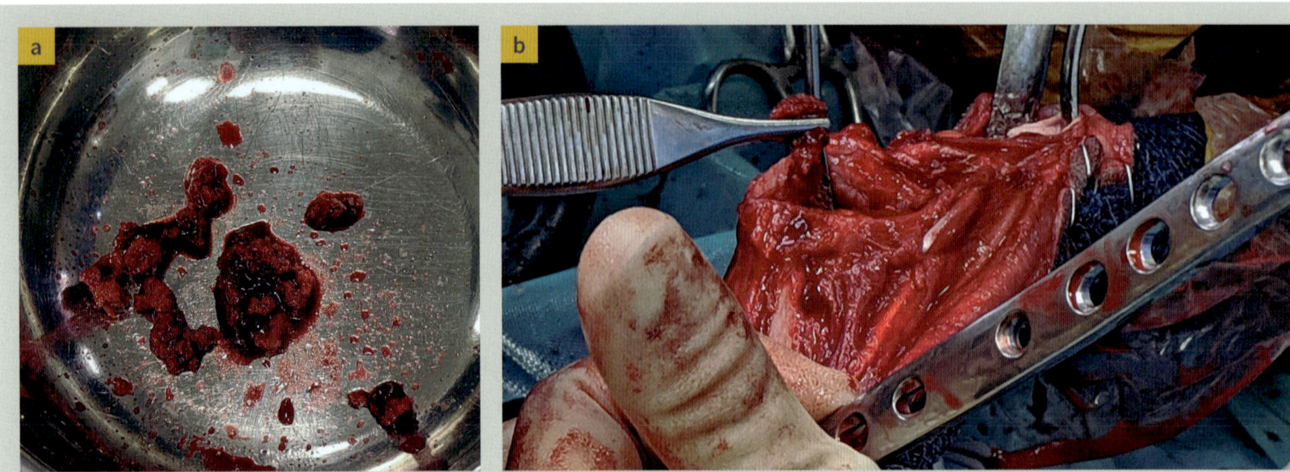

Figure 11. Harvesting of autogenous bone graft (a) and placement between the different joints (b).

The internal fixation plate selected for the patient is then applied. There are a large number of them designed specifically for this surgical procedure. These plates have a predetermined angle and are prepared for the placement of larger diameter screws in the distal part of the radius and smaller diameter screws in the metacarpal bones. Although most plates are designed to stabilise only the third metacarpal bone, there is a castless plate designed to simultaneously stabilise the third and fourth metacarpal bones. The design of the latter is intended to provide greater stability to the distal part of the pancarpal arthrodesis in order to avoid the use of postoperative bandages and minimise the incidence of metacarpal bone fractures in the postoperative period. The author routinely uses hybrid pancarpal arthrodesis plates, placing the screws as follows: the first screw is placed in the radiocarpal bones, and then the most distal screw of the plate is placed in the third metacarpal bone in a neutral position, to ensure that these two screws are centred in their respective bone. Next, the most proximal screw of the third metacarpal bone and the most distal screw of the radius are placed, both in compression mode and, finally, the rest of the screws are placed in the plate. All the screws are then tightened sequentially, ending with the screw in the radiocarpal bone (Clarke and Pink, 2018).

> To stabilise the plate in position (centred on the bone), it may be useful to place hypodermic needles in the interosseous muscles lateral and medial to the third metacarpal bone.

Occasionally, the plate does not sit correctly on the dorsal aspect of the carpus due to bony prominences or osteoarthritis. In these cases, the author uses a pneumatic burr to smooth the dorsal surface of the distal radius or the base of the third metacarpal in order to better place the plate on the bone.

In dorsal pancarpal arthrodesis, some surgeons place crossed Kirschner wires (or crossed cortical screws) for additional stabilisation (Fig. 12), which are inserted from the second and fifth metacarpal bones (Arnott et al., 2008). However, a biomechanical study (Arnott et al., 2008) has shown that, although the addition of this crossed stabilisation increases load resistance, its clinical relevance is not clear from a biomechanical point of view, as the group with dorsal hybrid plates withstands higher forces than a dog can exert in its daily activity.

For surgical closure, the common digital extensor muscle tendon is repositioned and the extensor carpi radialis muscle tendon is sutured to the remnants of the joint capsule (the author uses absorbable monofilament polydioxanone). The subcutaneous tissue is sutured in a routine fashion (the author uses absorbable monofilament poliglecaprone 25 in a simple continuous pattern), and the skin is sutured with nonabsorbable monofilament (nylon) or surgical staples. Finally, the author performs relaxing incisions around the surgical incision if excess skin tension is evident during closure (Fig. 13). The purpose of these relaxing incisions is twofold. On the one hand, they relieve tension in the surgical wound and facilitate wound healing; on the other hand, they prevent the formation of a tourniquet effect in the distal part of the limb. Relaxing incisions heal by secondary intention in 1–2 weeks.

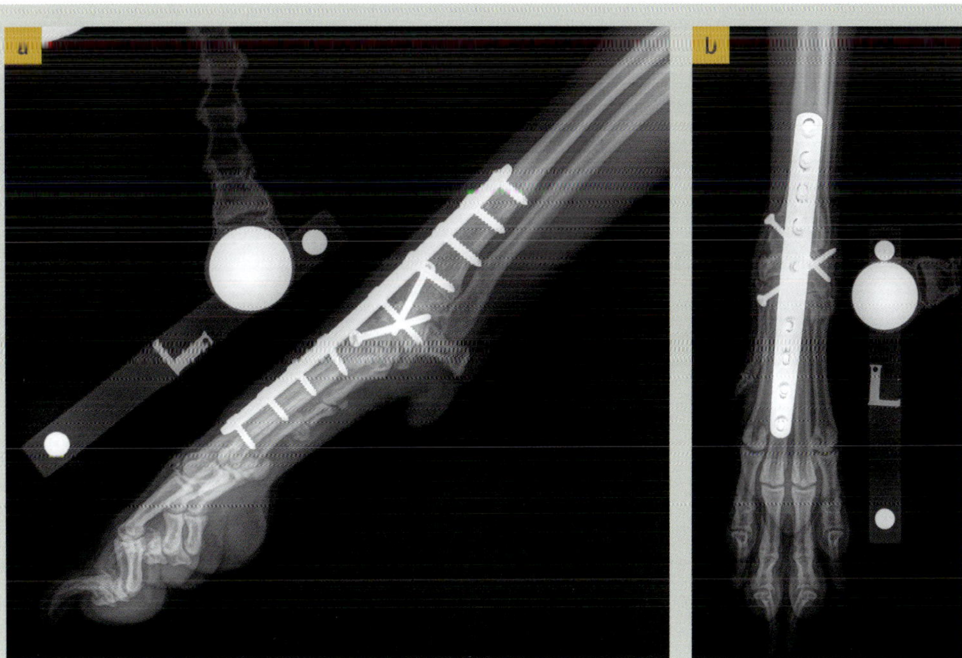

Figure 12. Mediolateral (a) and dorsopalmar (b) orthogonal radiographs of the stabilisation of a pancarpal arthrodesis using a hybrid plate.

> If excess skin tension is evident, it is advisable to make relaxing incisions around the surgical incision to facilitate healing.

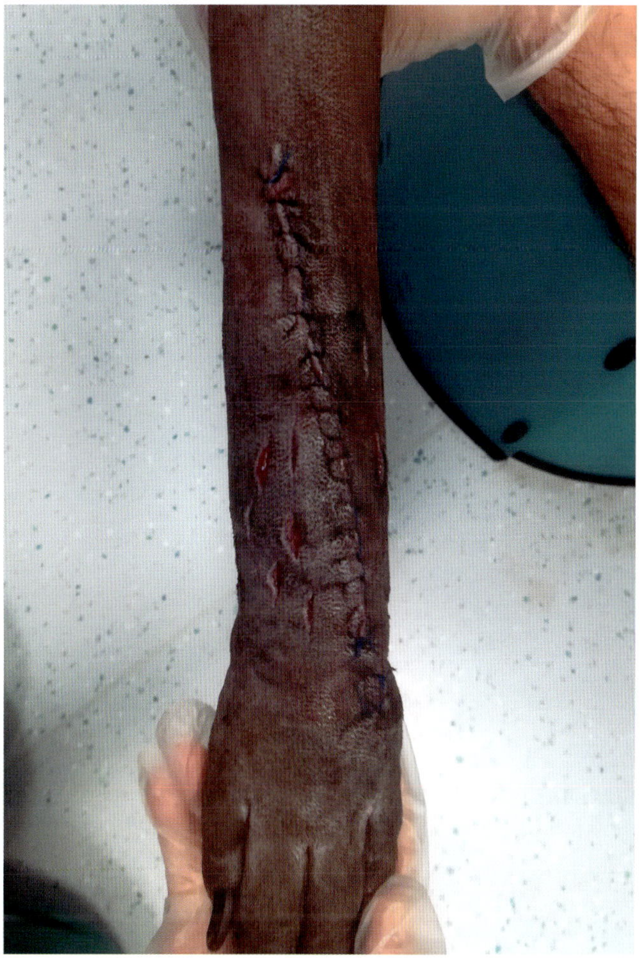

Figure 13. Relaxing incisions around the surgical wound in a pancarpal arthrodesis.

POSTOPERATIVE MANAGEMENT

Postoperative orthogonal radiographs are indicated to assess the anatomical reduction of the carpus and the position of the implants. If there are no contraindications, nonsteroidal anti-inflammatory drugs are prescribed for 2–3 weeks. The administration of postoperative antibiotics is controversial. Pancarpal arthrodesis is classified as a clean surgery and, therefore, postoperative antibiotic therapy would not be indicated. However, numerous studies describe this type of postsurgical treatment, varying between 0–25 % (Bristow et al., 2015; Ramírez and Macías, 2016) and 100 % (Tuan et al., 2019) of cases in these studies. Therefore, from this observation it follows that it is relatively common to prescribe postoperative antibiotic treatment for 7–10 days (usually amoxicillin and clavulanic acid, or a cephalosporin).

Bone healing can take up to 30 weeks to complete in a pancarpal arthrodesis (Michal et al., 2003) and postoperative follow-up radiographs are recommended every 6 weeks until consolidation of the arthrodesis is confirmed (Michal et al., 2003; Basa and Johnson, 2019), or earlier if the patient presents clinical deterioration. During this period, the patient should be confined and exercise restricted until there is radiographic evidence that bone healing is progressing. Owners are advised to be strict with the confinement of their pet for the first 6 weeks postoperatively, keeping the patient confined to a cage (or small room if the patient is large), with very brief walks on a short lead 3–4 times a day (5–10 minutes). In the event that arthrodesis is progressing adequately (evident on radiographs taken approximately 6 weeks after surgery), a gradual increase in the patient's exercise is instituted over the next 6 weeks. The author recommends increasing the duration of lead walks progressively. The duration of exercise is progressively increased until consolidation of the arthrodesis is confirmed by radiography, at which time the patient can resume normal activity.

Traditionally, it was recommended to apply a postoperative bandage with a splint for 3–9 weeks, but recent studies suggest that these bandages are not necessary (Woods et al., 2012; Bristow et al., 2015). A support dressing may be applied for the first 2–7 days following surgery to reduce postoperative swelling and improve the patient's postoperative comfort.

In cases where a bandage is placed for 3–9 weeks, it should be carefully monitored to avoid associated complications. The bandage should be changed frequently (at least every week) to examine the surgical area. The author does not apply these bandages after pancarpal arthrodesis.

> If a bandage is applied for a prolonged period, it should be changed at least weekly to examine the surgical area and avoid associated complications.

OUTCOME

The prognosis is good after pancarpal arthrodesis. Patients walk with an alteration in the flight phase of gait, leading to mild circumduction of the limb (Lewis et al., 2019). Some 73–91 % of patients have mild or no lameness in the long term (Bristow et al., 2015; Tuan et al., 2019) and 83 % of working dogs can return to the level of activity they had before the carpal injury (Jerram et al., 2009).

When owners' perceptions of their pets' functionality were assessed, 74 % of owners felt that their patients had no lameness, 97 % felt that their pets had improved after pancarpal arthrodesis and 94 % were satisfied with the results of the intervention (Parker et al., 1981).

The prognosis in cats is very similar to that of dogs, with 64 % of patients showing an excellent outcome and 36 % showing a satisfactory outcome after surgery (Calvo et al., 2009). The most significant difference with respect to the canine species was a decrease in jumping height and a reduced desire to jump or climb (Calvo et al., 2009).

COMPLICATIONS

An intraoperative complication rate of 12–30 % has been reported for pancarpal arthrodesis (Bristow et al., 2015; Clarke et al., 2009). In the canine species, mild and severe postoperative complications have been observed in 0–9 % and 22–41 % of patients, respectively (Kapatkin et al., 2018; Tuan et al., 2019; Ramírez and Macías, 2016; Bristow et al., 2015). In the feline species, the total complication rate is 35 % (Calvo et al., 2009). Excluding complications associated with bandages, the postoperative complication rate reported in the literature is 34–41 % (Bristow et al., 2015).

Postoperative infection is the most frequent complication in pancarpal arthrodesis. Incidence rates of postoperative infection of 7–66 % (Beierer, 2021) and 7–31 % (Tuan et al., 2019; Bristow et al., 2015) have been described. The reason for this high postoperative infection rate is unknown, but factors such as the duration of the surgical procedure, poor soft tissue protection at the surgical site or thermal necrosis during articular cartilage debridement have been proposed as probable causes (Beierer, 2021). A recent study evaluated the incidence of postoperative infections when increasing the rigidity of stabilisation, combining the use of dorsal locking plates and crossed cortical screws. Despite the increased rigidity of the stabilisation, the postoperative infection rate was very similar to that reported in previous studies (Tuan et al., 2019).

Other frequent complications are those associated with bandages (dermatitis, ulcers and skin necrosis with varying degrees of severity), when applied in the postoperative period, and significant swelling of the distal limb in the first 24–72 hours postoperatively (Fig. 14). A bandage-associated complication rate of 63 % has been reported (Meeson et al., 2011), of which 20 % are serious complications requiring specific wound management treatment (Meeson et al., 2011).

Other less frequent complications of pancarpal arthrodesis include metacarpal fractures in 8–19 % of patients (Whitelock et al., 1999; Clarke et al., 2009), loosening of implants in 0–26 % of patients (Denny and Barr, 1991; Clarke et al., 2009; Bristow et al., 2015), implant fracture in less than 1 % of cases (Bristow et al., 2015), migration of crossed Kirschner wires, nonconsolidation of arthrodesis, implant sensitivity and gait disturbance (Kapatkin et al., 2018; Basa and Johnson, 2019).

In summary, the complication rate in pancarpal arthrodesis is much higher than in other surgical procedures. Sometimes, it is necessary to remove the implants once the arthrodesis has consolidated. Implant removal after pancarpal arthrodesis has been reported in 21 % (Díaz-Bertrana et al., 2009) and 7–33 % of cases (Lotsikas and Radasch, 2006).

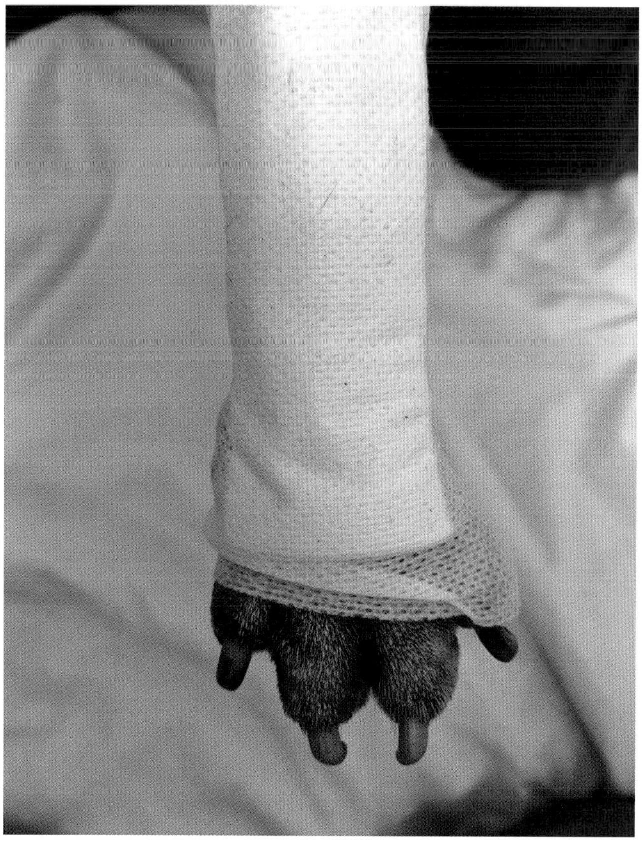

Figure 14. Swelling of the limb distal to the area of pancarpal arthrodesis.

REFERENCES AND FURTHER READING

FUNDAMENTALS AND PRACTICAL BASIS

ARTHROCENTESIS

Clements D, Arthrocentesis and synovial fluid analysis in dogs and cats, *In Practice*, 2006, 28(5):256–262.

Craig LE, Julian ME, Ferracone JD, The diagnosis and prognosis of synovial tumors in dogs: 35 cases, *Veterinary Pathology*, 2002, 39(1):66–73.

Hardie EM, Roe SC, Martin FR, Radiographic evidence of degenerative joint disease in geriatric cats: 100 cases (1994–1997), *Journal of the American Veterinary Medical Association*, 2002, 220(5):628–632.

Harris A, Santangelo K, Joint fluid analysis and collection considerations, In: *Canine Lameness*, 1st ed., Duerr FM (ed.), John Wiley & Sons, 2020, pp. 111–123.

Johnston SA, Osteoarthritis. Joint anatomy, physiology, and pathobiology, *Veterinary Clinics of North America: Small Animal Practice*, 1997, 27(4):699–723.

Johnston SA, Tobias KM, *Veterinary Surgery: Small Animal Expert Consult*, 2nd ed., Saunders-Elsevier, 2018.

MacWilliams PS, Friedrichs KR, Laboratory evaluation and interpretation of synovial fluid, *Veterinary Clinics of North America: Small Animal Practice*, 2003, 33(1):153–178.

Mielke B et al., Spontaneous septic arthritis of canine elbows: twenty-one cases, *Veterinary and Comparative Orthopaedics and Traumatology*, 2018, 31(6):488–493.

Miller JM et al., A guide to utilization of the microbiology laboratory for diagnosis of infectious diseases: 2018 update by the Infectious Diseases Society of America and the American Society for Microbiology, *Clinical Infectious Diseases*, 2018, 67(6):e1–e94.

Proot JL, de Vicente F, Sheahan DE, Analysis of lactate concentrations in canine synovial fluid, *Veterinary and Comparative Orthopaedics and Traumatology*, 2015, 28(5):301–305.

Steel CM, Pannirselvam RR, Anderson GA, Risk of septic arthritis after intra-articular medication: a study of 16,624 injections in Thoroughbred racehorses, *Australian Veterinary Journal*, 2013, 91(7):268–273.

Torres BT, Duerr FM, Arthrocentesis technique, In: *Canine Lameness*, 1st ed., Duerr FM (ed.), John Wiley & Sons, 2020, pp. 95–104.

ARTHROSCOPY

Beale BS et al., *Small Animal Arthroscopy*, Philadelphia (Pennsylvania), Saunders, 2003.

Danielson KC et al., Histomorphometry of fragmented medial coronoid process in dogs: a comparison of affected and normal coronoid processes, *Veterinary Surgery*, 2006, 35(6):501–509.

Farrell M et al., Does radiographic arthrosis correlate with cartilage pathology in Labrador Retrievers affected by medial coronoid process disease? *Veterinary Surgery*, 2014, 43(2):155–165.

Schulz KS, Arthroscopy, In: *Veterinary Surgery: Small Animal*, Tobias K, Johnston S (eds.), St Louis (Missouri), Saunders Elsevier, 2012, pp. 1135–1158.

GENERALITIES OF OSTEOCHONDRITIS DISSECANS

Breur GJ, Lambrechts NE, Osteochodrosis, In: *Veterinary Surgery: Small Animal: Volume 2*, Tobias KM, Johnston SA (eds.), St Louis (Missouri), Elsevier-Saunders, 2012, pp. 1178–1189.

Cook JL et al., Evaluation of synthetic osteochondral implants, *The Journal of Knee Surgery*, 2014, 27(4):295–302.

Danielski A, Farrell M, Use of synthetic osteochondral implants to treat bilateral shoulder osteochondritis dissecans in a dog, *Veterinary and Comparative Orthopaedics and Traumatology*, 2018, 31(5):385–389.

Egan P et al., Treatment of osteochondrosis dissecans of the canine stifle using synthetic osteochondral resurfacing, *Veterinary and Comparative Orthopaedics and Traumatology*, 2018, 31(2):144–152.

Fitzpatrick N et al., Osteochondral autograft transfer for treatment of osteochondritis dissecans of the caudocentral humeral head in dogs, *Veterinary Surgery*, 2010, 39(8):925–935.

Husby KA et al., Evaluation of a permanent synthetic osteochondral implant in the equine medial femoral condyle, *Veterinary Surgery*, 2016, 45(3):364–373.

Murphy SC, Egan PM, Fitzpatrick NM, Synthetic osteochondral resurfacing for treatment of large caudocentral osteochondritis dissecans lesions of the humeral head in 24 dogs, *Veterinary Surgery*, 2019, 48(5):858–868.

Olivieri M et al., Arthroscopic treatment of osteochondritis dissecans of the shoulder in 126 dogs, *Veterinary and Comparative Orthopaedics and Traumatology*, 2007, 20(1):65–69.

GENERAL CONCEPTS ABOUT ARTHRODESIS

De Camp CE et al., Principles of joint surgery, In: *Brinker, Piermattei, and Flo's Handbook of Small Animal Orthopedics and Fracture Repair*, 5th ed., Elsevier, 2016, pp. 211–229.

SHOULDER

TRAUMATIC SHOULDER LUXATION

BARBER LN et al., Long-term outcome following cranial biceps brachii tendon transposition in a dog with a traumatic cranial scapulohumeral luxation, *Open Veterinary Journal*, 2021, 10(4):400–406.

FITCH RB et al., Clinical evaluation of prosthetic medial glenohumeral ligament repair in the dog (ten cases), *Veterinary and Comparative Orthopaedics and Traumatology*, 2001, 14(4):222–228.

HUCK JL, BERGH MS, Traumatic craniolateral shoulder luxation and fracture of the lesser tubercle of the humerus in a dog, *Veterinary and Comparative Orthopaedics and Traumatology*, 2011, 24(6):474–477.

O'DONNELL EM et al., Treatment of medial shoulder joint instability in dogs by extracapsular stabilization with a prosthetic ligament: 39 cases (2008–2013), *Journal of the American Veterinary Medical Association*, 2017, 251(9):1042–1052.

POST C et al., Temporary transarticular stabilization with a locking plate for medial shoulder luxation in a dog, *Veterinary and Comparative Orthopaedics and Traumatology*, 2008, 21(2):166–170.

PUCHEU B, DUHAUTOIS B, Surgical treatment of shoulder instability. A retrospective study on 76 cases (1993–2007), *Veterinary and Comparative Orthopaedics and Traumatology*, 2008, 21(4):368–374.

RINGWOOD PB et al., Medial glenohumeral ligament reconstruction for ex-vivo medial glenohumeral luxation in the dog, *Veterinary and Comparative Orthopaedics and Traumatology*, 2001, 14(4):196–200.

SIDAWAY BK et al., Role of the tendons of the biceps brachii and infraspinatus muscles and the medial glenohumeral ligament in the maintenance of passive shoulder joint stability in dogs, *American Journal of Veterinary Research*, 2004, 65(9):1216–1222.

VASSEUR PB, MOORE D, BROWN SA, Stability of the canine shoulder joint: an in vitro analysis, *American Journal of Veterinary Research*, 1982, 43(2):352–355.

OSTEOCHONDRITIS DISSECANS OF THE SHOULDER JOINT

ADAMIAK Z, *Orthopedics and Traumatology of the Joints and Tendo-Muscular System of Dogs and Cats* [in Polish], Lodz (Poland), Galaktyka, 2007, pp. 10–12.

BIEZYŃSKI J et al., Assessment of treatment of osteochondrosis dissecans (OCD) of shoulder joint in dogs—the results of two years of experience, *Polish Journal of Veterinary Sciences*, 2012, 15(2):285–290.

FITZPATRICK N et al., Osteochondral autograft transfer for treatment of osteochondritis dissecans of the caudocentral humeral head in dogs, *Veterinary Surgery*, 2010, 39(8):925–935.

KUROKI K et al., Characterizing osteochondrosis in the dog: potential roles for matrix metalloproteinases and mechanical load in pathogenesis and disease progression, *Osteoarthritis and Cartilage*, 2005, 13(3):225–234.

LAFOND E, BREUR GJ, AUSTIN CC, Breed susceptibility for developmental orthopedic diseases in dogs, *Journal of the American Animal Hospital Association*, 2002, 38(5):467–477.

MURPHY SC, EGAN PM, FITZPATRICK NM, Synthetic osteochondral resurfacing for treatment of large caudocentral osteochondritis dissecans lesions of the humeral head in 24 dogs, *Veterinary Surgery*, 2019, 48(5):858–868.

OLIVIERI M et al., Arthroscopic treatment of osteochondritis dissecans of the shoulder in 126 dogs, *Veterinary and Comparative Orthopaedics and Traumatology*, 2007, 20(1):65–69.

PIERMATTEI DL, FLO GL, DECAMP CE, The shoulder joint, In: *Brinker, Piermattei, and Flo's Handbook of Small Animal Orthopedics and Fracture Repair*, 4th ed., Philadelphia (Pennsylvania), Saunders Elsevier, 2006, pp. 262–296.

RUDD RG, WHITEHAIR JG, MARGOLIS JH, Results of management of osteochondritis dissecans of the humeral head in dogs: 44 cases (1982 to 1987), *Journal of the American Animal Hospital Association*, 1990, 26(2):173–178.

VEZZONI A et al., A modification of the Cheli craniolateral approach for minimally invasive treatment of osteochondritis dissecans of the shoulder in dogs: description of the technique and outcome in 164 cases, *Veterinary and Comparative Orthopaedics and Traumatology*, 2021, 34(2):130–136.

WALL CR, COOK CR, COOK JL, Diagnostic sensitivity of radiography, ultrasonography, and magnetic resonance imaging for detecting shoulder osteochondrosis/osteochondritis dissecans in dogs, *Veterinary Radiology and Ultrasound*, 2015, 56(1):3–11.

INFRASPINATUS CONTRACTURE (FIBROTIC MYOPATHY)

DEVOR M, SØRBY R, Fibrotic contracture of the canine infraspinatus muscle: pathophysiology and prevention by early surgical intervention, *Veterinary and Comparative Orthopaedics and Traumatology*, 2006, 19(2):117–121.

Franch J et al., Simultaneous bilateral contracture of the infraspinatus muscle, *Veterinary and Comparative Orthopaedics and Traumatology*, 2009, 22(3):249–252.

Mikkelsen MA, Ottesen N, CT findings in a dog with subacute myopathy and later fibrotic contracture of the infraspinatus muscle, *Veterinary Radiology and Ultrasound*, 2021, 62(2):E11–E15.

Johnson KA, *Piermattei's Atlas of Surgical Approaches to the Bones and Joints of the Dog and Cat*, 5th ed., St Louis (Missouri), Saunders, 2014, p. 127.

BICEPS BRACHII TENDINOPATHY

Adamiak Z, Szałecki P, Treatment of bicipital tenosynovitis with double tenodesis, *Journal of Small Animal Practice*, 2003, 44(12):539–540.

Averbukh E et al., Gene expression of insulin-like growth factor-I, its receptor and binding proteins in retina under hypoxic conditions, *Metabolism*, 1998, 47(11):1331–1336.

Bardet JF, Lesions of the biceps tendon diagnosis and classification: a retrospective study of 25 cases in 23 dogs and one cat, *Veterinary and Comparative Orthopaedics and Traumatology*, 1999, 12(4):188–195.

Bergenhuyzen AL et al., Long-term follow-up after arthroscopic tenotomy for partial rupture of the biceps brachii tendon, *Veterinary and Comparative Orthopaedics and Traumatology*, 2010, 23(1):51–55.

Cook JL, Kenter K, Fox DB, Arthroscopic biceps tenodesis: technique and results in six dogs, *Journal of the American Animal Hospital Association*, 2005, 41(2):121–127.

DeCamp CE et al., *Brinker, Piermattei, and Flo's Handbook of Small Animal Orthopedics and Fracture Repair*, 5th ed., St Louis (Missouri), Elsevier-Saunders, 2015.

Farkas B et al., Increased chondrocyte death after steroid and local anesthetic combination, *Clinical Orthopaedics and Related Research*, 2010, 468(11):3112–3120.

Fransson BA, Gavin PR, Lahmers KK, Supraspinatus tendinosis associated with biceps brachii tendon displacement in a dog, *Journal of the American Veterinary Medical Association*, 2005, 227(9):1429–1433.

Fubini SL et al., Corticosteroids alter the differentiated phenotype of articular chondrocytes, *Journal of Orthopaedic Research*, 2001, 19(4):688–695.

Gilley RS, Wallace LJ, Hayden DW, Clinical and pathologic analyses of bicipital tenosynovitis in dogs, *American Journal of Veterinary Research*, 2002, 63(3):402–407.

Handa JT et al., Hypoxia precedes the development of experimental preretinal neovascularization, *Graefe's Archive for Clinical and Experimental Ophthalmology*, 1996, 234(1):43–46.

Kannus P, Natri A, Etiology and pathophysiology of tendon ruptures in sports, *Scandinavian Journal of Medicine & Science in Sports*, 1997, 7(2):107–112.

Leeman JJ et al., Extracorporeal shockwave therapy and therapeutic exercise for supraspinatus and biceps tendinopathies in 29 dogs, *Veterinary Record*, 2016, 179(15):385.

Lincoln JD, Potter K, Tenosynovitis of the biceps brachii tendon in dogs, *Journal of the American Animal Hospital Association*, 1984, 20(3):385–392.

Notarnicola A, Moretti B, The biological effects of extracorporeal shock wave therapy (ESWT) on tendon tissue, *Muscles Ligaments and Tendons Journal*, 2012, 2(1):33–37.

Ogden JA, Tóth-Kischkat A, Schultheiss R, Principles of shock wave therapy, *Clinical Orthopaedics and Related Research*, 2001, (387):8–17.

Slauson DO, Cooper BJ, Inflammation and repair, In: *Mechanisms of Disease: A Textbook of Comparative General Pathology*, 2nd ed., Baltimore (Maryland), Williams & Wilkins, 1990, pp. 177–178, 277.

Stobie D et al., Chronic bicipital tenosynovitis in dogs: 29 cases (1985–1992), *Journal of the American Veterinary Medical Association*, 1995, 207(2):201–207.

Venzin C et al., Extracorporeal shockwave therapy in a dog with chronic bicipital tenosynovitis, *Schweizer Archiv für Tierheilkunde*, 2004, 146(3):136–141.

Wall CR, Taylor R, Arthroscopic biceps brachii tenotomy as a treatment for canine bicipital tenosynovitis, *Journal of the American Animal Hospital Association*, 2002, 38(2):169–175.

SUPRASPINATUS TENDINOPATHY

Canapp SO et al., Supraspinatus tendinopathy in 327 dogs: a retrospective study, *Veterinary Evidence*, 2016a, 1(3).

Canapp SO Jr et al., The use of adipose-derived progenitor cells and platelet-rich plasma combination for the treatment of supraspinatus tendinopathy in 55 dogs: a retrospective study, *Frontiers in Veterinary Science*, 2016b, 3:61.

Fransson BA, Gavin PR, Lahmers KK, Supraspinatus tendinosis associated with biceps brachii tendon displacement in a dog, *Journal of the American Veterinary Medical Association*, 2005, 227(9):1429–1433.

Ho LK et al., Single ultrasound-guided platelet-rich plasma injection for treatment of supraspinatus tendinopathy in dogs, *The Canadian Veterinary Journal*, 2015, 56(8):845–849.

Lafuente MP et al., Surgical treatment of mineralized and nonmineralized supraspinatus tendinopathy in twenty-four dogs, *Veterinary Surgery*, 2009, 38(3):380–387.

Laitinen OM, Flo GL, Mineralization of the supraspinatus tendon in dogs: a long-term follow-up, *Journal of the American Animal Hospital Association*, 2000, 36(3):262–267.

Leeman JJ et al., Extracorporeal shockwave therapy and therapeutic exercise for supraspinatus and biceps tendinopathies in 29 dogs, *Veterinary Record*, 2016, 179(15):385.

Maddox TW et al., Comparison between shoulder computed tomography and clinical findings in 89 dogs presented for thoracic limb lameness, *Veterinary Radiology and Ultrasound*, 2013, 54(4):358–364.

McDougall RA, Canapp SO, Canapp DA, Ultrasonographic findings in 41 dogs treated with bone marrow aspirate concentrate and platelet-rich plasma for a supraspinatus tendinopathy: a retrospective study, *Frontiers in Veterinary Science*, 2018, 5:98.

Mistieri ML et al., Ultrasonographic evaluation of canine supraspinatus calcifying tendinosis, *Journal of the American Animal Hospital Association*, 2012, 48(6):405–410.

Spall BF et al., Tendon volume determination on magnetic resonance imaging of supraspinatus tendinopathy, *Veterinary Surgery*, 2016, 45(3):386–391.

DORSAL SCAPULAR LUXATION

Jones SC et al., Surgical management of dorsal scapular luxation in three dogs, *Veterinary and Comparative Orthopaedics and Traumatology*, 2017, 30(1):75–80.

SHOULDER ARTHRODESIS

Fitzpatrick N et al., Shoulder arthrodesis in 14 dogs, *Veterinary Surgery*, 2012, 41(6):745–754.

Herron MR, Scapulo-humeral arthrodesis: an evaluation of two techniques in 33 cases, *Veterinary Surgery*, 1989, 18:78.

Johnson A, Houlton J, Vannini R, *AO Principles of Fracture Management in the Dog and Cat*, Davos Platz (Switzerland), AO Publishing, 2005.

Oxley B, Bilateral shoulder arthrodesis in a Pekinese using three-dimensional printed patient-specific osteotomy and reduction guides, *Veterinary and Comparative Orthopaedics and Traumatology*, 2017, 30(3):230–236.

Piermattei DL, Flo GL, DeCamp CE, The shoulder joint, In: *Brinker, Piermattei, and Flo's Handbook of Small Animal Orthopedics and Fracture Repair*, 4th ed., Philadelphia (Pennsylvania), Saunders Elsevier, 2006, pp. 262–296.

Piermattei DL, Johnson KA, Approach to the cranio-lateral region of the shoulder joint, In: *An Atlas of Surgical Approaches to the Bones and Joints of the Dog and Cat*, 4th ed., Piermattei DL, Johnson KA (eds.), Philadelphia (Pennsylvania), Saunders Elsevier, 2004, pp. 112–118.

Vasseur PB, Arthrodesis for congenital luxation of the shoulder in a dog, *Journal of the American Veterinary Medical Association*, 1990, 197(4):501–503.

ELBOW

TRAUMATIC ELBOW LUXATION

Campbell JR, Nonfracture injuries to the canine elbow, *Journal of the American Veterinary Medical Association*, 1969, 155(5):735–744.

Campbell JR, Luxation and ligamentous injuries of the elbow of the dog, *Veterinary Clinics of North America*, 1971, 1(3):429–440.

Farrell M et al., In vitro validation of a technique for assessment of canine and feline elbow joint collateral ligament integrity and description of a new method for collateral ligament prosthetic replacement, *Veterinary Surgery*, 2007, 36(6):548–556.

Mitchell KE, Traumatic elbow luxation in 14 dogs and 11 cats, *Australian Veterinary Journal*, 2011, 89(6):213–216.

O'Brien MG, Boudrieau RJ, Clark GN, Traumatic luxation of the cubital joint (elbow) in dogs: 44 cases (1978–1988), *Journal of the American Veterinary Medical Association*, 1992, 201(11):1760–1765.

Sajik D et al., Multi-centre retrospective study of long-term outcomes following traumatic elbow luxation in 37 dogs, *Journal of Small Animal Practice*, 2016, 57(8):422–428.

Schaeffer IGF et al., Traumatic luxation of the elbow in 31 dogs, *Veterinary and Comparative Orthopaedics and Traumatology*, 1999, 12(1):33–39.

UNUNITED ANCONEAL PROCESS

Cawley AJ, Archibald J, Ununited anconal processes of the dog, *Journal of the American Veterinary Medical Association*, 1959, 134(10):454–458.

Ferrigno CRA et al., Treatment of ununited anconeal process in 8 dogs by osteotomy and dynamic distraction of the proximal part of the ulna, *Pesquisa Veterinária Brasileira*, 2007, 27(8):352–356.

Fox SM et al., Ununited anconeal process: lag-screw fixation, *Journal of the American Animal Hospital Association*, 1996, 32(1):52–56.

Gasch EG, Labruyère JJ, Bardet JF, Computed tomography of ununited anconeal process in the dog, *Veterinary and Comparative Orthopaedics and Traumatology*, 2012, 25(6):498–505.

Guthrie S, Some radiographic and clinical aspects of ununited anconeal process, *Veterinary Record*, 1989, 124(25):661–662.

Herron MR, Ununited anconeal process—a new approach to surgical repair, *Modern Veterinary Practice*, 1970, 51(6):30–34.

Krotscheck U, Böttcher P, Surgical diseases of the elbow, In: *Veterinary Surgery: Small Animal*, Tobias KM, Johnston SJ, (eds.), Elsevier, 2018, pp. 848–852.

Krotscheck U et al., Ununited anconeal process: lag-screw fixation with proximal ulnar osteotomy, *Veterinary and Comparative Orthopaedics and Traumatology*, 2000, 13(4):212–216.

Meyer-Lindenberg A, Nolte I, Fehr M, The ununited anconeal process: retro- and prospective investigations on surgical treatment, *Tierarztliche Praxis Ausgabe Kleintiere Heimtiere*, 1999, 27(5):309–320.

Meyer-Lindenberg A, Fehr M, Nolte I, Short- and long-term results after surgical treatment of an ununited anconeal process in the dog, *Veterinary and Comparative Orthopaedics and Traumatology*, 2001, 14(2):101–110.

Meyer-Lindenberg A, Fehr M, Nolte I, Co-existence of ununited anconeal process and fragmented medial coronoid process of the ulna in the dog, *Journal of the Small Animal Practice*, 2006, 47(2):61–65.

Pettitt RA et al., Effect of surgical technique on radiographic fusion of the anconeus in the treatment of ununited anconeal process, *Journal of Small Animal Practice*, 2009, 50(10):545–548.

Pritchard DL, Anconeal process pseudoarthrosis: treated by lag-screw fixation, *Canine Practice*, 1976, 3:18–23.

Roy RG, Wallace LJ, Johnston GR, A retrospective long-term evaluation of ununited anconeal process excision on the canine elbow, *Veterinary and Comparative Orthopaedics and Traumatology*, 1994, 7(3):94–97.

Sjöström L, Kasström H, Källberg M, Ununited anconeal process in the dog. Pathogenesis and treatment by osteotomy of the ulna, *Veterinary and Comparative Orthopaedics and Traumatology*, 1995,8(4):170–176.

Talcott KW et al., In vitro biomechanical study of rotational stabilizers of the canine elbow joint, *American Journal of Veterinary Research*, 2002, 63(11):1520–1526.

Turner BM et al., Dynamic proximal ulnar osteotomy for the treatment of ununited anconeal process in 17 dogs, *Veterinary and Comparative Orthopaedics and Traumatology*, 1998, 11(2):76–79.

Vezzoni A, How I treat ununited anconeal process, Proceedings of the 18th ESVOT congress, 2016, London, pp. 282–286.

Vezzoni A, Benjamino K, Canine elbow dysplasia: ununited anconeal process, osteochondritis dissecans, and medial coronoid process disease, *Veterinary Clinics of North America: Small Animal Practice*, 2021, 51(2):439–474.

MEDIAL COMPARTMENT DISEASE

Bayer K et al., Complications and short-to-midterm results in a case series of 52 CUE procedures using a modified caudo-medial approach, *Open Veterinary Journal*, 2019, 9(3):205–215.

Coghill FJ, Ho-Eckart LK, Baltzer WI, Mid- to long-term outcome after arthroscopy and proximal abducting ulnar osteotomy versus arthroscopy alone in dogs with medial compartment disease: thirty cases, *Veterinary and Comparative Orthopaedics and Traumatology*, 2021, 34(2):85–90.

Cook JL et al., Clinical outcomes associated with the initial use of the Canine Unicompartmental Elbow (CUE) Arthroplasty System®, The *Canadian Veterinary Journal*, 2015, 56(9):971–977.

Danielski A et al., Complications after proximal abducting ulnar osteotomy and prognostic factors in 66 dogs, *Veterinary Surgery*, 2022, 51(1):136–147.

Farrell M et al., Does radiographic arthrosis correlate with cartilage pathology in Labrador Retrievers affected by medial coronoid process disease? *Veterinary Surgery*, 2014, 43(2):155–165.

Fitzpatrick N, Bertran J, Solano MA, Sliding humeral osteotomy: medium-term objective outcome measures and reduction of complications with a modified technique, *Veterinary Surgery*, 2015, 44(2):137–149.

Fitzpatrick N et al., Techniques of application and initial clinical experience with sliding humeral osteotomy for treatment of medial compartment disease of the canine elbow, *Veterinary Surgery*, 2009, 38(2):261–278.

Franklin SP et al., Theory and development of a unicompartmental resurfacing system for treatment of medial compartment disease of the canine elbow, *Veterinary Surgery*, 2014, 43(7):765–773.

Mason DR et al., Measurement of humeroradial and humeroulnar transarticular joint forces in the canine elbow joint after humeral wedge and humeral slide osteotomies, *Veterinary Surgery*, 2008, 37(1):63–70.

Wendelburg KM, Beale BS, Medium and long term evaluation of sliding humeral osteotomy in dogs, *Veterinary Surgery*, 2014, 43(7):804–813.

OSTEOCHONDROSIS OF THE ELBOW JOINT

Bouck GR, Miller CW, Taves CL, A comparison of surgical and medical treatment of fragmented coronoid process and osteochondritis dissecans of the canine elbow, *Veterinary and Comparative Orthopaedics and Traumatology*, 1995, 8(4):177–183.

Danielski A, Farrell M, Use of synthetic osteochondral implants to treat bilateral shoulder osteochondritis dissecans in a dog, *Veterinary and Comparative Orthopaedics and Traumatology*, 2018, 31(5):385–389.

Egan P et al., Treatment of osteochondrosis dissecans of the canine stifle using synthetic osteochondral resurfacing, *Veterinary and Comparative Orthopaedics and Traumatology*, 2018, 31(2):144–152.

Husby KA et al., Evaluation of a permanent synthetic osteochondral implant in the equine medial femoral condyle, *Veterinary Surgery*, 2016, 45(3):364–373.

Mason TA et al., Osteochondrosis of the elbow joint in young dogs, *Journal of Small Animal Practice*, 1980, 21(12):641–656.

Minas T, Nehrer S, Current concepts in the treatment of articular cartilage defects, *Orthopedics*, 1997, 20(6):525–538.

Slater MR et al., Diet and exercise as potential risk factors for osteochondritis dissecans in dogs, *American Journal of Veterinary Research*, 1992, 53(11):2119–2124.

SHORT ULNA SYNDROME

Carwardine DR et al., Three-dimensional-printed patient-specific osteotomy guides, repositioning guides and titanium plates for acute correction of antebrachial limb deformities in dogs, *Veterinary and Comparative Orthopaedics and Traumatology*, 2021, 34(1):43–52.

Coggeshall JD et al., Arthroscopic-guided ulnar distraction for the correction of elbow incongruency in four dogs, *Journal of Small Animal Practice*, 2014, 55(1):46–51.

Crosse KR, Worth AJ, Computer-assisted surgical correction of an antebrachial deformity in a dog, *Veterinary and Comparative Orthopaedics and Traumatology*, 2010, 23(5):354–361.

DeCamp CE et al., *Brinker, Piermattei, and Flo's Handbook of Small Animal Orthopedics and Fracture Repair*, 5th ed., St Louis (Missouri), Elsevier-Saunders, 2015.

Deruddere KJ, Snelling SR, A retrospective review of antebrachial angular and rotational limb deformity correction in dogs using intraoperative alignment and type 1b external fixation, *New Zealand Veterinary Journal*, 2014, 62(5):290–296.

Fitzpatrick N, Yeadon R, Working algorithm for treatment decision making for developmental disease of the medial compartment of the elbow in dogs, *Veterinary Surgery*, 2009, 38(2):285–300.

Fitzpatrick N et al., The double-arch modified type-1b external skeletal fixator. Technique description and functional outcome for surgical management of canine antebrachial limb deformities, *Veterinary and Comparative Orthopaedics and Traumatology*, 2011, 24(5):374–382.

Fox SM, Premature closure of distal radial and ulnar physes in the dog. I. Pathogenesis and diagnosis, *The Compendium on Continuing Education for the Practicing Veterinarian*, 1984, 6(2):128–139.

Johnston SA, Tobias KM, *Veterinary Surgery: Small Animal Expert Consult*, 2nd ed., St Louis (Missouri), Elsevier-Saunders, 2017, Kindle edition.

Johnston SA, Tobias KM, *Veterinary Surgery: Small Animal Expert Consult*, 2nd ed., 2018, Saunders.

Longo F et al., Three-dimensional computer-assisted corrective osteotomy with a patient-specific surgical guide for an antebrachial limb deformity in two dogs, *Schweizer Archiv für Tierheilkunde*, 2019, 161(7):473–479.

Marcellin-Little DJ et al., Hinged Ilizarov external fixation for correction of antebrachial deformities, *Veterinary Surgery*, 1998, 27(3):231–245.

O'Brien TR, Morgan JP, Suter PF, Epiphyseal plate injury in the dog: a radiographic study of growth disturbance in the forelimb, *Journal of Small Animal Practice*, 1971, 12(1):19–36.

Oxley B, A 3-dimensional-printed patient-specific guide system for minimally invasive plate osteosynthesis of a comminuted mid-diaphyseal humeral fracture in a cat, *Veterinary Surgery*, 2018, 47(3):445–453.

Quinn MK et al., Realignment of the radius in canine antebrachial growth deformities treated with corrective osteotomy and bilateral (type II) external fixation, *Veterinary Surgery*, 2000, 29(6):558–563.

Ramadan RO, Vaughan LC, Premature closure of the distal ulnar growth plate in dogs—a review of 58 cases, *Journal of Small Animal Practice*, 1978, 19(11):647–667.

Worth AJ, Crosse KR, Kersley A, Computer-assisted surgery using 3D printed saw guides for acute correction of antebrachial angular limb deformities in dogs, *Veterinary and Comparative Orthopaedics and Traumatology*, 2019, 32(3):241–249.

CARPUS

ABDUCTOR POLLICIS LONGUS TENOSYNOVITIS

HITTMAIR KM, GROESSL V, MAYRHOFER E, Radiographic and ultrasonographic diagnosis of stenosing tenosynovitis of the abductor pollicis longus muscle in dogs, *Veterinary Radiology and Ultrasound*, 2012, 53(2):135–141.

MOORES AP, COMERFORD EJ, What is your diagnosis? Stenosing tenosynovitis of the tendon of the abductor pollicis longus muscle, *Journal of Small Animal Practice*, 2005, 46(1):41–43.

PANCARPAL ARTHRODESIS

ARNOTT JL et al., An in vitro comparison of a 2.7/3.5 mm hybrid plate alone and combined with crossed K-wires for canine pancarpal arthrodesis, *Veterinary and Comparative Orthopaedics and Traumatology*, 2008, 21(4):307–311.

BASA RM, JOHNSON KA, Management of feline carpal injuries: What are the options and when is arthrodesis indicated? *Journal of Feline Medicine and Surgery*, 2019, 21(9):809–823.

BEIERER LH, Canine carpal injuries: from fractures to hyperextension injuries, *Veterinary Clinics of North America: Small Animal Practice*, 2021, 51(2):285–303.

BRISTOW PC et al., Clinical comparison of the hybrid dynamic compression plate and the castless plate for pancarpal arthrodesis in 219 dogs, *Veterinary Surgery*, 2015, 44(1):70–77.

BROWN G et al., Highly comminuted, articular fractures of the distal antebrachium managed by pancarpal arthrodesis in 8 dogs, *Veterinary Surgery*, 2016, 45(1):44–51.

CALVO I et al., Carpal arthrodesis in cats. Long-term functional outcome, *Veterinary and Comparative Orthopaedics and Traumatology*, 2009, 22(6):498–504.

CHAMBERS JN, BJORLING DE, Palmar surface plating for arthrodesis of the canine carpus, *Journal of the American Animal Hospital Association*, 1982, 18(6):875–882.

CLARKE S, PINK J, The carpus, In: *BSAVA Manual of Canine and Feline Musculoskeletal Disorders*, 2nd ed., ARTHURS G, BROWN G, PETTITT R (eds.), 2018, British Small Animal Veterinary Association, pp. 330–346.

CLARKE SP, FERGUSON JF, MILLER A, Clinical evaluation of pancarpal arthrodesis using a CastLess plate in 11 dogs, *Veterinary Surgery*, 2009, 38(7):852–860.

DENNY HR, BARR ARS, Partial carpal and pancarpal arthrodesis in the dog: a review of 50 cases, *Journal of Small Animal Practice*, 1991, 32(7):329–334.

DÍAZ-BERTRANA C et al., The stepped hybrid plate for carpal panarthrodesis. Part II: a multicentre study of 52 arthrodeses, *Veterinary and Comparative Orthopaedics and Traumatology*, 2009, 22(5):389–397.

GUERRERO TG, MONTAVON PM, Medial plating for carpal panarthrodesis, *Veterinary Surgery*, 2005, 34(2):153–158.

GUILLOU RP et al., In vitro mechanical evaluation of a limited contact dynamic compression plate and hybrid carpal arthrodesis plate for canine pancarpal arthrodesis, *Veterinary and Comparative Orthopaedics and Traumatology*, 2012, 25(2):83–88.

JERRAM RM et al., Prospective evaluation of pancarpal arthrodesis for carpal injuries in working dogs in New Zealand, using dorsal hybrid plating, *New Zealand Veterinary Journal*, 2009, 57(6):331–337.

JOHNSON KA, Carpal arthrodesis in dogs, *Australian Veterinary Journal*, 1980, 56(12):565–573.

KAPATKIN AS, GARCÍA-NOLEN T, HAYASHI K, Carpus, metacarpus and digits, In: *Veterinary Surgery: Small Animal Expert Consult*, 2nd ed., JOHNSTON SA, TOBIAS KM (eds.), Saunders-Elsevier, 2018.

KOCH D, Screws and plates, In: *AO Principles of Fracture Management in the Dog and Cat*, JOHNSON AL, HOULTON JEF, VANNINI R (eds.), Switzerland, AO Publishing Davos, 2005.

LEWIS ST et al., Antebrachiometacarpal arthrodesis in five dogs, *Australian Veterinary Journal*, 2019, 97(4):122–127.

LOTSIKAS PJ, RADASCH RM, A clinical evaluation of pancarpal arthrodesis in nine dogs using circular external skeletal fixation, *Veterinary Surgery*, 2006, 35(5):480–485.

MEESON RL, DAVIDSON C, ARTHURS GI, Soft-tissue injuries associated with cast application for distal limb orthopaedic conditions. A retrospective study of sixty dogs and cats, *Veterinary and Comparative Orthopaedics and Traumatology*, 2011, 24(2):126–131.

MEESON RL, GOODSHIP AE, ARTHURS GI, A biomechanical evaluation of a hybrid dynamic compression plate and a CastLess arthrodesis plate for pancarpal arthrodesis in dogs, *Veterinary Surgery*, 2012, 41(6):738–744.

MICHAL U, FLÜCKIGER M, SCHMÖKEL H, Healing of dorsal pancarpal arthrodesis in the dog, *Journal of Small Animal Practice*, 2003, 44(3):109–112.

PARKER RB, BROWN SG, WIND AP, Pancarpal arthrodesis in the dog: a review of forty-five cases, *Veterinary Surgery*, 1981, 10(1):35–43.

PETAZZONI M, JAEGER GH, *Atlas of Clinical Goniometry and Radiographic Measurements of the Canine Pelvic Limb*, Milan (Italy), Merial, 2008.

PETAZZONI M, NICETTO T, Rapid prototyping to design a customized locking plate for pancarpal arthrodesis in a giant breed dog, *Veterinary and Comparative Orthopaedics and Traumatology*, 2014, 27(1):85–89.

RAMÍREZ JM, MACÍAS C, Pancarpal arthrodesis without rigid coaptation using the hybrid dynamic compression plate in dogs, *Veterinary Surgery*, 2016, 45(3):303–308.

TUAN J, COMAS N, SOLANO M, Clinical outcomes and complications of pancarpal arthrodesis stabilised with 3.5 mm/2.7 mm locking compression plates with internal additional fixation in 12 dogs, *New Zealand Veterinary Journal*, 2019, 67(5):270–276.

WHITELOCK RG, DYCE J, HOULTON JF, Metacarpal fractures associated with pancarpal arthrodesis in dogs, *Veterinary Surgery*, 1999, 28(1):25–30.

WININGER FA et al., Failure mode and bending moment of canine pancarpal arthrodesis constructs stabilized with two different implant systems, *Veterinary Surgery*, 2007, 36(8):724–728.

WOODS S, WALLACE RJ, MOSLEY JR, The effect of external coaptation on plate deformation in an ex vivo model of canine pancarpal arthrodesis, *Veterinary and Comparative Orthopaedics and Traumatology*, 2012, 25(6):439–444.